Laparoscopy

Laparoscopy

Editor-in-Chief

Jordan M. Phillips, M.D., F.A.C.O.G.
Associate Clinical Professor of Gynecology and Obstetrics
Chief of the Section of Gynecologic Endoscopy
University of California, Irvine
California College of Medicine
Irvine, California

President, American Asociation of Gynecologic Laparoscopists

Editorial Board

Stephen L. Corson, M.D., F.A.C.O.G.
Assistant Clinical Professor of Obstetrics and Gynecology
University of Pennsylvania School of Medicine
Chief of the Section of Gynecologic Endoscopy
Pennsylvania Hospital
Philadelphia, Pennsylvania

Louis Keith, M.D., F.A.C.O.G.
Professor of Obstetrics and Gynecology
Northwestern University Medical School and
Prentice Women's Hospital and Maternity Center
Professor of Obstetrics and Gynecology
Cook County Graduate School of Medicine
Chicago, Illinois

Treasurer, American Association of Gynecologic Laparoscopists

Carl J. Levinson, M.D., F.A.C.O.G.
Associate Professor of Obstetrics and Gynecology
Section of Gynecologic Endocrinology
Baylor College of Medicine
Texas Medical Center
Houston, Texas

A. Albert Yuzpe, M.D., M.Sc., F.R.C.S. (C), F.A.C.O.G.
Associate Professor of Obstetrics and Gynecology
University of Western Ontario Faculty of Medicine
London, Ontario
Canada

Williams & Wilkins Company
Baltimore

Made in the United States of America

Library of Congress Cataloging in Publication
Data

Main entry under title:

Laparoscopy.

  Includes bibliographies and index.
  1. Laparoscopy. 2. Gynecologic examination.
3. Gynecology, Operative. I. Phillips, Jordan M. II.
Corson, Stephen L. [DNLM: 1. Gynecologic diseases—Diagnosis. 2. Laparoscopy. WP141 L299]
RG107.5.L34L36   618.1'07'54   76-48208
ISBN 0-683-06876-8

Design by Don Moyer

Composed and printed at the
Waverly Press, Incorporated
Mount Royal and Guilford Aves.
Baltimore, Maryland 21202
U.S.A.

Acknowledgments

"You give but little when you give of your possessions. It is when you give of yourself that you truly give."

— Kahlil Gibran
The Prophet
1923

The completion of this book is followed by a most pleasant, yet difficult, task that of paying homage to and thanking all those who inspired, contributed or assisted in the production of this book.

The members of the Editorial Board, Stephen L. Corson, Louis Keith, Carl J. Levinson and A. Albert Yuzpe, contributed much time, effort and knowledge to specific chapters. Their individual experience has helped each author in his effort toward making this book as comprehensive and cosmopolitan as possible. My long-time friends and colleagues contributed forewords to this book, as well as continuous encouragement. All of these gentlemen are acknowledged world authorities.

I would like to thank Dr. Raoul Palmer, the father of laparoscopy; Dr. med. Hans Frangenheim, the creator of much instrumentation and many innovative techniques; Mr. Patrick C. Steptoe, author of the first English language monograph on the subject of laparoscopy; and Dr. Melvin R. Cohen, the modern American father of gynecologic laparoscopy.

The individual contributors are experts with vast expertise. Their careful observations and meticulous techniques have produced scholarly chapters.

Docteurs R. Legros and J. P. Abeille of Creteil, France, gave permission for the use of much of their outstanding color atlas for this book. Their use of intracorporeal flash lighting has created pictures of superb quality.

The Board of Trustees and the members of the AAGL have been unstinting in their support of this publication.

We gratefully acknowledge the cooperation and professionalism of Ms. Donna Kessel in her final editing of the text.

Mr. Dick Hoover of Williams & Wilkins had a very human approach to the difficult role of representing the publishers in the creation, publication and distribution of this book.

Our thanks to Ms. Wanda Rice Boineau for the comprehensive index and the painstaking effort to acquaint the reader with the wide variety of technical details demanded in laparoscopy.

We thank Mr. Don Moyer for his approach, ideas, and energy and for his art work, layout and divider pages.

Mr. Samuel N. Turiel, a friend and colleague and the first individual to receive the "Distinguished Friends Award" of the American Association of Gynecologic Laparoscopists, gave freely of his advice and support in helping to make the color atlas possible. The Searle Company helped underwrite the use of the Legros-Abeille color prints.

The following instrument manufacturers also helped by underwriting pages of the color atlas: Eder Instrument Co., Inc., Gynemed Inc., Karl Storz Endoscopy—America, Inc., and Richard Wolf Medical Instruments Corp.

It has been a great joy to be present at the conception, to witness the gestation of the multiple drafts, and attend the final birth of this book. This has been an outstanding experience in my life and in those of the editors and contributors. We are wiser for the interchange of ideas with our colleagues. We have all been enriched intellectually and scientifically by our efforts on behalf of this book.

We, the contributors, are most enthusiastic in the ever expanding utilization of this intriguing subject, laparoscopy. As knowledgeable readers, you will most certainly share this interest.

Jordan M. Phillips, M.D.
Editor-in-Chief

Preface

Gynecologists visiting Europe or receiving training there during the mid-1960s often brought back to America laparoscopic instruments and accounts of several decades' accumulated experience with the use of these instruments on the continent. My personal introduction to laparoscopy occurred in 1968, when I heard Dr. Melvin Cohen describe the operation. Shortly thereafter I purchased my first laparoscope and performed my first procedure. In those days one learned by the see-one, do-one method. A few excellent manuals were available from France, Italy and Germany; there was one from England in the English language. At first, reports of this new operation were slow in gathering, due in part to the fact that only a few gynecologists in even fewer medical centers were experimenting with this new diagnostic tool and in part to the time lag between experience and publication.

The American Association of Gynecologic Laparoscopists was formed in 1972. Since then, this organization has provided momentum for the rapid dissemination of information about gynecologic endoscopy, a platform for spirited debate and a fertile proving ground for the emergence of new experts. My association with this international group of physicians has given me several pleasant and stimulating years, and I count many of the members of this group as friends as well as respected colleagues. The enthusiasm and excitement of first a few hundred and now over 2,000 members is an index of that uniquely American spirit of sharing time, knowledge, expertise and techniques. We have carefully discussed and formulated methods, standards, instruction systems and ethics. Surveys and reports have been collected, and published. Already, more laparoscopic procedures are being performed in the United States than in any other country in the world. The decreased rate of serious complications suggests that a substantial degree of technical stability has been reached. Now the time has come to compile an account of the experience of experts into a current, clinical textbook.

Sometimes one writes to solidify or establish a method of learning. This book is written to abolish the method by which we, the authors, learned: no longer is the see-one, do-one technique adequate; the burden of teaching laparoscopy has shifted to medical centers and residency training programs. This volume has been prepared not only as a text for the trained and practicing laparoscopist but also as an adjunct to a training program. It is a book for reading and reference rather than a recipe book. Little that is old is presented here, yet the reader should know that even the new is in the process of being improved. We are ever vulnerable to the evolution of our craft. To be well trained is to be continually trained.

This textbook was written primarily for and by gynecologists, but it can very well be used by surgeons, urologists, gastroenterologists, oncologists or any other physicians investigating the abdominal and pelvic cavities. The book is not a treatise on pelvic anatomy, physiology or disease, although these subjects are discussed in part when applicable. A comprehensive index is included. Since we are describing one form of diagnostic and operative technique, discussion of treatment is presented only when performed through the laparoscope.

Laparoscopy has precisely fulfilled the goals set by its developers and has revolutionized the practice of gynecology. Physicians have grasped the concept that the laparoscope provides a picture window to what could only be palpated previously or seen through a large laparotomy incision. Patients have benefited from the rapid diagnostic and recovery time, minimal cosmetic injury, greatly reduced costs, elimination of sexual restriction, avoidance of the risks of major surgery and many fewer delays in treatment. Laparoscopy has eliminated the risk and frustration of clinical observation and has made possible immediate, definitive therapy for infertility, endometriosis, acute and chronic pelvic pain, blunt abdominal trauma, malignancies with and without metastases and congenital abnormalities. Laparoscopy is the method of choice for removing foreign bodies, such as intrauterine devices or peritoneal dialysis catheters, from the peritoneal cavity. It is an elegant procedure based on simple concepts but with a complex application of those concepts.

Laparoscopy requires the concerted efforts and skills of a team who must be taught, coordinated and supervised by the qualified laparoscopist, who must have a technical understanding of the instruments, photographic and optical principles, and the basic fundamentals of electricity and electrosurgical units. Care of the equipment is a vital part of laparoscopy, also, for one nonfunctioning part will make an exquisitely trained team useless. Scientific care is never casual.

The current challenges of laparoscopy are many. Sterilization operations make up 60% of the volume of laparoscopic practice and are becoming a precise and predictable procedure. Nonelectrical methods of sterilization are being perfected and should increase safety. Accidental bowel burns are the most compelling problem remaining to be solved. Diagnostic laparoscopy often requires exceptional visual and technical acumen, and there will be increased educational emphasis on this area in the future. New photographic techniques are being explored, and we will soon be able to document laparoscopic findings on a screen the same way the radiologist uses x-rays. Fertility studies and reproductive physiology studies will continue to produce needed answers to age-old questions. Instrument changes (improvements, we hope) continually make our latest purchase obsolete. Our learning and teaching are still uneven. We are now light-years away from where we began just a decade ago, but the word *laparoscopy* is entering some dictionaries just this year; it is not yet in the card catalog of some medical school libraries.

We are increasingly concerned about reports of a new boldness among some endoscopists: there have been disclosures of laparoscopic gymnastics that cannot be duplicated and probably should not be proposed or suggested. To do a major operation through a minor incision is not heroic but foolhardy and reckless. The risk/benefit ratio must be carefully weighed for each patient before surgery is done.

The excellence of the individual chapters of this book made my editorial task a delight. My special appreciation goes to the editorial board and contributors for the time and attention they gave. I prize my time and association with these people.

Jordan M. Phillips, M.D.
Downey, California

Contributors

Docteur J. P. Abeille
Attaché du Service de Gynécologie
du Centre Hôspitalier de Créteil
Créteil, France

Satoski Ariga, M.D.
Lecturer
Department of Obstetrics and Gynecology
Hokkaido University School of Medicine
Sapporo, Japan

Robert H. Bartlett, M.D.
Associate Professor of Surgery
University of California, Irvine
California College of Medicine
Irvine, California

George Berci, M.D., F.C.S.H.
Assistant Clinical Professor of Surgery
University of California, Los Angeles
School of Medicine
Director, Department of Endoscopy
Cedars-Sinai Medical Center
Los Angeles, California

Willard H. Boynton, M.D., M.P.H.
Deputy Director
Office of Population
Agency for International Development
Department of State
Washington, D.C.

Philip G. Brooks, M.D., F.A.C.O.G.
Assistant Clinical Professor
Department of Obstetrics and Gynecology
University of Southern California School of Medicine
Los Angeles, California

Edwin S. Bronstein, M.D., M.P.H., F.A.C.O.G.
Professor of Obstetrics and Gynecology
Medical College of Georgia
Augusta, Georgia

Diogene Cloutier, M.D., F.R.C.S. (C)
Associate, Department of Obstetrics and
    Gynecology
Laval University Faculty of Medicine
Chief of Gynecology
Le Centre Hôspitalier de L'Université Laval
Quebec City, Quebec, Canada

Docteur Michel Cognat
Chef de Clinique à la Faculté de Lyon
Lyon, France

Melvin R. Cohen, M.D., F.A.C.O.G.
Professor of Obstetrics and Gynecology
Northwestern University School of Medicine
Director, Fertility Institute, Ltd.
Chicago, Illinois

Stephen L. Corson, M.D., F.A.C.O.G.
Assistant Clinical Professor of Obstetrics and
    Gynecology
University of Pennsylvania School of Medicine
Chief of the Section of Gynecologic Endoscopy
Pennsylvania Hospital
Philadelphia, Pennsylvania

Norman G. Courey, M.D., C.M., F.A.C.O.G.
Clinical Professor of Obstetrics and Gynecology
State University of New York at Buffalo
Director of Obstetrics and Gynecology
E. J. Meyer Memorial Hospital
Buffalo, New York

Rafael G. Cunanan, Jr., M.D.
Clinical Assistant Professor
Department of Gynecology and Obstetrics
State University of New York at Buffalo
Buffalo, New York

W. Richard Dukelow, Ph.D.
Professor and Director
Endocrine Research Unit
Michigan State University
East Lansing, Michigan

W. Dow Edgerton, M.D., F.A.C.O.G.
Clinical Assistant Professor of Obstetrics and
    Gynecology
University of Iowa, Iowa City
Director of Obstetrics and Gynecology
St. Luke's Hospital
Davenport, Iowa

Tibor Engel, M.D.
Associate Clinical Professor of Obstetrics and
    Gynecology
University of Colorado Medical Center
Denver, Colorado

John Esposito, M.D., F.A.C.O.G.
Assistant Clinical Professor of Obstetrics and
    Gynecology
State University of New York
Downstate Medical Center
Brooklyn, New York

John I. Fishburne, Jr., M.D., F.A.C.O.G.
Associate Professor of Obstetrics and Gynecology
    and of Anesthesiology
Bowman Gray School of Medicine
Wake Forest University
Winston-Salem, North Carolina

Dr. med. Hans Frangenheim
Chefarzt der Stadtischen Frauenklinik
Konstanz, Germany

Alan B. Gazzaniga, M.D.
Associate Professor of Surgery
University of California, Irvine
California College of Medicine
Irvine, California

Dorothy N. Glenn, M.D., F.A.C.O.G.
Technical Services Branch
Family Planning Services Division
Office of Population
Agency for International Development
Department of State
Washington, D.C.

Arthur I. Goldstein, M.D.
Assistant Professor of Gynecology and Obstetrics
University of California, Irvine
California College of Medicine
Irvine, California

Victor Gomel, M.D., F.R.C.S. (C)
Clinical Assistant Professor of Obstetrics and
    Gynecology
University of British Columbia
Vancouver, British Columbia, Canada

John E. Gunning, M.D., F.A.C.O.G.
Assistant Clinical Professor of Obstetrics and
    Gynecology
University of California, Los Angeles
School of Medicine and Harbor General Hospital
Torrance, California

H. M. Hasson, M.D.
Clinical Associate of Obstetrics and Gynecology
Northwestern University Medical School
Chicago, Illinois

Arthur J. Horowitz, M.D.
Assistant Clinical Professor of Obstetrics and
    Gynecology
University of Minnesota Medical School
Minneapolis, Minnesota

Keim T. Houser, M.D.
Clinical Associate of Obstetrics and Gynecology
Northwestern University Medical School
Chicago, Illinois

Barbara Hulka, M.D.
Associate Professor of Epidemiology
University of North Carolina
School of Public Health
Chapel Hill, North Carolina

Jaroslav F. Hulka, M.D.
Associate Professor
Department of Obstetrics and Gynecology
University of North Carolina School of Medicine
Chapel Hill, North Carolina

Robert Israel, M.D., F.A.C.O.G.
Associate Professor of Obstetrics and Gynecology
Section of Reproductive Biology
University of Southern California School of Medicine
Chief, Section of Gynecology
Los Angeles County/University of Southern
    California Medical Center
Los Angeles, California

Donald Keith, M.B.A.
Fellow of the Society of Logistics Engineers
Reston, Virginia

Louis Keith, M.D., F.A.C.O.G.
Professor of Obstetrics and Gynecology
Northwestern University Medical School and
Prentice Women's Hospital and Maternity Center
Professor of Obstetrics and Gynecology
Cook County Graduate School of Medicine
Chicago, Illinois
Treasurer, American Association of Gynecologic
    Laparoscopists

Richard K. Kleppinger, M.D., F.A.C.O.G., F.A.C.S.
Chairman, Section of Obstetrics
Reading Hospital and Medical Center
Temple University Health Sciences Center
Philadelphia, Pennsylvania

Docteur R. Legros
Chef de Service du Centre
Hôspitalier de Créteil
Créteil, France

David Leisten, M.D.
Gynecology, Obstetrics and Infertility
Forest Hills, New York

Carl J. Levinson, M.D., F.A.C.O.G.
Associate Professor of Obstetrics and Gynecology
Section of Gynecologic Endocrinology
Baylor College of Medicine
Texas Medical Center
Houston, Texas

Franklin D. Loffer, M.D., F.A.C.O.G.
Department of Obstetrics and Gynecology
Maricopa County General Hospital
Phoenix, Arizona

Jaroslav J. Marik, M.D., F.A.C.O.G.
Assistant Clinical Professor of Obstetrics and
    Gynecology
University of California, Los Angeles School of
    Medicine
Associate Director, Tyler Clinic
Los Angeles, California

John Marlow, M.D., F.A.C.O.G.
Assistant Professor
George Washington University School of Medicine
Program Director for the Columbia Hospital for
    Women
Washington, D.C.

Docteur Raoul Palmer
Ancien Interne des Hôpitaux de Paris
Ex-Chef des Travaux de Gynécologie à la Faculté
     de Médecine
Paris, France

A. Jefferson Penfield, M.D., F.A.C.O.G.
Assistant Clinical Professor of Obstetrics and
     Gynecology
Upstate Medical Center
Syracuse, New York

David Pent, M.D., F.A.C.O.G.
Associate, Department of Obstetrics and
     Gynecology
University of Arizona School of Medicine
Phoenix, Arizona

Jordan M. Phillips, M.D., F.A.C.O.G.
Associate Clinical Professor of Gynecology and
     Obstetrics
Chief of the Section of Gynecologic Endoscopy
University of California, Irvine
California College of Medicine
Irvine, California
President, American Association of Gynecologic
     Laparoscopists

Robert Quint
Product Manager
American Cystoscope Makers, Inc.
Stamford, Connecticut

R. T. Ravenholt, M.D., M.P.H.
Director of the Office of Population
Agency for International Development
Department of State
Washington, D.C.

Jacques-E. Rioux, M.D., F.R.S.H., F.A.C.O.G.
Associate Professor of Obstetrics and Gynecology
Laval University Faculty of Medicine
Quebec City, Quebec, Canada
Secretary, American Association of Gynecologic
     Laparoscopists

Maxwell Roland, M.D., F.A.C.O.G., F.A.C.S.
Professor of Obstetrics and Gynecology
French and Polyclinic Medical School and Health
     Center
New York, New York

Alvin M. Siegler, M.D., D.Sc.
Clinical Professor of Obstetrics and Gynecology
State University of New York
Downstate Medical Center
Brooklyn, New York

Burton H. Smith, M.D.
Professor of Medicine
University of California, Irvine
California College of Medicine
Director of Endoscopy, Gastroenterology
     Department
Orange County Medical Center
Irvine, California

Richard M. Soderstrom, M.D., F.A.C.O.G.
Mason Clinic
Associate Clinical Professor of Obstetrics and
     Gynecology
University of Washington
Seattle, Washington
Vice President, American Association of Gyneco-
     logic Laparoscopists

J. Joseph Speidel, M.D., M.P.H.
Chief, Research Division
Office of Population
Bureau for Population and Humanitarian Assistance
Agency for International Development
Department of State
Washington, D.C.

William W. Stanton, M.D.
Assistant Professor
Department of Surgery
University of California, Irvine
California College of Medicine
Irvine, California

Patrick C. Steptoe, F.R.C.S., F.R.C.O.G.
President, British Fertility Society
Oldham, Lancashire, England

Gerold V. van der Vlugt, M.D., Dr.P.H., F.A.C.P.M.
Population Advisor
Family Planning Services Division
Office of Population
Agency for International Development
Department of State
Washington, D.C.

Clifford R. Wheeless, Jr., M.D.
Assistant Professor
Obstetrics and Gynecology
Johns Hopkins University School of Medicine
Baltimore, Maryland

Andrew T. Wiley, M.D., M.P.H.
Chief of the Technical Services Branch
Family Planning Services Division
Office of Population
Agency for International Development
Department of State
Washington, D.C.

Gerald Winfield, Sc.D.
Chief, Manpower and Institutions Division
Office of Population
Agency for International Development
State Department
Washington, D.C.

InBae Yoon, M.D., F.A.C.O.G.
Assistant Professor of Gynecology
Johns Hopkins University
Baltimore, Maryland

A. Albert Yuzpe, M.D., M.Sc., F.R.C.S. (C),
    F.A.C.O.G.
Associate Professor of Obstetrics and Gynecology
University of Western Ontario Faculty of Medicine
London, Ontario, Canada

Contents

Section 1   **Introduction**

Jordan Phillips   Preface

Melvin Cohen   1   Forewords
Hans Frangenheim   2
Raoul Palmer
Patrick Steptoe

John Gunning   2   History of Laparoscopy
                                              6

Section 2.   **Instruments**

Robert Quint   3   Physics of Light and Image Transmission
                                              18

Jacques Rioux   4   Basic Principles of Electrosurgery
Diogene Cloutier   24

Richard Soderstrom   5   Contemporary Instruments
                                              34

Tibor Engel   6   Instrument Maintenance and Personnel
                                              Training
                                              46

Section 3.   **Preparation**

Philip Brooks   7   Indications and Contraindications
John Marlow   52

Edwin Bronstein   8   Informing and Counseling Patients
                                              60

John Fishburne   9   Anesthesia
Louis Keith   69

Section 4.   **Fundamentals**

    Stephen L. Corson   10   Operating Room Preparation and Basic
                                                       Techniques
                                                       88

Section 5.   **Diagnostic Procedures**

    Hans Frangenheim   11   Pelvic Pain
                                                       104

    Alan Gazzaniga   12   Blunt and Penetrating Injuries to the Abdo-
    William Stanton   men
    Robert Bartlett   113

    Victor Gomel   13   Oncologic Laparoscopy
    Stephen Corson   119

Section 6.   **Operative Procedures**

    Alvin Siegler   14   Operative Laparoscopy: An Overview
                                                       130
    A. Albert Yuzpe   Ovarian Biopsy   133
    Robert Israel   Removal of Extrauterine Intrauterine
                                                       Devices   140
    H. M. Hasson   Open Laparoscopy   145
    Jaroslav Marik   Uterine Suspension   150
    John Esposito   Ectopic Pregnancy Management   155

    Richard Soderstrom   15   Operative Sterilization: An Overview   159
    Jaroslav Hulka   The Spring Clip   167
    InBae Yoon   The Silicone Ring   174
    Richard Soderstrom   The Snare Method   179
    Norman G. Courey
    Arthur Horowitz   Sterilization Combined with Abortion
    Rafael G. Cunanan   182
    Louis Keith
    Keim Houser   Puerperal Sterilization   187

Section 7   **Diagnosis and Management of Infertility**

Stephen L. Corson   Introduction
                                                       192

Melvin Cohen   16   Laparoscopy and Infertility
                                                       194

Maxwell Roland   17   Diagnosis of Infertility
David Leisten   200

John Esposito   18   Infertility Management
                                                       207

Victor Gomel   19   Fertility Surgery
                                                       212

Section 8   **Complications**

Carl J. Levinson   20   Complications
                                                       220

Clifford R. Wheeless   21   Thermal Gastrointestinal Injuries
                                                       231

A. Jefferson Penfield   22   Trocar and Needle Injuries
                                                       236

Franklin D. Loffer   23   Statistics
                                                       242

Section 9.   **Systems for Instruction**

Franklin Loffer   24   Self-Instruction
David Pent   248

David Pent   25   Teaching Laparoscopy
Franklin Loffer   252

George Berci   26   Development of an Endoscopy Unit
                                                       259

W. Dow Edgerton   27   Laparoscopy in a Community Hospital
Richard Kleppinger   265

Clifford Wheeless   28   Laparoscopy in an Academic Training
                                                       Program
                                                       275

R. T. Ravenholt   29   Worldwide Program Experiences for
Willard H. Boynton   US Agency for International Develop-
Dorothy N. Glenn   ment
J. Joseph Speidel   281
Gerold van der Vlugt
Andrew T. Wiley
Gerald Winfield

Section 10.
Special Aspects

Michel Cognat
30
Pediatric Laparoscopy
294

Melvin Cohen
31
Photography
300

A. Albert Yuzpe
32
Television
306

Jordan Phillips
33
Legal Liability
313

Burton Smith
Arthur Goldstein
34
Nongynecologic Laparoscopy
324

Section 11.
Research and New Developments

W. R. Dukelow
Satoski Ariga
35
Laparoscopy in Nonhuman Primates
334

Section 12.
State of the Art

Jordan M. Phillips
Donald Keith
Jaroslav Hulka
Barbara Hulka
Louis Keith
36
Survey of Laparoscopy, 1971–1975
342

Jaroslav Hulka
37
Summary of the State of the Art
353

Atlas of Color Plates

Index to Color Figures

Normal   Panoramic view of pelvis   1

Ovulation   Early follicle   2
                  Developing follicle   3
                  Pre-ovulatory follicle   4
                  Corpus luteum   5

Pelvic Pain   **Endometriosis**
                  Bladder   6
                  Cul-de-sac   7
                  Ovary   8
                  Adhesions   9

                  PID
                  Hydrosalpinx   10
                  Pyosalpinx   11

                  Adhesions
                  Omental to abdominal wall   12
                  Bridal veil   13
                  Peritubal   14

                  Hernia
                  Inguinal   15
                  Incarcerated   16

                  Ectopic
                  Ampullary   17
                  Isthmic   18
                  Chronic ectopic   19
                  Surgical excision   20

                  Miscellaneous
                  Allen-Masters syndrome   21
                  Pelvic varicosities   22
                  Cystic structure Biopsy: endometriosis   23
                  Appendix—normal   24
                  Appendicitis—acute   25
                  Appendicitis—chronic   26
                  Infarction of para-ovarian cyst   27

Infertility   Adhesions, pelvic   28
                  Adhesions, pelvic   29
                  Adhesions, myoma, patent tubes   30
                  Adhensions, PID, patent tubes   31
                  Corpus hemorrhagicum. Fimbrial dye   32
                  Hydrosalpinx plus dye   33
                  TB tube   34
                  Polycystic ovarian disease (Stein-Levinthal
                    syndrome)   35
                  Polycystic ovary   36
                  Endometrioma   37
                  Intramural cornual myoma   38

	Periovarian adhesions	39
	Gall bladder and liver with adhesions to diaphragm	40
	Hydatid of Morgagni plus chromopertubation	41
	Division of omentum from uterus	42
	Double uterus	43
Malignancy	Catheter placed for infusion of chromic phosphate P32; inspection of underside of liver	44
	Advanced carcinoma of the ovary	45
	Liver with metastasis	46
	Omentum with metastasis	47
	Carcinoma of the bladder with metastasis	48
	Ovarian carcinoma and cul-de-sac metastasis	49
	Metastasis to tube	50
	Metastasis to abdominal wall	51
Anomalies	Turner's syndrome	52
	Streak ovary	53
	Rokitansky-Kuster-Hauser syndrome	54
	Bicornuate uterus	55
	Double uterus separated by urinary bladder	56
	Hypoplasia of uterus—panhypopituitarism	57
Masses	Myomata, cystic left ovary	58
	Myomata	59
	Ovary—dermoid cyst	60
	Tubo-ovarian abscess	61
	Hyperstimulation of ovary	62
Sterilization	**Cautery**	
	Normal anatomy	63
	Grasp	64
	First burn	65
	Late burn	66
	Cut	67
	End product	68
	Clip	69
	Clip	70
	Ring	71
	Ring	72
	Ring	73
	Spontaneous reanastamosis of tube after Pomeroy procedure	74
	Appearance of tube (2 years after cautery)	75
Miscellaneous	Aspiration of ovarian cyst	76
	Suspension of uterus—suture in round ligament	77
	Suspension of uterus	78

Uterosacral ligament resection 79
IUD—lying free 80
  —imbedded, string free 81
  —removal 82
Removal of tubal splint 83
Assessment of tube for tuboplasty following
  previous Pomeroy 84
Extraperitoneal insufflation 85
Ovarian stromal luteinization (menopause) 86
Perihepatitis 87
Normal liver and gallbladder 88
Incisional hernia with extruded omentum 89
Ovarian biopsy 90
Snare Technique 91

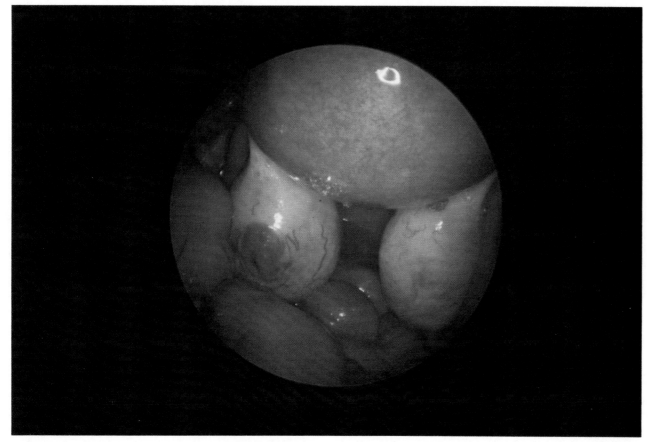

1

M. Cohen

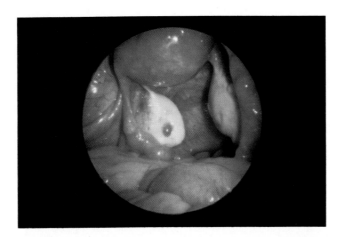

2   M. Cohen

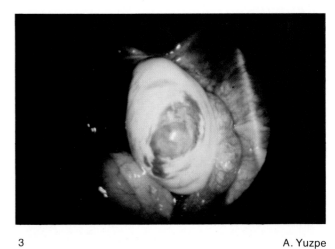

3   A. Yuzpe

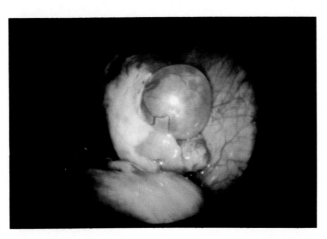

4   A. Yuzpe

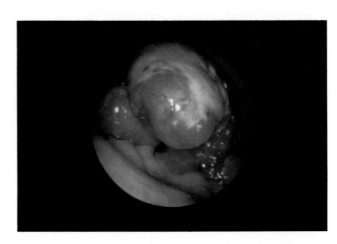

5   M. Cohen

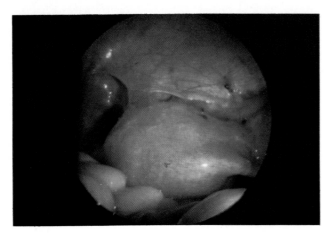

6   M. Cohen

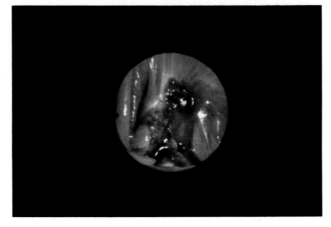

7   M. Cohen

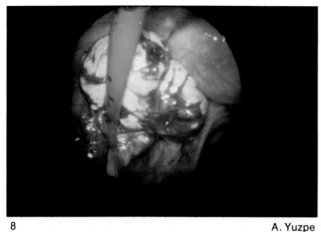

8   A. Yuzpe

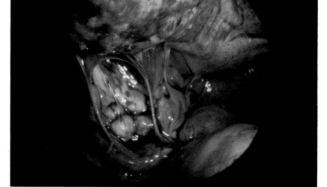

9   M. Cohen

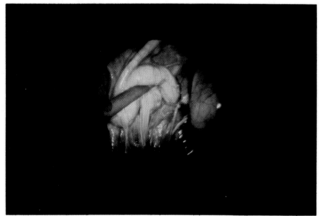

10   A. Yuzpe

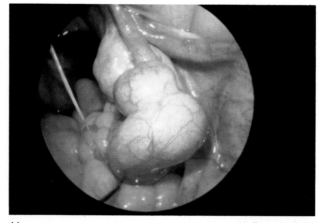

11   H. Frangenheim

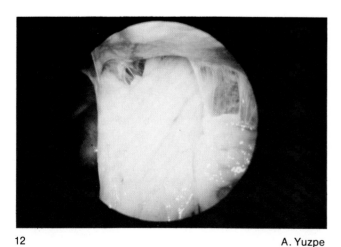

12   A. Yuzpe

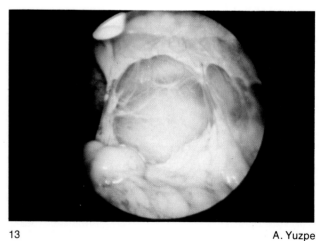

13   A. Yuzpe

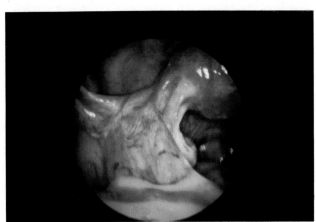

14   A. Yuzpe

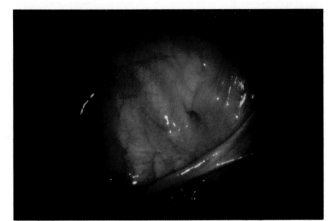

15   M. Cohen

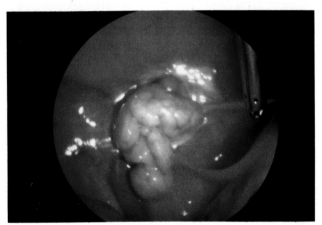

16   H. Frangenheim

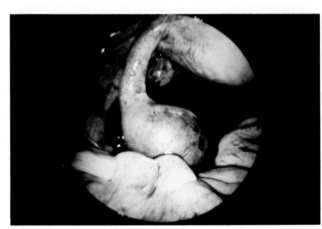

17   A. Yuzpe

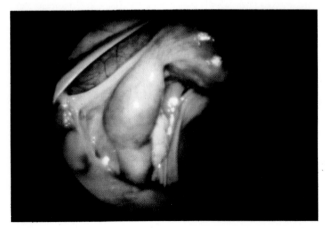

18   A. Yuzpe

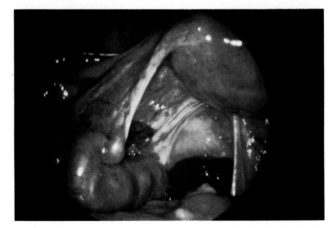

19   H. Frangenheim

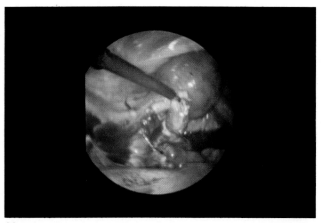

20 V. Gomel

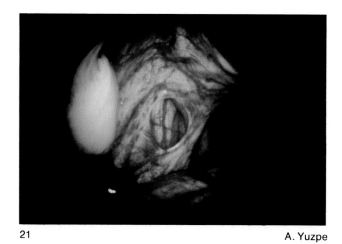

21 A. Yuzpe

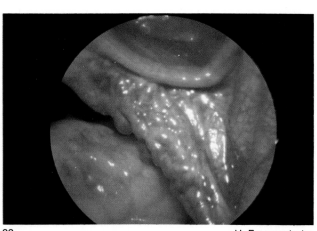

22 H. Frangenheim

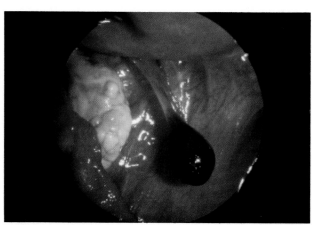

23 M. Cohen

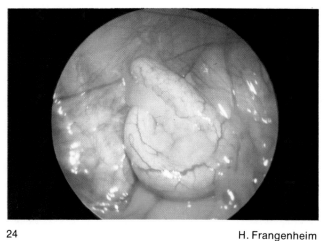

24 H. Frangenheim

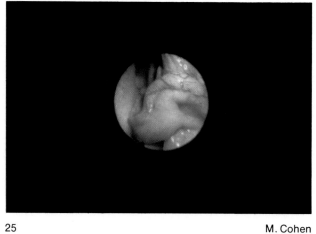

25 M. Cohen

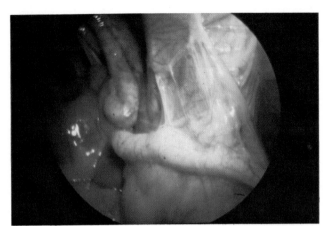

26   H. Frangenheim

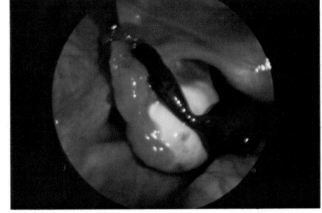

27   H. Frangenheim

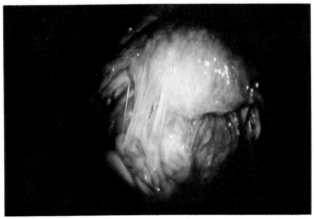

28   A. Yuzpe

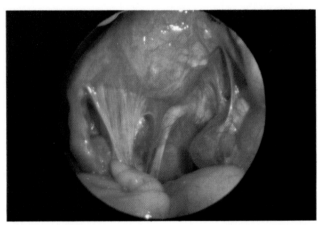

29   M. Cohen

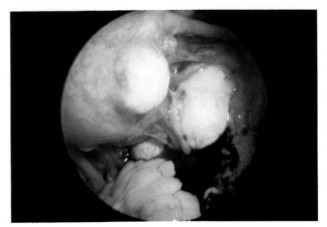

30   M. Cohen

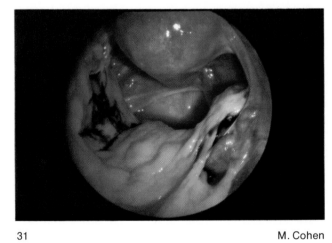

31   M. Cohen

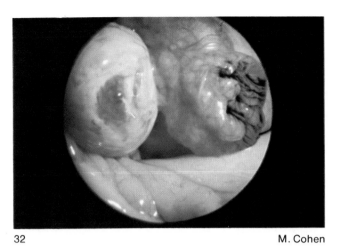

32   M. Cohen

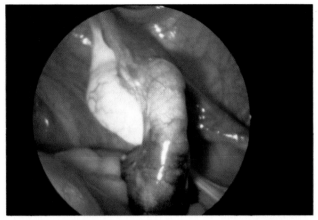

33   H. Frangenheim

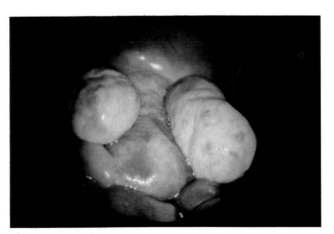

34   R. Legros/J. Abeille

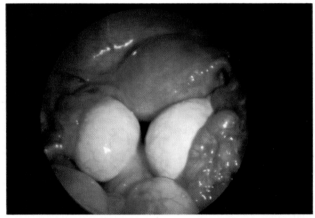

35   M. Cohen

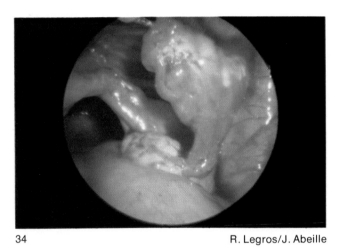

36   A. Yuzpe

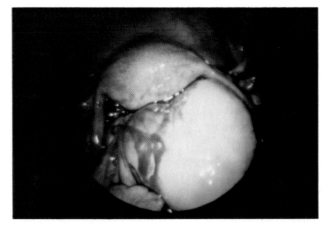

37   A. Yuzpe

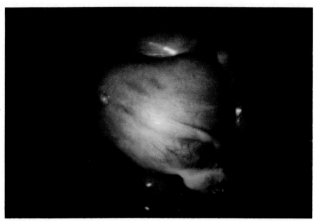

38   A. Yuzpe

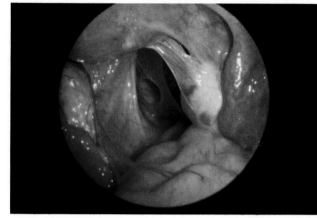

39   M. Cohen

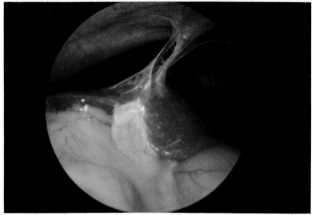

40   M. Cohen

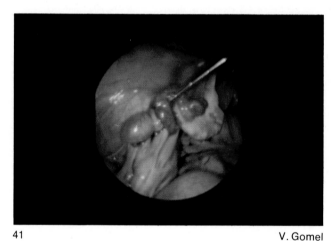

41   V. Gomel

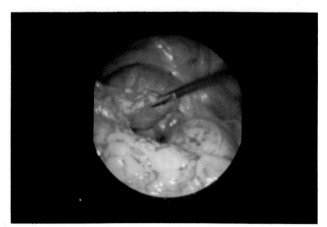

42   V. Gomel

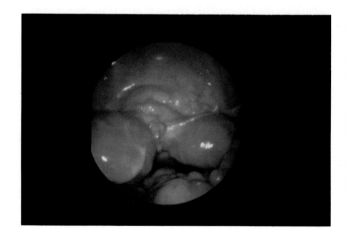

43   V. Gomel

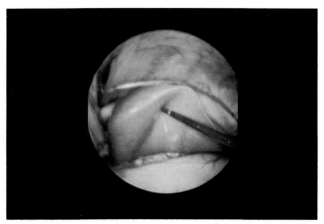

44 V. Gomel

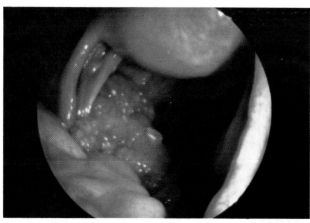

45 H. Frangenheim

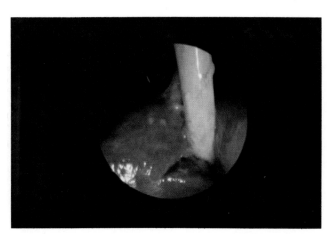

46 R. Legros/J. Abeille

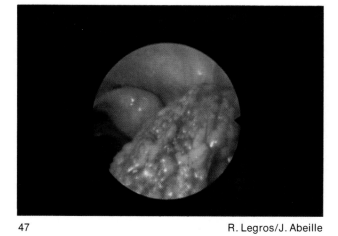

47 R. Legros/J. Abeille

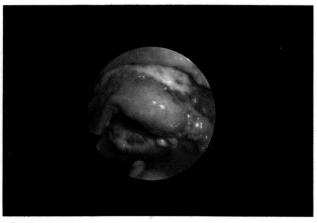

48 H. Frangenheim

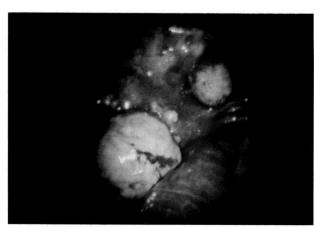

49 A. Yuzpe

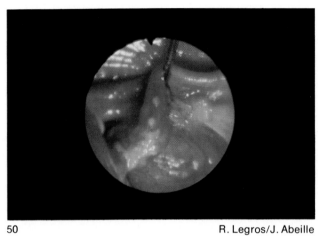

50   R. Legros/J. Abeille

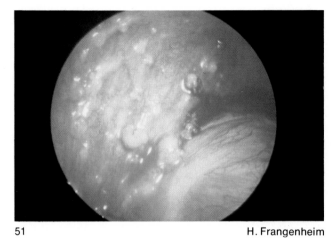

51   H. Frangenheim

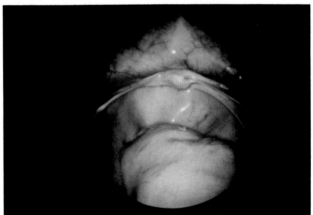

52   A. Yuzpe

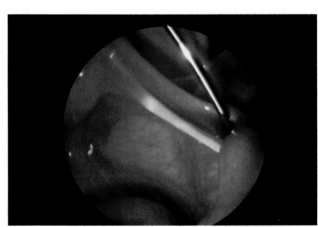

53   H. Frangenheim

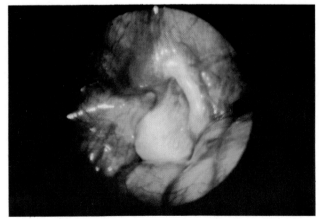

54   A. Yuzpe

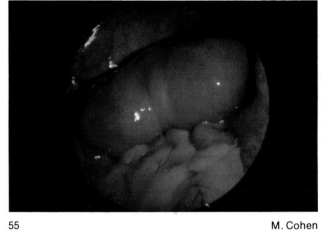

55   M. Cohen

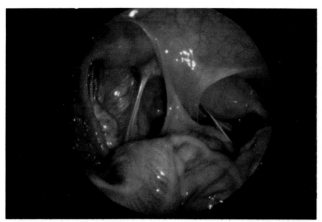

56   M. Cohen

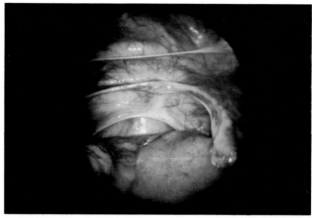

57   A. Yuzpe

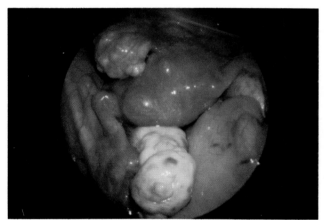

58   M. Cohen

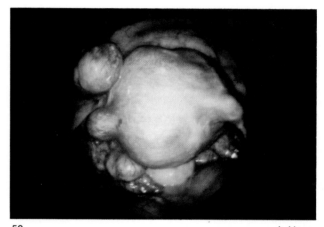

59   A. Yuzpe

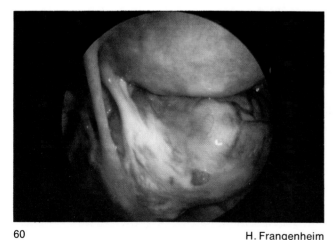

60   H. Frangenheim

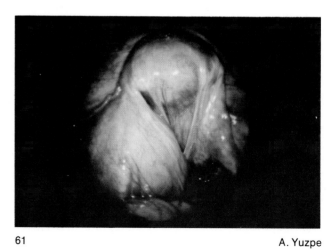

61   A. Yuzpe

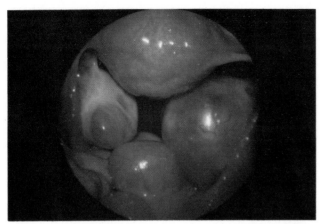

62   R. Legros/J. Abeille

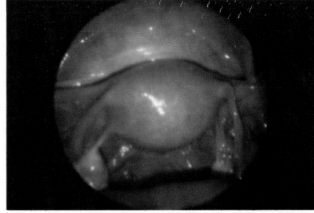
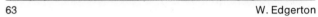

63   W. Edgerton

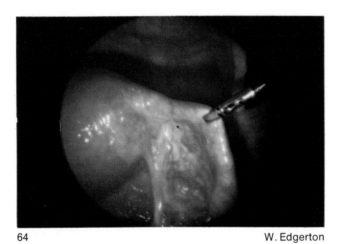

64   W. Edgerton

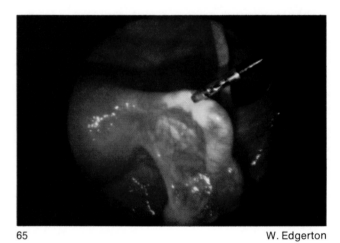

65   W. Edgerton

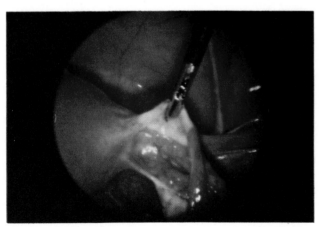

66   W. Edgerton

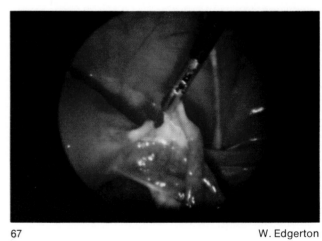

67   W. Edgerton

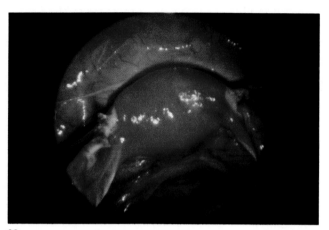

68   W. Edgerton

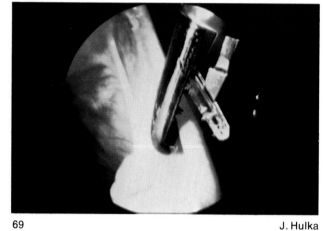

69   J. Hulka

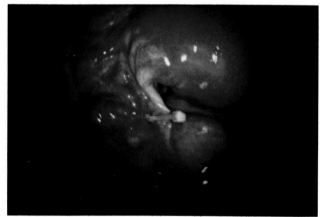

70   J. Phillips

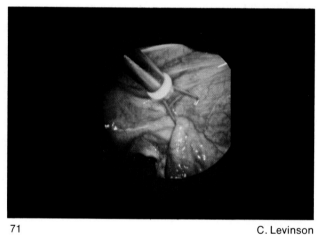

71   C. Levinson

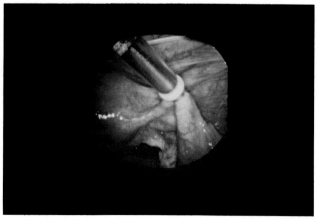

72   C. Levinson

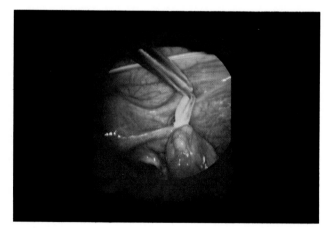

73   C. Levinson

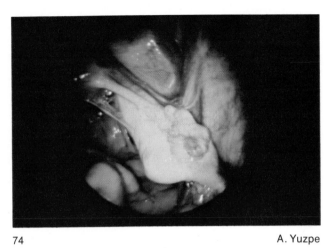

74   A. Yuzpe

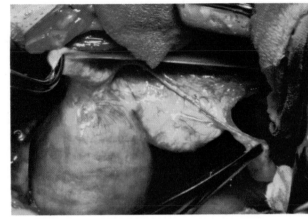

75   A. Yuzpe

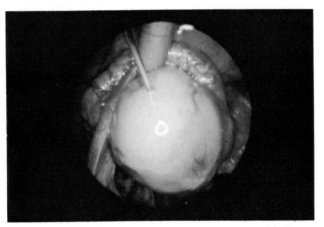

76   A. Yuzpe

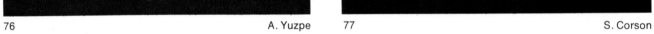

77   S. Corson

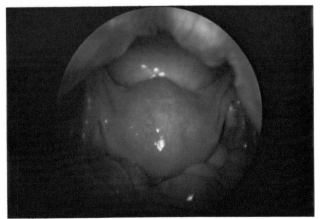

78   S. Corson

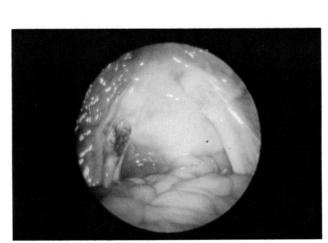

79   A. Yuzpe

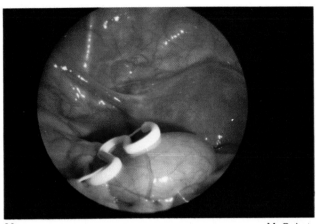

80   M. Cohen

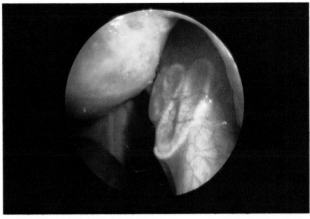

81   H. Frangenheim

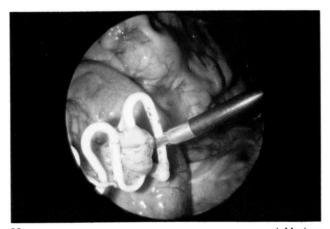

82   J. Marlow

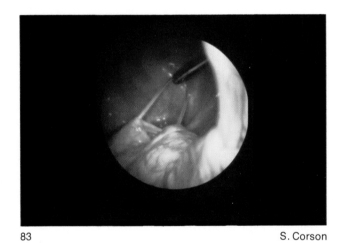

83   S. Corson

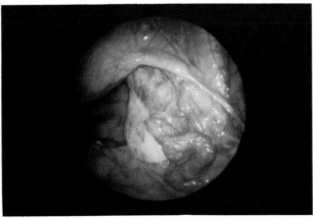

84   A. Yuzpe

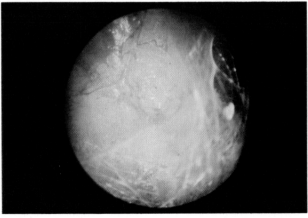

85   A. Yuzpe

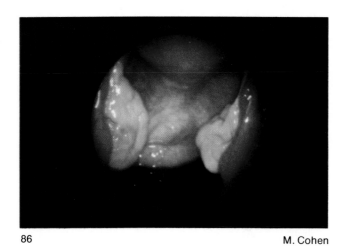

86   M. Cohen

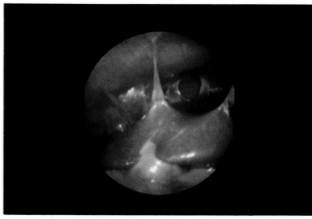

87   V. Gomel

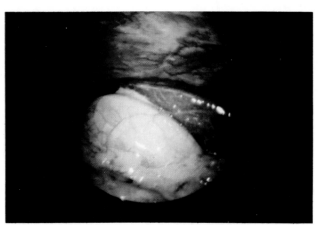

88   A. Yuzpe

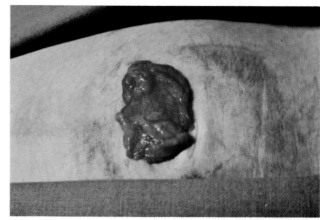

89   H. Frangenheim

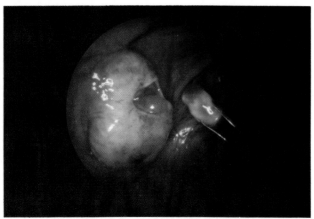

90   H. Frangenheim

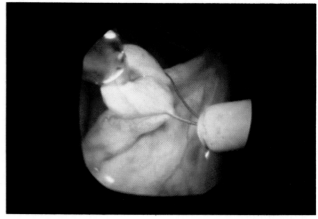

91   R. Soderstrom

Section 1

Introduction

Chapter 1

Forewords

Melvin R. Cohen, M.D.
Hans Frangenheim, M.D.
Raoul Palmer, M.D.
Patrick C. Steptoe, M.D.

Gynecologic laparoscopy has "come a long way" during the past ten years, and this new book is testimony to what has been accomplished during this brief period. This volume, so ably compiled by Dr. Jordan M. Phillips and the Editorial Board, is replete with discussions of indications, contraindications and complications of laparoscopy. The subject is discussed from many points of view, and the reader has the benefit of the collective experience of experts. However, some of the more exotic techniques—such as new methods of sterilization, both permanent and temporary, laparoscopic ovarian resection for the polycystic ovarian syndrome, retrieval of preovulatory ova for *in vitro* fertilization, salpingectomy for an unruptured tubal pregnancy, round ligament shortening and uterosacral ligament denervation—might be considered to be in the realm of human experimentation. As such, they should be approved by appropriate hospital committees as well as by the patient—a medicolegal must.

As a senior gynecologic laparoscopist, I would like to sound a word of warning to all present and future laparoscopists. A review of laparoscopy since 1900 demonstrates that this technique was discarded periodically, only to be rediscovered every ten years or so. Laparoscopy has shown periods of great enthusiasm followed by condemnation, the latter because of catastrophic complications. Excellent instruments, safe sources of gas, safe power supplies, greatly improved electrosurgical units, coupled with superb anesthesia by trained physician anesthesiologists: all are safety factors. However, no technique is foolproof, and certain techniques are not for everybody. Remember, the two chief indications for laparoscopy are (1) diagnosis of obscure pelvic disease, and (2) tubal sterilization. Even the experienced laparoscopist should not tackle a procedure that is better treated by laparotomy.

Melvin R. Cohen, M.D.
Chicago, Illinois

In the past century perhaps no examination method has revolutionized the diagnostic and therapeutic procedures of gynecologists and, with certain limitations, of surgeons and pediatricians as has endoscopy. At the head of all procedures stands gynecologic laparoscopy. In the 1950s and 1960s the clinical testing of the many indications and the trying out of the first operative procedures lay in the hands of a few pioneers. At first it was difficult to conquer prejudices and convince the world that laparoscopy was a method in every respect superior to the many other diagnostic and therapeutic ones. It took more than 15 years of intensive effort until this procedure was generally accepted. In the United States the superiority of laparoscopy over culdoscopy was fully recognized at the end of the 1960s and beginning of the 1970s, and now a trend in the history of laparoscopy is being set.

Whereas diagnostic laparoscopy with its ramified indications was the center of interest in Europe, the main attention in the United States was directed almost exclusively—a few practitioners (researchers, experimenters) excepted—toward laparoscopic tubal sterilization.

The American Association of Gynecologic Laparoscopists has guided this development and influenced it immeasurably through the enormous efforts of its executive committee, under the direction of Dr. Jordan Phillips. Extension courses, educational literature, international meetings of the highest level and, above all, the analysis of the complications committee have contributed to the general acceptance of the 20-year European experience with laparoscopy and to the large-scale clinical application of the procedure in the United States in less than five years.

This text, which has been compiled through the experience of experts around the world, will be a standard work and long outlive its time. I would like to extend my best wishes to its initiator, Jordan Phillips, and his associates Louis Keith and Jaroslav Hulka.

Dr. med. Hans Frangenheim
Konstanz, West Germany

The extraordinary boom of laparoscopy in the USA in the last six years is mostly explainable by its extensive use in female sterilization. At the moment it is still the most effective, most rapid, most elegant and least disagreeable method of female sterilization—except for the complications and costs. The complications can nearly always be avoided by a continuous surveillance during all stages of the procedure. The costs are acceptable if the complex, fragile and expensive set of instruments is fully employed and well maintained. I am not sure that laparoscopic sterilization is the best method for developing countries, except for the university centers, where the laparoscopist is not performing sterilizations exclusively.

In France, laparoscopy has been a recognized tool of advanced gynecology since 1946 and a must in sterility work for the last 20 years. In Europe, it spread rapidly to Italy, England and Germany when cold-light optics appeared; laparoscopy often permits a better view of the adnexa than laparotomy does. I believe that laparoscopic operations will be used more and more in the treatment of such conditions as sterility and pelvic pain.

However, to be efficient and sure, laparoscopists must remain an elite of people with good skill, continuous attention, innate curiosity and adequate preparation for scientific investigation.

Raoul Palmer
Paris, France

The art and science of laparoscopy is now established beyond all doubt as a diagnostic and operative technique of paramount importance to the modern practitioner of gynecology. It is largely due to the dedication of Dr. Jordan M. Phillips and his colleagues of the American Association of Gynecologic Laparoscopists that the teaching, training and uses of laparoscopy in the United States of America have been based on thoroughly sound principles. They have disseminated knowledge of the indications, contraindications, diagnostic and operative details, the difficulties and dangers involved, types of anesthesia used with due regard to the safety of the patient and the goal of her ultimate benefit. The difficulty of achieving precise diagnosis of many gynecologic disorders is now overcome, and diagnostic laparotomies are no longer necessary. Not only do the patients benefit from the sound teaching, but the would-be practitioner of gynecologic endoscopy does, also, for if he follows the precepts advocated within these pages he will be able to defend himself "right valiantly," should he be accused of malpractice.

During the past ten years there have been numerous international and national meetings in gynecology, infertility and endoscopy, so many expert practitioners have exchanged notes on their experiences. The editorial board of this new textbook of laparoscopy has collected a number of such contributors, who describe the present position of laparoscopy, its extended indications and developing techniques. The clinical results of the use of laparoscopy in gynecology have now reached such proportions that they can be subjected to critical appraisal, and the reader will be able to benefit from expert analysis.

The real value of laparoscopy lies not only in the field of operative female sterilization but also in that of accurate diagnosis and management of infertility, amenorrhea, pelvic and abdominal pain, genital malignancy, intrapelvic bleeding, the differential diagnosis of small masses, acute and chronic pelvic inflammatory disease, endocrine disturbances, dysmenorrhea, endometriosis, congenital anomalies and trauma. It also provides new opportunities for research into the complex physiology of human reproduction. Dr. Jordan M. Phillips and the Editorial Board are to be complimented on their choice of contributions, each of which plays a valuable part in the teaching and practice of laparoscopy. The instrument makers can provide us with superb equipment, but those who use them must be properly trained. This book will be a source of inspiration to all of those engaged in the practice of laparoscopy.

Patrick C. Steptoe
Oldham, England

Chapter 2

History
of
Laparoscopy

John E. Gunning, M.D.

The people and events of history cast long shadows that fall, if only faintly, on the things that we enjoy today and call our own. So it is with the past and present in respect to gynecologic laparoscopy. Look as long as we might, it will be hard to point to any major development or individual without acknowledging a debt to some of the early pioneering developments and ingenuity. Gynecologic laparoscopy is a spin-off of abdominal endoscopy, which in itself is a spin-off of cystoscopy. The pioneers of bygone days would indeed be astounded at how far some of their concepts have progressed in the modern world.

Bozzani (1805) was the first to attempt to visualize the interior of a body cavity. He visualized the human urethra in a living subject for the first time using candlelight and a cumbersome tube as an endoscope. Segalas (1826) refined the technique of urethroscopy by adding a cannula to the endoscopic tube as an obturator to facilitate introduction and a system of mirrors to reflect light into the cavity. Desormeaux (1853) developed the first serviceable urethroscope and cystoscope using mirrors to reflect light of a kerosene lamp. Nitze (1877) added a lens system to the endoscopic tube which magnified the area being examined, and this lens system is the forerunner of the optical system of modern cystoscopes and all other endoscopes. Edison (1880) invented the incandescent lamp, and Newman (1883) described an instrument using the incandescent lamp as a light source. Boisseau de Rocher (1889) separated the ocular part of the cystoscope from the sheath, thus allowing the use of multiple telescopes, which provided greater latitude of observation and made manipulation through the sheath possible. At the close of the 19th century cystoscopy and other open cavity endoscopic procedures such as bronchoscopy, laryngoscopy and esophagoscopy were well established and in daily clinical use.

Ott (1901) introduced endoscopic inspection of the abdominal cavity. He inspected the abdominal cavity with the help of a headmirror and a speculum, which was introduced through a small abdominal wall incision. He also used the same technique to visualize the pelvis by making a vaginal cul-de-sac incision with the patient in the Trendelenburg position. Kelling (1901) demonstrated the use of closed cavity endoscopy for the first time. He first inserted a needle into the peritoneal cavity of living dogs and distended it with air. He then inserted a Nitze cystoscope at another site for viewing. Jacobaeus (1910) was the first to report the use of pneumoperitoneum and the inspection of the abdominal cavity with a cystoscope in human beings. He did not use any special pneumoperitoneum needle, as Kelling had, but introduced the air through a cystoscope trocar sheath and then introduced the cystoscope. Bernheim (1911) inserted a proctoscope through a small abdominal wall incision for direct viewing of the contents.

Between 1901 and 1911 four investigators from different parts of the world reported their attempts to visualize the abdominal organs by methods not requiring major surgery. Ott and Bernheim utilized a small incision through which a speculum or proctoscope was inserted. This method is closed cavity endoscopy utilizing an open technique. Kelling introduced filtered air through a needle into the abdominal cavity and then, at a separate site, introduced a cystoscope. Jacobaeus used a trocar tube with a trapdoor to introduce filtered air and then inserted a cystoscope through the same trocar. This method is closed cavity endoscopy utilizing a closed technique. Kelling's original report described his work on dogs. In 1910 he published a reply to Jacobaeus stating that he had used his method on humans and in 1923 addressed the German Surgical Society concerning his experience on humans. Unfortunately, Kelling did not publish his experiences with humans. Both Kelling and Jacobaeus utilized a Nitze cystoscope, with the advantages of its lens system. Ott and Bernheim used a speculum or proctoscope without a lens system and introduced it through an incision. Kelling and Jacobaeus are the "fathers" of what we know today as *laparoscopy*. It would also be fair to say that Ott and Bernheim are the "fathers" of what we know today as the *minilaparotomy*, although neither suggested that operative procedures could be performed using their techniques.

Nordentoft (1912), using a method identical to that of Kelling and Jacobaeus, described viewing the female pelvis in a cadaver which had been placed in deep Trendelenburg position. Orndoff (1920) developed a sharp, pyramidal point on the trocar to facilitate puncture of the abdominal cavity after a pneumoperitoneum had been created. He also developed an automatic trocar sheath valve to prevent the escape of gas. Unverricht (1922) built a larger endoscope with a wider angle of vision and a stronger light to improve the visual image. Zollikofer (1924) was the first to use carbon dioxide as the gas of choice for insufflation because it was easily and quickly absorbed. A fore-oblique (135 degrees) lens viewing system was developed and introduced by Kalk in 1929. Kalk also was the first to use a second puncture for controlled liver biopsies. He used abdominal endoscopy extensively and thus encouraged many Europeans to use this technique. He published 29 papers between 1929 and 1959. Fervers (1933) developed techniques and instruments to cauterize abdominal adhesions and biopsy abdominal tissues.

Ruddock (1934) developed his own single puncture operating peritoneoscope and biopsy instruments. Hope (1937) suggested the use of abdominal endoscopy in the differential diagnosis of ectopic pregnancy and reported ten cases. This was the first report in the literature to date to be directed exclusively to the diagnosis of gynecologic diseases. Ruddock (1937) reported his experience with 900 cases, including 58 cases of ectopic pregnancies. Anderson (1937) reported his experiences with peritoneoscopy and suggested that his work would be of special interest to gynecologists. By using his special electrode and endothermic coagulation, sterilization of the female can be performed. He does not mention having done this procedure, nor does he subsequently report having done female sterilization utilizing his cautery method. Veress (1938) introduced a new type of pneumoperitoneum needle with a spring-loaded blunt probe surrounded by a sharp outer sleeve. This needle offered additional safety in preventing intraabdominal, soft tissue perforations.

Orndoff (1920), a radiologist, mentioned abdominal endoscopy as being of value in diagnosing ectopic gestation and ovarian cysts; however, his reported cases deal primarily with other abdominal conditions. Beling (1941) reviewed and listed the indications for peritoneoscopy. Included in his nine indications are: suspected pelvic neoplasms including endometriosis, old chronic inflammatory disease of any pelvic organ and suspected ectopic pregnancy. Powers and Barnes (1941), using a Ruddock peritoneoscope and the techniques of Ruddock, fulgurated the fallopian tubes using high frequency, high voltage pulsating current. Using a biopsy forceps they grasped the tube near the cornua and applied the fulgurating current until a segment of tube about 1 cm in length was blanched. They performed it both on dogs and humans and published histologic photographs of tubes removed six weeks following fulguration. Neither the number of cases performed nor that of the follow-ups is stated. They felt that this method warranted further study and clinical trial because it appeared to present certain advantages over various other generally accepted procedures. Donaldson (1942) used the Ruddock peritoneoscope and described a technique for performing an Olshausen uterine suspension without an open abdominal incision.

Decker (1944) indicated that he had used abdominal endoscopy but found that visualization of the pelvis gave uniformly unsatisfactory results. In an effort to improve the usefulness of the endoscope in pelvic diagnosis he became interested in the vaginal route and introduced culdoscopy. He demonstrated that in the knee-chest position, puncture of the cul-de-sac creates a spontaneous pneumoperitoneum, and an endoscope can be inserted safely through the thin rectovaginal septum and the pelvic organs visualized. At about the same time Palmer began utilizing abdominal endoscopy with the patients in deep Trendelenburg position. He preferred the abdominal route and subsequently used this route exclusively. Palmer (1946) reported his experiences with 250 cases of gynecologic diagnostic coelioscopy, many of which dealt with infertility. Palmer developed an endouterine cannula to move the uterus and to inject dye through the fallopian tubes while viewing them.

Historically, it is difficult to detemine ex-actly when gynecologic endoscopy became a specialty unto itself. In 1901 Ott, a Russian gynecologist, developed his technique of introducing a speculum through a cul-de-sac puncture with the patient in the lithotomy and Trendelenburg position. He also used the same technique of introducing a speculum through a small abdominal incision. The majority of subsequent investigators were primarily interested in liver and stomach disorders. Orndoff, a radiologist, reported, in 1920, his experiences utilizing the technique of Jacobaeus in the differential diagnosis of ovarian cysts, ectopic pregnancy and other abdominal diseases. Hope (1937) published the first papers specifically dealing with a gynecologic disease entity when he reported using peritoneoscopy for the diagnosis of ectopic pregnancy. Ruddock, a general surgeon, had 58 ectopic pregnancies included in 900 cases of peritoneoscopy, on which he published a paper in 1939. Powers and Barnes, in 1941, reported a technique of tubal cauterization for sterilization utilizing Ruddock's peritoneoscope. Palmer reported specifically on 250 gynecologic cases in 1947, and it probably can be said that he is the "father" of "modern gynecologic laparoscopy," although he refers to the procedure as gynecologic coelioscopy. Palmer subsequently developed many ancillary instruments for diagnostic and surgical treatment of gynecologic disorders.

Endoscopy procedures, in general, were revolutionized in 1952 when Fourestier, Gladu and Valmier introduced a new apparatus. They developed a method of transmitting an intense light along a quartz rod from the proximal to the distal end of the telescope. Previous light sources consisted of lamps located at the distal end of the endoscope. The development immediately removed the danger of accidents due to electrical faults and heat and provided intense light to be concentrated at the distal end of the endoscope so that photographs could be taken. The light bulb is placed at the proximal end of the telescope and cooled by a cooling tube which leads to a fan. Also in 1952 Hopkins and Kapany introduced fiber optics to the field of endoscopy. Their work was in developing a fiber optic gastroscope; however, the use of fiber optics was to have a dramatic and lasting effect on all endoscopic procedures. Following this development many investigators in

France, Italy and Germany published works on the subject. Endoscopic colored films were produced, and in 1959 a closed-circuit television program was first produced using a Fourestier, Gladu and Valmier apparatus.

Frangenheim (1957) began publishing his experiences with gynecologic laparoscopy and stressed improvement of technique. He delineated complications and methods in order to help others avoid those complications. He was a particularly strong proponent of general anesthesia as a preferred anesthetic agent rather than local anesthesia, which was used by most previous investigators. He likewise refined the optical instruments, and the laparoscope of Frangenheim is one of the standard optical instruments available today. He published the first textbook on gynecologic laparoscopy in 1959.

Utilization of gynecologic laparoscopy began to spread throughout Europe in the late 1940s. Palmer made a significant contribution in infertility investigation using laparoscopy. He developed the Palmer drill biopsy forceps for ovarian biopsy and was quick to develop laparoscopes utilizing the Fourestier, Gladu and Valmier apparatus. He began utilizing electrocoagulation of the tube for sterilization in 1962. Frangenheim's contributions, likewise, stimulated the growth of gynecologic laparoscopy in the European countries. He began utilizing diathermy for tubal sterilization in 1963 and developed laparoscopes utilizing fiber optics in conjunction with the Richard Wolf Company in 1965. Textbooks on gynecologic laparoscopy were published in France by Thoyer and Rozat and in Italy by Albano and Cittadini in 1962.

Gynecologic laparoscopy was a well established diagnostic and therapeutic procedure throughout the majority of European countries by 1965. Ancillary instruments and procedures were being developed and researched. Sjovall (1964) reported on ten years' experience using laparoscopy to diagnose acute salpingitis, a condition considered by most to be a contraindication to laparoscopy. De Brux (1967–68) reported his five-year experiences on the cytologic diagnosis of fluid aspirated from ovarian cysts and peritoneal fluid aspirated at laparoscopy.

In England and America, during almost three decades after Ruddock's extensive experiences, there was little interest in laparoscopy. In 1939 Meigs published a report on gynecologic medical progress in the *New England Journal of Medicine*. Two paragraphs are devoted to peritoneoscopy. He states, "The worth of the peritoneoscope is beginning to be appreciated," and "There are many possible uses for this instrument and its value for making accurate diagnosis in pelvic conditions is certain to increase." Marshall (1943), president of the Royal Society of Medicine, stated in his address to the society on peritoneoscopy, "It is of value in the diagnosis of lesions of the pelvic organs, particularly of the fallopian tubes and ovaries and it is especially valuable in the diagnosis of ectopic pregnancy." In 1935 there were two or three peritoneoscopes in America, and by 1941 there were over 300 in use. This change was most likely due to the influence of Ruddock. Why the popularity of the new procedure decreased in America during the next two-and-a-half decades, especially since it was endorsed by such an outstanding gynecologist as Meigs, is difficult to pinpoint. England experienced the same lack of interest in spite of Marshall's enthusiasm. No doubt World War II had some effect, as did the popularity of culdoscopy as the pelvic endoscopic procedure of choice in the United States.

In 1967 Steptoe published the first textbook on laparoscopy in the English language. Frangenheim, who authored the chapter on diagnosis of sterility, believes the laparoscope to be superior to all other methods of examination. Steptoe describes his method of sterilization utilizing coagulation and then division. The publication of this book had great impact in England and America, and the gynecologists in both countries rediscovered this marvelous tool.

It should be remembered that the instruments had undergone considerable change since the days of Ruddock. Lens improvements, fiber optics, automatic CO_2 machines and ancillary instruments were improved greatly, and the view of the pelvis seen at laparoscopy was most exciting. Some acknowledgment must be given to the Eder Company, Karl Stortz Company, Richard Wolf Company, and others for their contribution to these magnificent improvements.

Cohen and Fear both published articles on laparoscopy in the May 1968 issue of *Obstetrics and Gynecology,* which stimulated the reawakening of interest in the United States. These were the only two publications to appear in the American literature in 1968.

In 1969 Alexander published an article on the systemic effects of CO_2 pneumoperitoneum. Jacobson used laparoscopy to make an objective diagnosis of acute pelvic inflammatory disease. Steptoe reported combining therapeutic abortion with laparoscopic sterilization. Smith reported using the laparoscope for the first time to remove an ectopic intrauterine device (IUD). Both Neuwirth and Wheeless reported experiences with laparoscopic sterilization. Interest in laparoscopy was increasing rapidly, and many investigators as well as practicing gynecologists began to learn and utilize the technique.

In 1970 numerous reports appeared in the literature, and postgraduate courses on laparoscopy were offered in a few teaching institutions. Coltart found a 50% error in hysterosalpingography tubal patency tests when compared to laparoscopic evaluation. Steptoe and Edwards recovered viable human oocytes utilizing laparoscopy. Liston and associates reported their results in 760 laparoscopic sterilizations. Neuwirth reported his experiences in 155 cases, Peterson and Behrman their experiences in 538 cases, and Siegler and Garret their experiences utilizing ancillary procedures in 214 cases of gynecologic laparoscopy. Wheeless reported his experiences with laparoscopic sterilization as an outpatient procedure and pointed out the safety and low cost when compared to other methods. Steptoe reported his results in 500 cases of laparoscopic sterilization.

The utilization of gynecologic laparoscopy and the expansion of ancillary procedures and techniques continued in 1971. Soderstrom and Smith reported a new technique of tubal sterilization utilizing a rectal polyp snare. The frequency of sterilization procedures in the United States was rising dramatically due to public, professional and legal liberalization. This fact alone can account for increasing popularity and utilization of laparoscopy. As experiences increased, so the indications for laparoscopy broadened. Prior contraindications were tested and found to be invalid in the hands of some investigators. Keith and his colleagues reported their preliminary results using laparoscopy for puerperal sterilization. Hasson introduced new instruments and techniques for open laparoscopy which in principle are much like Ott's but with the advantages of better instruments, lighting and optics.

By 1972 laparoscopy was a well accepted and frequently used procedure in the United States and Canada. It was taught in most obstetrics and gynecology residency programs, and numerous postgraduate courses were given. Over 150 scientific papers appeared in the world literature in 1972 dealing with gynecologic laparoscopy. Series of cases, experimental procedures in laboratory animals, technique modifications, new instruments and complications were among the many subjects. Wheeless reintroduced the single puncture technique under local anesthesia for sterilization which, aside from CO_2 utilization, was little different from the technique used by Ruddock. Clarke introduced instruments for tubal ligation, and Hulka reported on the use of clips for tubal sterilization. Popular debate took place about the sterilization cautery technique to use — cautery at three sites, cautery at two sites, cautery plus division or cautery plus division with removal of a segment of tube.

Phillips founded the American Association of Gynecologic Laparoscopists in 1972, and in November of that year the Association held their first annual meeting in Las Vegas, Nevada, with an attendance of over 600. A committee on complications, chaired by Hulka, gave their first annual report. A flying doctors group was formed to teach laparoscopy in developing countries.

By 1973 gynecologic laparoscopy was a routine operating-room procedure in most major hospitals in every city in the United States. The world literature contains over 175 scientific papers on the subject. Considerable effort was expended to develop methods which would avoid the small but significant number of complications, especially the burns, by using a bipolar cautery, which eliminated the current's passing through the patient's body to a ground plate. Thompson and Wheeless reported a review of 3,600 laparoscopic sterilizations.

The second annual meeting of the American Association of Gynecologic Laparoscopists was held in New Orleans in November 1973 in conjunction with the First International Congress of Gynecologic Laparoscopy. The attendance was 600, with representation from England, France, Germany, Thailand, Japan, Austria, the Netherlands, Canada and Mexico. Distinguished experts were present: Palmer, Steptoe, Frangenheim, Behrman, Cohen, Cognat and Semm, to name just a few. The second annual report on complications was presented, as well as many papers on all aspects of laparoscopy. The proceedings were published in 1974.

The year 1974 continued with the same enthusiasm as that of 1973. Over 100 scientific papers appeared. Follow-up experiences on previous reports and reviews of experiences were numerous. For sterilization Yoon began using a silastic ring, which fits tightly around a knuckle of tube, and developed an applicator to fit an operating laparoscope.

A survey of gynecologic laparoscopy, covering numerous aspects of techniques, anesthesia, individual experiences and complications, was conducted by the American Association of Gynecologic Laparoscopists. The data represents the experiences of 886 physicians who do laparoscopy. Active membership in the American Association of Gynecologic Laparoscopists was now 1,750 and 800 were in attendance at their annual meeting, held in Anaheim, California.

By 1975 gynecologic laparoscopy had withstood the test of time. The review of hundreds of thousands of cases and the experiences of thousands of operators verified this fact. It is now a very important diagnostic and therapeutic modality for the gynecologist. No doubt minor debates will continue over single- or two-puncture techniques, local or general anesthesia, carbon dioxide or nitrous oxide pneumoperitoneum, cautery or other techniques for sterilization. Instruments will continue to improve, additional safety in cautery equipment will evolve and newer techniques undoubtedly will make sterilization safer as well as utilized more often. The growth and development of gynecologic laparoscopy in the last ten years has been phenomenal and one would trust that the faint shadows cast by our colleagues who preceded us will be recognized.

Summary of Historical Contributions to Gynecologic Laparoscopy

Year	Contributor	Contribution
1805	Bozzani (Germany)	Visualized urethra with a simple tube and candlelight.
1826	Segalas (France)	Added cannula to urethroscope tube and utilized mirrors to reflect candlelight.
1853	Desormeaux (France)	Presented first serviceable urethroscope and cystoscope. Utilized mirrors to reflect kerosene lamplight.
1877	Nitze (Germany)	Added lens system to endoscopic tube, thus allowing magnification of area viewed.
1880	Edison (USA)	Invented incandescent lamp bulb.
1883	Newman (Scotland)	Developed a cystoscope using a small incandescent light bulb at distal end.
1889	Boisseau de Rocher (France)	Separated ocular part from sheath. Used different telescopes through sheath. Used part of sheath for ancillary manipulation.
1901	Ott (Russia)	Viewed abdominal cavity with speculum through small incision (ventroscopy).
1901	Kelling (Germany)	Created pneumoperitoneum in dogs using a needle and then inserted a Nitze cystoscope (coelioscopy).
1910	Jacobaeus (Sweden)	Created pneumoperitoneum in humans using a trocar and then introduced a Nitze cystoscope through the same trocar (laparoscopy).
1911	Bernheim (USA)	Inserted proctoscope through a small abdominal incision (organoscopy).
1920	Orndoff (USA)	Developed sharp pyramidal point on the trocar to facilitate puncture and automatic trocar sheath valve to prevent escape of air (peritoneoscopy).
1924	Zollikofer (Switzerland)	Used carbon dioxide instead of air to create pneumoperitoneum.
1929	Kalk (Germany)	Developed foroblique (135 degrees) lens system. Published 29 papers (1929–1959). Introduced second puncture for controlled liver biopsy.

Summary — *Continued*

Year	Contributor	Contribution
1933	Fervers (Germany)	Developed biopsy instruments and cauterized intraabdominal adhesions.
1934	Ruddock (USA)	Developed single-puncture operating peritoneoscope.
1937	Hope (USA)	Used Ruddock's peritoneoscope to diagnose ectopic pregnancy.
1937	Anderson (USA)	Suggested endothermic coagulation of fallopian tube as a method of sterilization.
1939	Ruddock (USA)	Published results of 900 peritoneoscopies. 100% diagnostic accuracy in 58 cases of ectopic pregnancy.
1941	Beling (USA)	Reviewed and listed indications for peritoneoscopy. Listed suspected pelvic neoplasm including endometriosis, chronic PID and suspected ectopic pregnancy, along with others.
1941	Powers and Barnes (USA)	Sterilization by means of peritoneoscopic tubal fulguration.
1942	Donaldson (USA)	Performed peritoneoscopic Olshausen uterine suspension.
1944	Decker (USA)	Introduced and preferred culdoscopy.
1947	Palmer (France)	Published results of 250 cases of gynecologic coelioscopy. Introduced endouterine cannula for moving uterus and for tubal patency test.
1952	Fourestier, Gladu and Valmier (France)	Developed quartz rod and external light source.
1952	Hopkins and Kapany (England)	Introduced fiber optics to endoscopy.
1959	Frangenheim (Germany)	Published German textbook on gynecologic laparoscopy.
1962	Thoyer and Rozat (France)	Published French textbook on gynecologic coelioscopy.
1962	Albano and Cittadini (Italy)	Published Italian textbook on gynecologic laparoscopy.

Summary—*Continued*

Year	Contributor	Contribution
1962	Palmer (France)	Utilized electrocoagulation for tubal sterilization by laparoscopy.
1963	Frangenheim (Germany)	Utilized diathermy for tubal sterilization by laparoscopy.
1964	Sjovall (Sweden)	Reported on laparoscopic diagnosis of acute salpingitis.
1967	Steptoe (England)	Published English textbook on gynecologic laparoscopy.
1968	Cohen and Fear (USA)	Constituted first American publication on gynecologic laparoscopy in almost 30 years.
1969	Smith (USA)	Removed ectopic IUD with laparoscopy.
1970	Cohen (USA)	Published American textbook on gynecologic laparoscopy.
1970	Coltant (England)	Found 50% salpingogram tubal patency error compared to laparoscopic evaluation.
1970	Steptoe and Edwards (England)	Recovered oocyte with the laparoscope.
1970	Wheeless (USA)	Reported on outpatient laparoscopic tubal sterilization.
1971	Keith (USA)	Reported on puerperal laparoscopic tubal sterilization.
1972	Clarke (USA)	Introduced instruments for tubal ligation by laparoscopy.
1972	Hulka (USA)	Used clips for tubal sterilization by laparoscopy.
1972	Phillips (USA)	Founded American Association of Gynecologic Laparoscopists.
1972	Hulka (USA)	Chaired first annual report of Complications Committee of American Association of Gynecologists and Laparoscopists.
1973	Rioux (Canada)	Developed and used bipolar cautery for tubal sterilization by laparoscopy.
1974	Yoon (USA)	Used silastic rings for tubal sterilization by laparoscopy.

Additional Reading

1. Alexander GD, Noe FE, Brown EM: Anesthesia for pelvic laparoscopy. Anesth Analg 48:14, 1969

2. Anderson ET: Peritoneoscopy. Am J Surg 35:136, 1937

3. Balin H, Wan LS, Istale SL: Recent advances in pelvic endoscopy. Obstet Gynecol 72:30, 1966

4. Beling CA: Selection of cases for peritoneoscopy. Arch Surg 42:872, 1941

5. Belt AE, Charnock DA: The history of the cystoscope. In *Modern Urology*. (H. Cabot, Ed.) Lea & Febiger, Philadelphia, 1936

6. Bernheim BM: Organoscopy. Ann Surg 53:764, 1911

7. Clarke HC: Laparoscopy: new instruments for suturing and ligation. Fertil Steril 23:274, 1972

8. Cohen MR: Culdoscopy vs peritoneoscopy. Obstet Gynecol 31:310, 1968

9. Cohen MR: *Laparoscopy, Culdoscopy and Gynecography.* WB Saunders Co, Philadelphia, 1970

10. Coltart TM: Laparoscopy in the diagnosis of tubal patency. J Obstet Gynaecol Br Commonw 77:69, 1970

11. De Brux JA, Dupre-Froment J, Mintz M: Cytology of the peritoneal fluids sampled by coelioscopy or by cul-de-sac puncture: its value in gynecology. Acta Cytol 12:395, 1968

12. De Brux JA, Palmer R, Mintz M: Cytology of para-uterine tumors punctured under celioscopy. J Int Fed Gynaecol Obstet 5:247, 1967

13. Decker A, Cherry TH: Culdoscopy. A new method in the diagnosis of pelvic disease—preliminary report. Am J Surg 64:40, 1944

14. Donaldson JK, Sanderlin JH, Harrell WB, Jr: A method of suspending the uterus without open abdominal incision. Am J Surg 55:537, 1942

15. Fear R: Laparoscopy: a valuable aid in gynecological diagnosis. Obstet. Gynecol. 31:297, 1968

16. Hope RB: Differential diagnosis of ectopic gestation by peritoneoscopy. Surg Gynecol Obstet 64:229, 1937

17. Hulka JF, Omraru KF: Comparative tubal occlusion: rigid and spring loaded clips. Fertil Steril 23:633, 1972

18. Hulka JF, Soderstrom RM, Corson SL, Brooks PG: Complications Committee of the American Association of Gynecological Laparoscopists, first annual report. J Reprod Med 10:301, 1973

19. Jacobson L, Westrom L: Objectivized diagnosis of acute pelvic inflammatory disease. Diagnostic and prognostic value of routine laparoscopy. Am J Obstet Gynecol 105:1088, 1969

20. Jones HW, JR., Jones GS: Editorial comment. Obstet Gynecol Surv 27:385, 1972

21. Keith L, Houser K, Webster A, Lash AF: Puerperal tubal sterilization using laparoscopic technique: a preliminary report. J Reprod Med 6:133, 1971

22. Liston WA, Downie J, Bradford W, Kerr MG: Female sterilization by tubal electrocoagulation under laparoscopic control. Lancet 1:683, 1970

23. Marshall G: Peritoneoscopy. Proceedings of the Royal Society of Medicine. 36:445, 1943

24. Meigs JV: Gynecology. N Engl J Med 220:242, 1939

25. Nadeau OE, Kampmeier OF: Endoscopy of the abdomen: abdominoscopy. A preliminary study, including a summary of the literature and a description of the technique. Surg Gynecol Obstet 41:259, 1925

26. Neuwirth RS: Recent experience with diagnostic and surgical laparoscopy. Am J Obstet Gynecol 160:119, 1970

27. Neuwirth RS, Cejas M: Sterilization by tubal cauterization and transection at laparoscopy. Am J Obstet Gynecol 105:632, 1969

28. Orndoff BH: The peritoneoscope in diagnosis of diseases of the abdomen. J Radiol 1:307, 1920

29. Peterson EP, Behrman SJ: Laparoscopy of the infertile patient. Obstet Gynecol 36:363, 1970

30. Phillips JM: Personal communication.

31. Phillips JM, Keith D, Keith L, Hulka J, Hulka B: Survey of gynecologic laparoscopy for 1974. J Reprod Med 15:45, 1975

32. Power FH, Barnes AC: Sterilization by means of peritoneoscopic tubal fulguration: a preliminary report. Am J Obstet Gynecol 41:1038, 1941

33. Rioux JE, Cloutier D: A new bipolar instrument for laparoscopic tubal sterilization. Am J Obstet Gynecol 119:737, 1974

34. Ruddock JC: Application and evaluation of peritoneoscopy. California Med 71:110, 1949

35. Ruddock JC: Peritoneoscopy. Southern Surgeon 8:113, 1939

36. Ruddock JC: Peritoneoscopy. Surg Gynecol Obstet 65:623, 1937

37. Ruddock JC: Peritoneoscopy. West J Surg 42:392, 1934

38. Ruddock JC: Peritoneoscopy: a critical clinical review. Surg Clin North Am 37:1249, 1957

39. Siegler AM: Trends in laparoscopy. Am J Obstet Gynecol 109:794, 1971

40. Siegler AM, Berenyi KJ: Laparoscopy in gynecology. Obstet Gynecol 34:572, 1969

41. Siegler AM, Garret M: Ancillary technics with laparoscopy. Fertil Steril 21:763, 1970

42. Smith BD, Dillon TF: Laparoscopy. Fertil Steril 21:193, 1970

43. Smith DC: Removal of an ectopic IUD through the laparoscope. Am J Obstet Gynecol 105:285, 1969

44. Soderstrom RM, Smith MR: Tubal sterilization: a new laparoscopic method. Obstet Gynecol 38:152, 1971

45. Steptoe PC: *Laparoscopy in Gynaecology.* E & S Livingston Ltd, Edinburgh, 1967

46. Steptoe PC, Edwards RG: Laparoscopic recovery of preovulatory human oocytes after priming of ovaries with gonadotrophins. Lancet 1:683, 1970

47. Thompson BH, Wheeless CR: Outpatient sterilization by laparoscopy: a report of 666 cases. Obstet Gynecol 38:912, 1971

48. Wheeless CR: A rapid, inexpensive and effective method of surgical sterilization by laparoscopy. J Reprod Med 3:65, 1969

49. Wheeless CR: Elimination of second incision in laparoscopic sterilization. Obstet Gynecol 39:134, 1972

50. Wheeless CR: Outpatient sterilization under local anesthesia. Obstet Gynecol 39:767, 1972

51. Wheeless CR, Thompson BH: Laparoscopic sterilization: review of 3600 cases. Obstet Gynecol 42:751, 1973

52. Wittman I: *Peritoneoscopy.* Publishing House of the Hungarian Academy of Sciences. Budapest, 1966

53. Yoon IB, King TM: A preliminary and intermediate report on a new laparoscopic tubal ring procedure. J Reprod Med 15:54, 1975

Section 2

Instruments

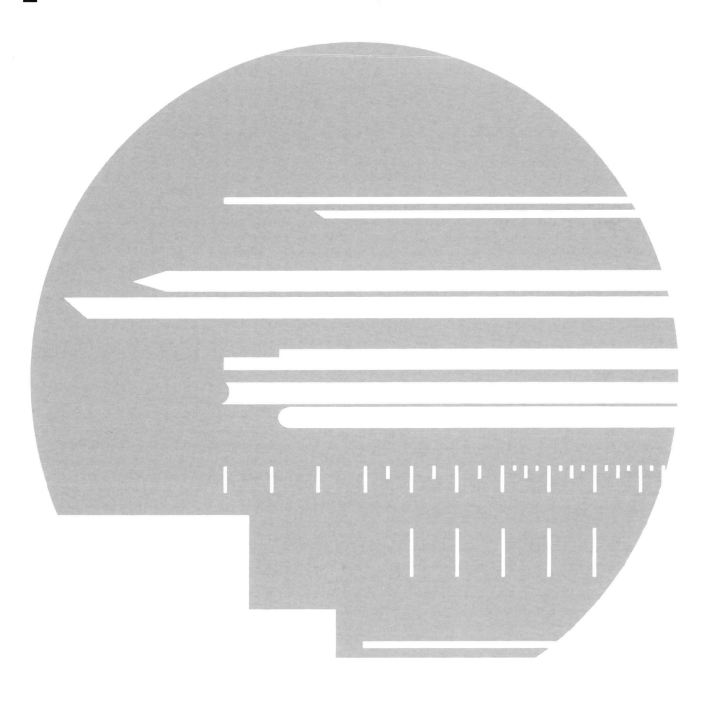

Chapter 3

Physics of Light and Image Transmission

Robert H. Quint

Types of Endoscopes

Endoscopes are devices utilized for visualization of interior body cavities. As such, they can be divided into two main groups—direct view and indirect view endoscopes.

The direct view endoscope is one which has no optical elements interposed between the tissue and the viewer. With devices of this type, that which can be seen can be seen well. However, the problems associated with direct view instruments are obvious. As with any simple tube, the angle of view is limited by the ratio of the luminal diameter to its length. As a result, indirect view instruments which contain optical elements have evolved to provide the operator with wide-angle information under variable magnification. *Indirect* here means that because optical elements are used, optical distortions occur which are absent in direct view devices. Examples of these types of endoscopes are listed below.

Direct view—The speculum, amnioscope and mini-lap devices.

Indirect view—The laparoscope, culdoscope and hysteroscope.

Indirect endoscopes can be grouped into two general subclasses according to type of relay system.

Types of Relay Systems

Relay systems (Figure 1) may be categorized as either refractive or reflective. Both contain an objective, the purpose of which is to form an image of the object. Both use an ocular at the proximal end of the instrument which allows the observer to see the image formed by the objective. In the first type the purpose of the relay system is to transfer the image by refraction from the objective end to the eye. Another purpose of the relay is to give the optical designer a means to correct some of the optical distortions and aberrations which occur in the objective.

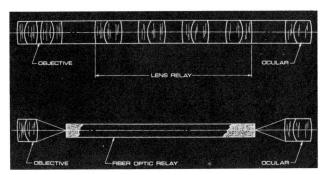

Figure 1
Refractive relay system (*top*).
Reflective relay system (*bottom*).

LENS SYSTEMS

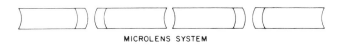

MICROLENS SYSTEM

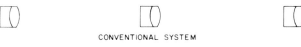

CONVENTIONAL SYSTEM

Figure 2
New and old refractive relay system.
Rod lens system (*top*).
Conventional doublet (*bottom*).

(DIFFERENT FIELDS OF VIEW)

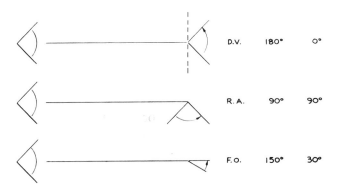

Figure 3
Classification of fields of view according to:
1st column — ACMI
2nd column — Wolf/Eder
3rd column — Storz

The second type of relay system uses a fiber optic device which permits flexion of the telescope as with a gastroscope or colonoscope. Fiber optic visualization systems have not been used to any great extent by gynecologists. The flexible fiber optic endoscope is very similar in optical design to the refractive type. There is an objective whose purpose is to form an image of the object on the distal end of the fiber bundle. Instead of refracting the image as a whole as the lens relay system does, the image is broken up into a spatial arrangement of dots of light by a fiber bundle which may contain 100,000 fibers of approximately 10μ diameter. It is obvious that each individual fiber supplies only a small part of the information contained in the image.

If this image bundle is coherent, that is, if there is a one-to-one relationship between the location of each individual fiber at the distal end and at the proximal end, the spots of light which are transferred by reflection to the proximal end of the image bundle will produce an image by means of the ocular, which is focused on the proximal end. The image is formed by means of the fusion of the dots of light.

Gynecologic Endoscopes

Older endoscopes employ a relay system with a few doublets spaced rather widely apart. In the late fifties Harry Hopkins, of the Imperial College of Science and Technology in London, developed a new system using long rod lenses (Figure 2). Since that time all manufacturers have moved in this direction because of the improved quality of the image which can be so obtained.

Improvements which accrue from this design include increased angle of view, brightness and contrast. The last is obtained by multicoating each one of the several lens surfaces. The original endoscopes used uncoated lenses. Coated lenses reduce the back reflection of incident energy. As a result, the image obtained with the conventional system was dark compared to what could be obtained with a multicoated system.

Compared with the old system, reflection loss in the multicoated system presently used has been reduced from 4% per surface to about 0.5% per surface.

Different manufacturers designate the inclination or obliquity of the field of view of their scopes as follows (Figure 3):

Endoscope	ACMI*	Eder or Wolf	Storz
Laparoscope	Direct	180°	0°
Hysteroscope	Foreoblique	130°–160°	30°
Culdoscope	Right angle/lateral	90°	70°

* American Cystoscope Makers, Inc.

It must be understood that the numerical system adapted gives no information whatsoever about the actual size of the field of view but only about its direction with respect to the shaft of the telescope. Manufacturers provide fields of view which can vary from 50° to 90°. The wider the field, the greater the distortion at the edges of the visual field. In a wide angle endoscope there is usually less magnification at the edges than in the center of the field. The ideal is a flat field or one with zero magnification change. With the angular size of the field mentioned above it is extremely difficult, if not impossible, to provide the flatness desired together with uniformity of brightness across the field. Uniformity of brightness can be considered a design prerequisite for a high-quality endoscope. A further concomitant in dealing with field of view is that with greater field angle there is a minification of detail. This means that the wider field scopes tend to decrease the size of small detail within the field, thus requiring closer proximity of the scope to the tissue.

The size of the image seen in the endoscope, the apparent field, is usually in proportion to the diameter of the optics:[3] specifically, the field stop size and the magnification of the ocular. Ideally, a 4 mm system might produce an image half the diameter of an 8 mm optical system, assuming the field stop size was in proportion to the dimensions of the optics and the magnifications were the same (Figure 4).

One of the big advantages of the direct (180° or 0°) scope is that the apparent field is co-linear with the true field. This has made this scope popular in laparoscopy. The right-angled scope used in culdoscopy can present confusion to the novice. The manufacturer provides a key to the user to indicate where the scope is looking by positioning the fiber optic port in such a direction that it is mechanically oriented in the same direction as the field of view. The foreoblique telescope has the advantage of being able to look out forward and obliquely at an angle. This capability is extremely useful in hysteroscopy and in certain situations encountered during laparoscopy.

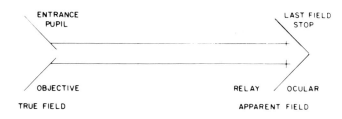

VISUAL MAGNIFICATION = INSTRUMENTAL MAGNIFICATION X ANGULAR OCULAR MAG

INSTRUMENTAL MAGNIFICATION = DIAMETER OF LAST FIELD STOP ÷ OBJECT SIZE

$$\text{VISUAL MAGNIFICATION} = \frac{250}{f} \times \text{INSTRUMENTAL MAGNIFICATION}$$

Figure 4
Schematic of endoscope, showing position of last field stop and magnification factors.

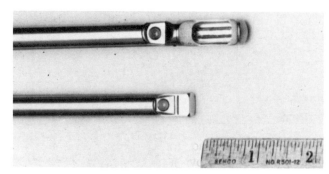

Figure 5
Endoscopic illumination systems.
Distal lamp (*top*).
Fiber optic (*bottom*).

The direct vision scope has the advantage that when it is rotated about its long axis, the same view is always seen. This is not the case with the foreoblique and the right angle scopes, rotation of which changes the view.

Problems In Vision

Analysis of what one sees through an endoscope is complicated by the physical relationship of the target to the direction of the field of view and the distance to the scope. A good practical demonstration relates to the difference in visibility of a probe when passed through an operating laparoscope (in line object) to that when the same probe is passed through a second incision (transverse object). The size and motion of the probe in the latter mode varies inversely with the distance of the probe from the optical system. In the former, because of the proximity to the optical system, the variation in size and speed is much more marked. As the probe extends into the field of view of the operating scope, it appears to be moving at a speed which is considerably greater than the speed with which it is actually being advanced by the operator. As the probe advances further into the field, the tip appears to slow down. At a certain distance it is impossible to see it advance even though the operator continues to move it. In the two-incision system this illusion does not exist. For both systems the only way to measure true dimension in the endoscopic domain is by means of a calibrated probe.

Illumination

Prior to the invention of fibers for transmitting illumination (Figure 5) the only way of providing vision endoscopically was by means of a distal or proximal lamp. Proximal lamps transmitted light through the agency of quartz rods which in themselves were fragile. Usually, bulky cooling devices had to be provided to reduce the temperature of the bulb, which was contained in a housing mounted to the telescope. The more commonly employed distal bulb not only projected into the physical space in front of the optical system, thereby reducing clearance for the scope, but also offered the possibility of burning tissue because of its high operating temperature. Fiber transmission of light solved both these problems at once and, further, allowed for higher levels of illumination not possible with distal lamps by means of intense projection sources, both tungsten and arc, mounted in housings flexibly connected to the endoscope.

Index of Refraction

Another complication in the use of instruments in the hands of a beginner is the variation in the index of refraction[2] of the medium through which one looks. This particularly holds true for hysteroscopy. In laparoscopy and culdoscopy the medium is gas. In hysteroscopy one can work in a gas or in a variety of solutions. The index of refraction of air is unity by definition. All other optical media are measured against air. The index of refraction of water is about 33% higher. As such, viewing in a bodily cavity which has a liquid medium decreases the total angle of view of the scope. On the other hand, the magnification of small detail and the depth of field are increased.

Fiber Optics

Both transmission of information (coherent) and illumination only (incoherent) by means of fibers function on the identical principle. Coherent transmission demands an identical arrangement of the distal and proximal fiber end surfaces in space. By this arrangement a pattern may be duplicated. When the coherent arrangement is scrambled, a true image cannot be transferred. However, illumination may be transferred equally well by an incoherent as by a coherent arrangement of fibers. Usually illumination is transferred by larger-diameter fibers, which are more effective than smaller fibers for this purpose. The inverse is true for imaging. In this case the smaller the fibers, the higher the resolving power of the endoscope, or its ability to discern small points as being discrete.

Fiber systems are of two general types, those using fibers composed of a core whose index of refraction is greater than the index of the sheath material and those using a core whose index varies with its radius, thus eliminating the requirement for a sheath, as in the first type. The purpose of the sheath is to keep the light in the core. It is obvious that when a group of fibers is packaged in any regular configuration, there will be interstices between individual fibers which transmit no light. The sheath of the first type transmits no light, so it is clear that the second type is more efficient than the first type in its overall light transmission. At present, type two is unavailable in flexible format.

Present-day commercial fibers suffer further from attenuation of incident energy by about 40% to 50% for two meter long fibers. They are selective as far as different wave lengths are concerned, favoring the red area of the spectrum to the blue. In this respect, refractive endoscopes are more highly transmittable, are more faithful in their reproduction of the entire spectrum and give a sharper, higher quality image.

Endoscopic Photography

Endoscopic photography is complicated by the wide variations in cameras, lenses and photoelectric metering systems employed in the camera computers. The size of the photographic image is proportional to the focal length of the lens; that is, by doubling the focal length of the lens, the exposed image doubles in diameter for a given endoscope. Its size relative to the visual image seen through the scope is the ratio of the focal length of the lens in millimeters divided by 250. Most endoscopic photography does not fill the film plane; therefore, the camera computer in automatic cameras must be so advised since in regular usage it functions properly only on the basis of the full frame exposure.

The endoscopic photographer's equation[1] shows that $t \, \alpha \, \dfrac{F^2 D^2}{B \sum_{eff}}$ for an average weighted photoelectric registering automatic camera where:

t = exposure time calculated by computer of camera
F = focal length of camera lens
D = distance
B = brightness of fiber source
$\sum_{eff}$ = film speed for an automatic exposure camera. Its value is related to the film and the ratio of the weighted value of the distribution of intensity in the total film plane to the weighted value of the exposed portion of the film plane.
$\sum_{film}$ = ASA nominal index

Quantitatively, the exposure time quadruples with doubling of the focal length of the lens. It quadruples with doubling of distance of the tissue to the endoscope. Doubling the brightness halves the exposure, as does doubling the film speed.

$\sum_{eff}$ is the value which must be inserted into the camera speed index dial in order for the computer to respond properly to the fact that the film plane is only partially filled. If the film plane were filled, then $\sum_{eff}$ would equal $\sum_{film}$. $\sum_{eff}$ is normally larger then $\sum_{film}$, and the relationship is approximately a hyperbolic one with size of exposed image. Another major factor is the transmission loss through the optical system. If, in a specific situation, the exposure time so determined is longer than desirable, say greater than a thirtieth of a second, then the exposed film sent to the processor must be "pushed." $\sum_{push}$ can be two to three times greater than $\sum_{film}$. Unless the processor is advised about this latter factor, assuming he/she has the capability, he/she will not do it.

Automatic movie cameras function similarly. The frame rate is analogous to the exposure time of the still camera. The reader is referred to other chapters in this text dealing with photographic and television considerations.

Conclusions

To summarize the characteristics of an endoscope: it is a monocular instrument, which makes it a little more difficult to learn how to use because operators are used to working with both eyes at laparotomy. Indirect view scopes possess a large angle of view whereas the direct view endoscope has a very small angle of view. Indirect endoscopes have a very small entrance pupil, which provides an extremely large depth of field without which endoscopy would be of little value. Endoscopes have magnification properties which vary the size of the target to be seen as the scope moves in and out with respect to the tissue.

References

1. Hett JH, and Quint RH: T/Numbers of endoscopes. Photographic Science and Engineering 13:210, 1969

2. Quint RH: The rigid hysteroscope. In *Hysteroscopic Sterilization.* (JJ Sciarra, JC Butler, Jr, JJ Speidel, Eds.) Stratton Intercontinental Medical Book Corp, New York, 1974, p 11

3. Taylor HW: A comparative evaluation of the 5 mm laparoscope in gynecological endoscopy. J Reprod Med 15:65, 1975

Chapter 4

Basic Principles of Electrosurgery

Jacques-E. Rioux, M.D.
Diogene Cloutier, M.D.

Introduction

The laparoscope has become an essential diagnostic tool of the gynecologist. Of equal importance is the array of operative procedures which can be performed in the course of laparoscopy.[7, 18] Many of them can be performed with the use of electrical current delivered as high frequency radio waves. Moreover, many operative procedures which do not require electrical current as their primary agent can be performed only because such a current is available in the event of complication.[12, 19] It is therefore most important that any gynecologist using electrical current in the course of an operation remember that he or she is adding a new dimension to the procedure and know the basic principles involved.[13]

Therefore, we will successively *define* high frequency current, *discover* the principles involved in different electrosurgical units generating it, *analyze* the types of waveforms in which it is produced, *evaluate* the methods of delivery and, finally, *apply* our newly acquired knowledge to the field of laparoscopy.

1. High Frequency Current

To be used efficiently in the human body, electrical current must be delivered at a frequency sufficiently high to avoid faradic stimulation. Below frequencies of 10,000 cycles per second, current stimulates (at the neuromuscular junction) involuntary movements which cannot be prevented even with deep anesthesia.

Figure 1 represents various electrical frequency patterns. The frequencies used therapeutically in electrosurgery lie in the kilohertz and megahertz range. Earlier electrosurgical units relied upon lower frequencies, but the newer generators employ frequencies at which the current oscillates between 2.5×10^5 and 3×10^6 times per second. Clinically there seems to be no difference, and no scientific medical research has ever determined the superiority of one frequency over another within this range.

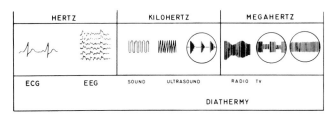

Figure 1
Frequencies used in diathermy

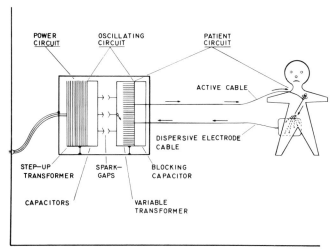

Figure 2
Spark gap generator

2. Electrosurgical Units

Historically and technically, electrosurgical units can be divided into three groups: spark gap generators, vacuum tube generators and solid-state generators. The main difference among them resides in the manner in which the oscillating circuit is made.

Spark Gap Generators: the first generators used for fulguration were of the spark gap type (Figure 2). They consist of (a) a *power supply circuit* in which a step up transformer boosts the line voltage (110–220 v); (b) an *oscillating circuit* to produce the high frequency from the 60-cycle alternating current. The high voltage coming out of the transformer charges the capacitors; when they reach sufficiently high tension, they will discharge through the spark gap, and current will flow through. Repeated charging and discharging produces a series of damped oscillations. The wider the spark gap, the higher the charge (i.e., voltage) accumulating in the capacitors and the longer the rest period between discharges. The frequency, however, remains constant. The third element, (c) the *patient's circuit*, delivers the current thus produced. This has to be done through a blocking capacitor which passes only the high frequency voltages. It is necessary to block the low frequency voltage as a safety precaution in case of breakdown of the apparatus. A breakdown would allow ordinary wall outlet current to pass through, giving the patient a shock or burn.[5]

In summary, the spark gap unit consists of a transformer and high voltage capacitors which discharge through a certain number of gaps of fixed spacing. This requires a precise adjustment to obtain the correct gap opening. Through them the current sparks or jumps at a very high frequency, thus producing a pulsating type of output. These gaps must be compensated for in order to maintain an original setting regardless of temperature variations. The newer spark gap oscillators are of tungsten for durability. They generate a highly damped current which, when pure, is hemostatic, without a cutting effect. For that reason they are called *coagulators*.

Vacuum Tube Generators: to add a smoother cutting current while making the generators more dependable (i.e., less prone to variations secondary to temperature and relative humidity changes), the vacuum tubes were introduced.

These generators also have three principal components (Figure 3): (a) a *power supply circuit*, which has a transformer and a rectifier to provide low voltage alternating current to light the filament of the oscillator tubes and some high voltage direct current for the plates of the same tubes; (b) an *oscillating circuit*, which produces high frequency current by the use of oscillators which are tuned at radio frequency and operate within a vacuum. It would be beyond the scope of this chapter to explain in detail the working of these radio tubes. The principle, simply put, is that the grid between the filament and the plate changes potential, thus alternatively passing and blocking the passage of electrons between the heated filament and the plate. The capacitor, by being charged and discharged at a very high rate, is responsible for these changes of potential in the grid and ultimately the production of an undamped current which flows to the patient via the (c) *patient's circuit* and produces, when pure, a cutting effect with very little coagulation effect.[5]

Solid-State Generators: Introduced in 1970, solid-state units are completely transistorized. Here again, one can recognize three principal divisions (Figure 4): (a) a *power supply circuit*, which transforms the current from the outlet into a usable form by the (b) *oscillating circuit*, which is composed of different types of electronic gadgetry which cycle the generator off and on at a very rapid rate to produce a damped current and, by pulsing oscillators, conductors, relays, capacitors, resistors, circuit boards, etc., to produce undamped current and a combination of the two (blended); (c) the *patient's circuit*, with the appropriate blocking capacitors and variable transformers, which will deliver the high frequency current to the patient.

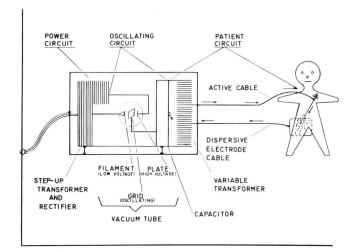

Figure 3
Vacuum tube generator

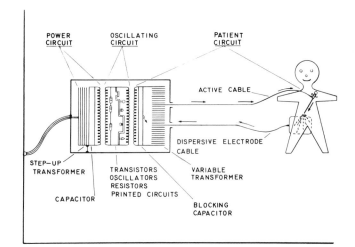

Figure 4
Isolated solid-state generator

Discussion: When one reviews the array of generators in use, it becomes clear that the spark gap principle is not utilized in the latest models. Likewise, one can see that the vacuum tubes are being phased out in favor of solid-state circuiting. However, one must realize that many modern units employing tubes are very good, and it is erroneous to assume that to have superior performance and better quality one must switch to transistors. Nevertheless, if the trend continues, only solid-state units will be manufactured in the United States within the next few years. That, as a whole, should be an improvement since the solid-state generators seem more versatile. They are much smaller than conventional units, yet they can generate as much, and often more, current. Their design is such that they incorporate more and better safeguards, such as isolated to ground circuitry.[14]

3. Output Waveforms

Three types of current within the high frequency spectrum are employed surgically. They can be identified by the wave patterns they display on an oscilloscope.

Coagulating Current: This highly damped current causes cellular dehydration. Its effect is mainly hemostatic. When used in its pure form, this type of current has very little cutting effect and will char the tissue completely when applied over a longer period. It is more likely to spark than is cutting current and, therefore, carries an inherent danger. On the oscilloscope (Figure 5) it is characterized by bursts of rapidly decreasing current separated by gaps when no current passes.

Cutting Current: This current is undamped and produces a cutting effect primarily by exploding cells, an effect secondary to the intense heat generated within the tissue itself. When a pure form of this current is used, very little hemostasis is obtained, and bleeding may occur. On the oscilloscope (Figure 6) it is characterized by a constant flow of oscillations of equal amplitude and a frequency between 250 kilohertz and 3 megahertz.

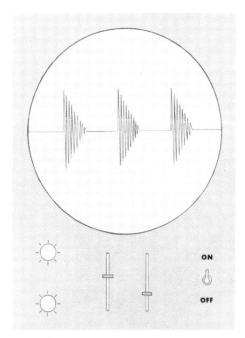

Figure 5
Highly damped current (coagulating)

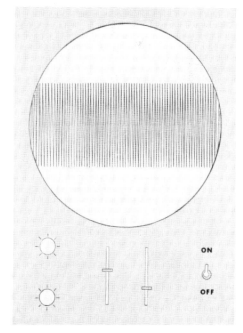

Figure 6
Undamped current (cutting)

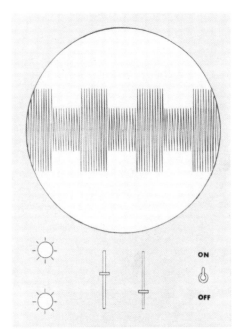

Figure 7
Blended current (it can be more or less damped
according to the amount of hemostasis desired)

Blended Current: By definition this is a combination of the two types of waves discussed above and results in both cutting and coagulating effects. On the oscilloscope (Figure 7) it is characterized by a wavy but continuous type of current, i.e., without gaps.

Discussion: Obviously, for the sake of simplification we are not trying to explain in detail why a *pure* coagulating current (highly damped) will have mostly a coagulating effect while a *pure* cutting current (undamped) will cut sharply and why a *blended* current will combine both effects.[4] In practice the laparoscopist should know very well what kind of waveforms his or her electrosurgical unit produces and when to use each one if there is a choice.[14]

4. Methods of Diathermy

Literally, the term *diathermy* is made from two Greek words *dia*, or through, and *therme*, or heat. It is therefore to be expected that the therapeutic effect of diathermy would be produced by heat going through the tissues to which it is applied. This is true of all methods of diathermy, but the principles involved differ drastically among the different forms.

Nonsurgical

An alternating electrical current of high frequency can be passed through parts of the body via two broad electrodes with no effect other than the production of heat, which is a direct result of the resistance offered to its passage by the body tissues (Figure 8). The electrodes themselves do not become hot but merely pick up the heat after the tissue is warmed by the current. Because of the broad electrodes the current density is very low, and there is no destruction of tissue. As with high frequency, there is no stimulation of nerves or muscles. This is the principle of medical diathermy.

Surgical Diathermy

When cell destruction or coagulation of vessels is desired, a much smaller instrument has to be used in order to select precisely the site where the therapeutic effect is desired. Heat again is the agent, but its application differs.

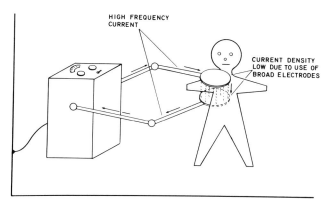

Figure 8
Nonsurgical diathermy

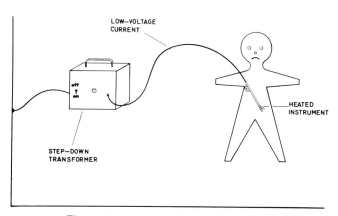

Figure 9
Electrocautery

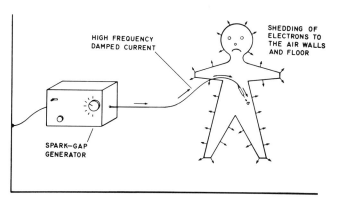

Figure 10
Monoterminal electrodessication
(electrofulguration)

Electrocautery: Here the heat is delivered by a red-hot wire. The apparatus consists of an insulated holder carrying at its tip a wire which is heated by a low-voltage high-amperage alternating current produced by a step down transformer. A variable resistor controls the intensity of the current. Treatment is administered selectively by actually burning the lesion using a blade or a wire in a loop. The histologic evaluation of the tissue so treated shows "amorphous material with loss of most structure alternating with small spaces representing areas of steam formation and carbon."[5] A good example of this method is cauterization of the cervix.

However, a modern application of this principle has been introduced recently in laparoscopic tubal sterilization (Figure 9). Semm of Germany has devised a tubal cautery forceps which uses heat as the primary therapeutic agent.[17] The instrument itself is introduced through a separate trocar and, after having grasped the tube, is rapidly heated to a predetermined degree (140 C) during a fixed length of time after which the instrument is cooled automatically. During the cooking period a sound is heard which is replaced by a different one while cooling. A very low voltage is used by the generator, and little or no current flows through the patient via the instrument. In other words, the heat is transferred directly to the tissue from the heated tip. We will see later that, in electrosurgery, the heat is generated within the tissue by the resistance offered to the passage of electrical currents.

Electrodessication (Electrofulguration): The very first use of electrical current as a therapeutic agent on the human body was of a *monoterminal* type. Here a high frequency damped current produced by a spark gap generator is delivered to the tissue using one active electrode (Figure 10). "That electrode may actually touch the tissue or may be held at a slight distance from the tissue causing a visible spark. A higher voltage is required since there is no ground plate and since the patient's circuit is completed by a shedding of electrons to the air, walls and floor about the patient."[5] However, should the patient be actually touching a ground, a preferred path would be established. Also, since that current is highly damped with greater voltage, it is intrinsically more dangerous as far as electrical accidents are concerned and without the benefits obtained when a similar apparatus is used in the biterminal fashion.

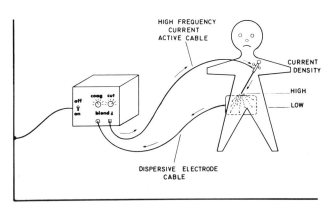

Figure 11
Surgical diathermy—unipolar

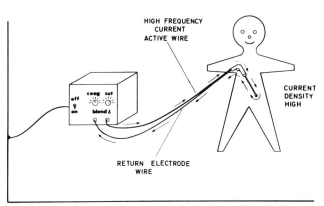

Figure 12
Surgical diathermy—bipolar

The figures have been executed by Phillip Eubanks
of Berkeley, California under the guidance of J.-E.R.

A typical use of that method in gynecology is the removal of vulvar condylomata under local anesthesia with a Hyfracator (trademark of the Birtcher Corp.). It is to be noted that this type of generator, which is quite handy in the office, is not for operating room use and certainly not for any kind of intraabdominal procedure.

Electrosurgery (Electrocoagulation and Electrosection): In order to make the procedure safer and broaden the range of surgical interventions, a ground plate was introduced to complete the circuit. This is the *biterminal* type since we have one active and one return electrode.

Unipolar System: Here, a high frequency current is presented at the site of the active electrode, which, being small, concentrates and thus achieves a high density current which can destroy the cells by dissolution of their molecular structure. From the point where it is applied the current must return to the generator via the return electrode, where the density must be low (since the electrode is large) in order to prevent a second site of tissue destruction (Figure 11).

The integrity of the circuit is essential since if the return electrode is not connected properly, the current would by necessity search out another avenue or route of escape, and any point at which the patient's body happened to be grounded would suffice, as, for example, via electrocardiogram (ECG) electrodes, where skin burns would occur at the point of contact.[2]

Bipolar System: Here the return electrode is not dispersive but acts as a return by being placed in close approximation to the active. The current, therefore, does not have to travel through the entire body of the patient to complete the circuit but only through a very small area, i.e., that between the electrodes, destroying the tissue or coagulating the vessels interposed between them in the process (Figure 12). The area of destruction is strictly limited to the space between the forceps, and injury to the surrounding tissues is impossible unless they are grasped inadvertently. For this reason such a technique is ideal for neurosurgeons[16] and plastic surgeons because of the limited area of coagulation without spreading along the vessels to deeper tissues. Also, because of the discrete locus, less current is needed in bipolar electrosurgery compared to unipolar. Whatever the method, technique, system or approach, current is used, and current is "hot." There is no such thing as "cold current."

5. Laparoscopic Uses of Diathermy

Grounded System – Unipolar

The classic method of using the various forms of current produced by all types of generators in laparoscopic diathermy is the grounded unipolar system. Here, the active electrode delivers the therapeutic current to the site at which it is required in the patient, and a ground plate collects the current as it leaves the patient's body. As we have seen previously, the integrity of such a system is of the utmost importance since the current thus deposited in the patient must return to the generator via the ground plate or find another path, which could be dangerous.[1, 2, 6]

With such a setup many laparoscopic interventions can be done by combining different instruments with different types of current. Also, these instruments can be used either with an operative laparoscope or a simple laparoscope and a second trocar.[7, 18]

Isolated System – Unipolar

In the isolated (floating) system the patient plate is not a ground. Here again, the current deposited into the patient must return to the generator via the return plate, which is not ground-seeking. The chassis of the generator is grounded via the three-way plug, but the generator inside is completely isolated. With the patient forming part of the circuit, a complete loop of current results which is also isolated from the ground and the generating current. Such a unit will not function if the return electrode is placed improperly or not connected. The current therefore will not be released by the active electrode if the return electrode is ineffective.

Theoretically this arrangement is ideal, and it is, in fact, possible at low power. However, at high frequencies and low voltage the radio frequency (RF) current can be transmitted without conductors, and there is always a small amount of leakage, which varies according to the electrosurgical unit and the instrument used.

Isolated System – Bipolar

The added security procured by the isolated system has made possible the development of bipolar forceps for tubal coagulation. Here there is no patient's plate since the return electrode is in the instrument itself and in close proximity to the active electrode. The patient is not part of the circuit: only the tissue grasped between the two prongs is used to complete the electrical circuit; therefore, the path of the current is limited to the space between the uninsulated forceps surfaces, and so is the burn, which has no spread.

In March of 1973 we developed the first bipolar instrument for laparoscopic tubal sterilization.[8, 9, 10, 11] This instrument was demonstrated to the "Flying Doctors Teaching Team of the American Association of Gynecologic Laparoscopists" during a postgraduate course on laparoscopy held at Le Centre Hospitalier de l'Université Laval in July 1973. At the same meeting Corson presented a paper in which he described an ideal instrument, which he had thought of independently, and which was of a similar description to the one we had been using since March 1973.[3]

Discussion: In the *grounded unipolar system*, the current must return to ground and the generator. That fact is so important that all kinds of systems have been devised to ensure the integrity of the ground circuit, including the common ground approach, which has merits in a grounded situation.

The *isolated output* offers, in our opinion, a much safer environment. Here, the current is not ground-seeking, and the unit is built in such a way that current will be delivered only if the circuit is complete. That safety factor makes the unipolar system safer and the bipolar approach possible.

However, one should remember that RF current has an inherent tendency to travel wirelessly, making a total isolation impossible in spite of the nonconductivity of insulating material. Moreover, the phenomenon of *capacitance* by which electrical energy can be stored by means of an electrostatic field and then released without suspicion may be responsible for some of the previously mentioned accidents.

6. Safety Recommendations

With the preceding in mind, the following precautions should be exercised:

1. Be sure that the wiring in the operating suite is adequate for the equipment now in use.
2. Be certain that the ground in the wall outlet is indeed a ground.
3. Check that all the equipment has the three-pronged plug.
4. Determine that the extension cords are intact, without multiple outlets.
5. Inspect the dials and settings of generators prior to each case.
6. Allow the activation of the circuit to be controlled only by the surgeon.
7. Schedule the entire system for a periodic inspection by the hospital engineers.
8. Have some control over the purchasing of good equipment and maintenance of same.
9. Know what to expect from the generator, and do not increase the output when the results are not within your expectations.
10. Read and follow the instructions accompanying every piece of equipment and instrumentation.

References

1. Atkin DH, Orkin LR: Electrocution in the operating room. Anesthesiology 38:181, 1973

2. Battig CG: Electrosurgical burn injuries and their prevention. JAMA 204:1025, 1968

3. Corson SL, Patrick H, Hamilton T, Bolognese RJ: Electrical consideration of laparoscopic sterilization. J Reprod Med 11:159, 1973

4. Honig WM: The mechanism of cutting in electrosurgery. IEEE Trans Biomed Eng 22:58, 1975

5. Jackson R: Basic principles of electrosurgery: a review. Can J Surg 13:354, 1970

6. Phillips J, Keith D, Keith L, Hulka J, Hulka B: Survey of gynecologic laparoscopy for 1974. J Reprod Med 15:45, 1975

7. Rioux J-E: Operative laparoscopy. J Reprod Med 10:249, 1973

8. Rioux J-E, Cloutier D: Laparoscopic tubal sterilization: sparking and its control. Vie Med Can Francais 2:760, 1973

9. Rioux J-E, Cloutier D: Bipolar cautery for sterilization by laparoscopy. J Reprod Med 13:6, 1974

10. Rioux J-E, Cloutier D: A new bipolar instrument for laparoscopic tubal sterilization. Am J Obstet Gynecol 119:737, 1974

11. Rioux J-E, Cloutier D: True bipolar electrosurgery for tubal sterilization by laparoscopy. In *Gynecological Laparoscopy: Principles and Techniques.* (JM Phillips, L Keith, Eds.) Stratton Intercontinental Book Corp, New York, 1974, p 315

12. Rioux J-E, Cloutier D, LaRochelle A: La biopsie d'ovaire perlaparoscopique: une etude de 130 cas et une classification. Union Med Can 120:1552, 1973.

13. Rioux J-E, Yuzpe AA: Electrosurgery untangled. Contemp Obstet Gynecol 4:118, 1974

14. Rioux J-E, Yuzpe AA: Know thy generator. Contemp Obstet Gynecol 6:15, 1975

15. Rioux J-E, Cloutier D: Bipolar electrosurgery for laparoscopic sterilization. In *Advances in Female Sterilization Techniques.* (JJ Sciarra, Ed.) (In press)

16. Robinson JL, Davies NJ: Bipolar diathermy. Can J Surg 17:287, 1974

17. Semm K: Tubal sterilization finally with cauterization or temporary with ligation via pelviscopy. In *Gynecological Laparoscopy: Principles and Techniques.* (JM Phillips, L Keith, Eds.) Stratton Intercontinental Book Corp, New York, 1974, p 337

18. Yuzpe AA: Operative laparoscopy. J Reprod Med 13: 27, 1974

19. Yuzpe AA, Rioux J-E: The value of laparoscopic ovarian biopsy. J Reprod Med 15:37, 1975

Editorial Comments

Rioux and I have shared an interest in electrosurgical correlates of laparoscopic surgery for some time. Working independently, we have reached a similar conclusion, namely, that the bipolar approach to laparoscopic surgery affords safety not possible with unipolar systems.

This chapter should serve to whet one's appetite for further knowledge in this area. With a plethora of new instrumentation on the medical scene, medical schools should include bioengineering courses in the curriculum.

Two additional references of interest are given below. They serve to demonstrate that there are still many areas of disagreement concerning the basic processes associated with electrosurgical laparoscopic procedures.

S.L.C.

References

1. Corson SL: (Mod) Panel Discussion—Electrosurgery in laparoscopy. In *Gynecological Laparoscopy: Principles and Techniques.* (JM Phillips, L Keith, Eds.) Stratton Intercontinental Book Corp, New York, 1974, p 433

2. Engel T, Harris FW: The electrical dynamics of laparoscopic sterilization. J Reprod Med 15:33, 1975

Chapter 5

Contemporary Instruments

Richard M. Soderstrom, M.D., F.A.C.O.G.

The purpose of this chapter is to review the basic instruments used in diagnostic and operative laparoscopy. Because of the highly specialized nature of this field, it is impossible to include a discussion of all the innovations and modifications of different laparoscopic tools now available. In fact, the keen interest in endoscopy in general means that some of the instruments may well become obsolete in the near future. The reader is encouraged to review, thoroughly, the brochures and operating instructions provided with all laparoscopy equipment before using the equipment.

The basic physics of the modern laparoscope can be found in Chapter 3. The surgeon must have working knowledge of these physical properties in order to appreciate fully each type of laparoscope, and to determine the minimum and maximum needs of any laparoscopic procedure. For instance, a laparoscope designed with an operating channel may have to sacrifice the lighting capabilities and total visual field that are available with a purely diagnostic endoscope. The angle of vision provided by a foreoblique laparoscope may facilitate the viewing of certain intraabdominal recesses not seen with the more popular, straight, end-on viewing scope (Figure 1, Tables 1 and 2).

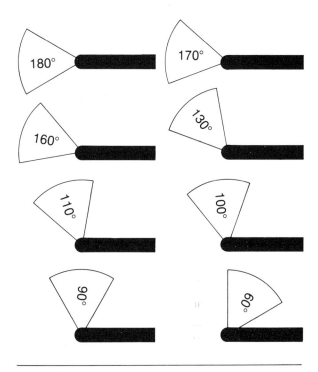

Figure 1
The multiple angles of view available in endoscopes.

Table 1*
Specifications of Viewing or Diagnostic Laparoscopes*

	Scope OD Trocar Size	Field of View	Viewing Angle	Insulation	Steam Autoclavable	Photo
ACMI	9–10 mm 5–6 mm	63° 70°	180°	Eyepiece	No	Yes
Eder	5–6 mm 8–9 mm 10–11 mm	70° 70° or 90° 70° or 90°	180° 180°–135° 180°–135°	Eyepiece	No	Yes
KLI	8–9 mm 10–11 mm	70°	180°	Eyepiece	No	Yes
Storz	2.7–4 mm 5.8–7 mm 6.5–7 mm 5.8–11 mm	68° 90°	135° 135° 135° 135°	Eyepiece	No	Yes
Winter & IBE	10–11 mm 5–6 mm	55–60°	180° 168°	Eyepiece	No	Yes
Wolf	5–6 mm 8–9 mm 10–11 mm	65° 65° 65°	180°, 160°, 130° 180°, 130° 180°, 160°, 130°	Eyepiece	Yes 8 mm & 10 mm	Yes

* Courtesy of Preston Williams, M. D.

Table 2
Specifications of Operating Telescopes*

	Scope OD Trocar size	Eyepiece Angle	Viewing Angle	Field of View	Insulation	Instrument Channel
ACMI	10–11.8 mm	Parallel-Offset	180°	70°	Sheath Scope Eyepiece	3.6 mm
Eder	10–11 mm	Parallel-Offset & Right Angle	180° or 90°	70°	Eyepiece Instrument Channel	3 or 5 mm
KLI	10–11 mm	Parallel-Offset	180°	70°	Eyepiece	3 mm
Storz	5 mm 10 mm 11 or 12 mm	0° 45°	135°	90°	Sheath Eyepiece	5 mm
Winter & Ibe	5 mm 10 mm 11 mm	0° 45°	168° 168°	45°	Eyepiece	5 mm
Wolf	10–11 mm 8–9 mm	Parallel-Offset	170°	65°	Eyepiece Instrument Channel	3 mm 5 mm

* Courtesy of Preston Williams, M.D.

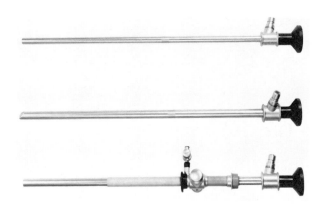

Figure 2
Diagnostic endoscopes are available in sizes ranging from 2.2 through 10 mm in diameter.

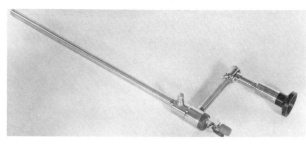

Figure 3
Bayonet type operating laparoscope with 3 mm operating channel.

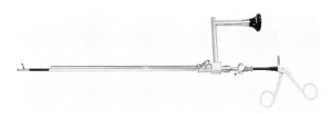

Figure 4
This 10 mm operating telescope has a 5 mm operating channel considered advantageous for more adequate biopsy procedures. A larger blind spot is noted with its use.

Any operator who wishes to utilize and coordinate light sources and photography must understand the physics of fiber optics. The principles of electricity can affect the safety of operative laparoscopy if improper or incompatible equipment is used. Before practicing laparoscopy or purchasing laparoscopic equipment, the reader should consult Chapters 4, 5, 7 and 10.

The Viewing Laparoscope

Viewing or diagnostic laparoscopes are essentially similar to any cystoscope. The major difference is usually more light capability and a wider angle of view. In fact, some institutions use their existing cystoscopes for purely diagnostic purposes.

These scopes vary in diameter size up to 10 mm. As the size of the laparoscope increases, so does the availability of light and usually the size of the image. The field of vision becomes wider and there is less distortion. Photographic capabilities improve with increasing size. The larger the laparoscope, however, the larger the incision. Also, as the size increases, the trocar tip becomes longer, which results in deeper penetration upon entry into the abdomen.

Most laparoscopists agree that if a smaller scope will accomplish the mission, then it should be used. When there is some question as to needs (photography, lighting, etc.), it is preferable to use a larger scope (Figure 2).

The Operating Laparoscope

The purpose of the operating laparoscope is to add versatility to the laparoscopic procedure, with or without the introduction of secondary instruments through a secondary trocar sleeve. The operating laparoscope is particularly popular for those using local anesthesia in tubal sterilization procedures. It is ideal for retrieving foreign objects, such as intraabdominal IUDs and large, resected specimens. Unfortunately, the operating laparoscope has been categorized as a one-hole instrument, which implies that all procedures must be done through the operating channel. This is inaccurate since the second-trocar method—or two-hole technique—can be used whenever necessary while using an operating scope. Most authorities feel, in fact, that all persons performing laparoscopy should become skilled in two-hole techniques before operating through an operating laparoscope. Once the operator becomes proficient, the additional operating channel can offer many technical advantages to the operation. An example is the ability to stabilize a structure through the operating channel while taking a biopsy or lysing an adhesion through the secondary trocar sleeve. Because of their operating channels, however, the diameter size of these scopes must be 8 to 10 mm.

Figures 3 and 4 show the most commonly used "bayonet type" operating laparoscope. It is available with 3 mm and 5 mm operating channels. Caution should be exercised when applying electrosurgery through these channels since a portion of the visual field may be obscured by the operating instrument. Electrical capacitance or charge can be transferred to the laparoscope sheath, creating a potential hazard. In order to prevent this from happening, the Richard Wolf Company has introduced a current "bleed off" attachment to the scope. The American Cystoscope Company has introduced a fully insulated operating laparoscope, which protects even more, provided that the insulation is intact. The Eder and Storz companies offer an angled eyepiece to reduce the number of prisms necessary, thus increasing light perception and clarity of image (Figure 5).

The Flexible Laparoscope

The Machida flexible laparoscope introduces a new dimension to peritoneoscopy (Figure 6). The flexible end rotates 90° in either direction and can be locked in place by a proximal dial control. The scope itself has a focusing ability which enables most people to shed their eyeglasses. Finally, the system features integrated fiber optics with the light cable bundles contiguous with the telescope, thereby increasing the efficiency of light transfer. The instrument, which has a narrow operating channel (2.6 mm), affords little advantage over classic telescopes for routine pelvic exploration, but may be invaluable for diagnostic and biopsy procedures in the upper abdomen and in difficult-to-visualize recesses of the entire abdominal cavity.

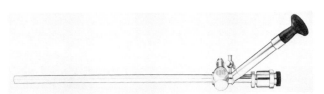

Figure 5
The oblique angle of this operating scope simplifies the optical prism system and ensures clarity of vision.

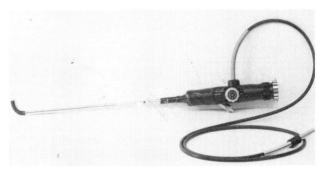

Figure 6
A newly designed flexible laparoscope found particularly useful in exploration of difficult-to-view recesses of the abdominal cavity.

Insufflation Equipment

Insufflation of the abdominal cavity is generally accomplished with a regulating insufflator, any type of flexible tubing and an insufflation needle. Most insufflators can insufflate either carbon dioxide or nitrous oxide gas. Hand pumps using room air have been effective in developing countries.

The Veress needle is most commonly employed (Figure 7). It is a double-cannula needle, with a blunt cannula movable within an outer sharp cannula. The blunt cannula protrudes beyond the sharp outer cannula to reduce the chance of laceration of the abdominal viscera. The hub of the needle contains a spring to allow the inner cannula to retract during insertion through the tough abdominal fascia. In order to prevent too rapid an insufflation, the internal diameter of the needle should not exceed 16 gauge. Other needle alternatives include the Touhey needle, the plastic Rochester catheter or, in the obese patient, a long spinal needle.

All insufflators have three basic requirements. The first is a regulator to control pressure and flow rate of the insufflating gas. Since the physiologic hazard of overinsufflation is increased pressure, insufflation must be monitored visually. Another desirable feature is a maximum pressure mechanism which shuts off the gas automatically at the recommended intraabdominal pressure. A meter for measuring the volume of gas insufflated is available on most insufflators; it adds an extra margin of safety by indicating possible overinsufflation, but, unfortunately, leakage during laparoscopy makes the meter reading highly inaccurate. The key to safety is monitoring intraabdominal pressure (usually 15 to 20 mm Hg).

The second requirement is, therefore, an accurate pressure gauge. Some insufflator gauges indicate actual pressure and fluctuations (Wysap, K.L.I.). Other insufflators have an automatic shutoff system which allows the physician to set the maximum pressure (Ohio, Carboflater). Many authorities prefer the fluctuating gauge to aid them in diagnosing misplacement of the needle (i.e., properitoneal space).

The third requirement is a flow ball to indicate system patency. The height of the floating ball can be used to indicate needle placement problems.

Figure 7
The Veress needle, assembled with its inner, blunt cannula protruding through the sharp-tipped outer sheath.

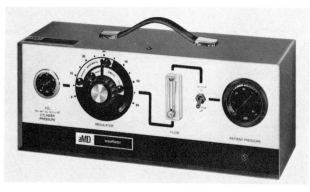

Figure 8
This insufflator contains the three basic requirements of all insufflators—a pressure regulator, a flow ball, and a patient pressure gauge.

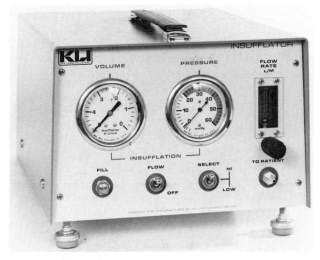

Figure 9
This insufflator provides a meter for measurement of gas insufflation with controls for low or high volume flow rate.

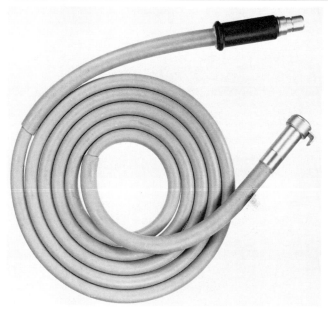

Figure 10
Standard large-bore fiber optic light bundle for
maximum light transfer.

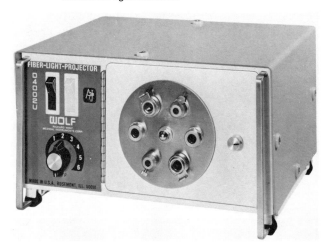

Figure 11
A 150-watt light for routine laparoscope with a turret
adaptor to accommodate various sizes and makes of
fiber optic light cables.

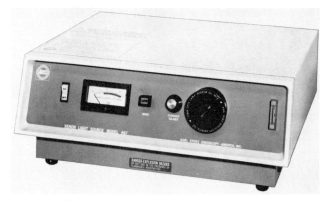

Figure 12
A high-powered xenon light source most suitable for
accurate color lighting in photography and for use
with teaching attachments.

In summary, any insufflator with a reliable
pressure regulator, pressure gauge, and flow ball is
adequate for safe insufflation (Figure 8). Other features, such as volume meter, storage tank meter,
and manual-automatic insufflation valves, are
found beneficial by many laparoscopists (Figure 9).

Light Sources and Cables
Any endoscopic light source is sufficient
for laparoscopy, provided that the adaptors for
connection of scope, light cord, and source are
compatible. The standard light bulb produces 150
watts and requires a light cord of at least 4 mm
diameter (Figures 10 and 11). As the cord diameter
increases, so does the efficiency of light transmission, until the fiberglass bundle exceeds those
found in the endoscope. One company attaches
two light cords to its scope to increase light transmission and still use smaller cords.

Light transmission is reduced almost 50%
when one fiber optic bundle is connected to another. Therefore, some scopes are made with integrated fiberglass bundles of scope and cord to
increase transmission of light, particularly beneficial in photographs. Special 1,000 watt and xenon
light sources for cinephotography are available and
advantageous where teaching sidearms are being
used (Figure 12).

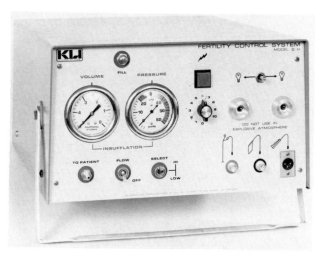

Figure 13
A combination "support" unit for insufflation, light source and electrocoagulation, found most useful when mobility is needed.

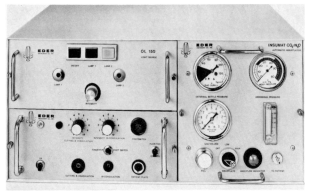

Figure 14
A combination laparoscopy unit with modular components to facilitate easy repair.

Combined Laparoscopic Units

Combination laparoscopic units which incorporate the light source, electrocoagulator and insufflator are available. One unit includes a storage container for basic laparoscopy instruments. These combined units are designed for increased mobility and for the traveling laparoscopist (Figure 13). A modular component unit is available to simplify repairs, which means that the replacement modules can be used (Figure 14). This permits the combination unit to be retained in the operating theater rather than causing the whole unit to be returned to the manufacturer when only one component fails. Lighter and more portable units are being designed.

Laparoscopic Trocars and Trocar Sleeves

Most laparoscopists prefer pyramidally-tipped trocars because of their ease of entry through the abdominal walls. Each company has its own laparoscopic trocar and trocar sleeve, and except for a few, they are not compatible with other companies' laparoscopes of similar size. All laparoscopic trocar sleeves have a valve to prevent gas leakage when the laparoscope is removed from the abdomen. These valves are of two basic types. The more popular is the trumpet valve type, which allows manual opening and closing of the valve. This is particularly helpful when an operating laparoscope is being used to remove intraabdominal IUDs or large resected specimens from the abdomen (Figure 15). The second type, an automatic flap valve, is much easier to maintain, but will not allow removal of objects from the abdomen (Figure 16).

Most trocar sleeves are made of fiberglass to reduce electrical conductivity. They are more fragile than metal sleeves and require careful maintenance. I prefer the older, metal sleeve; it penetrates the tissue with less resistance, and gas insufflation through the sleeve is more efficient when the laparoscope is contained within the sleeve. *However,* metal trocar sleeves should never be used unless the electrocoagulation source is of the low-voltage, high-frequency type. Some newer trocar sleeves, including their valve systems, are totally insulated.

Figure 15
Trumpet valve trocar sleeve; metal and fiberglass
sheaths, and pyramidally-tipped trocar.

Figure 16
Flap valve trocar sleeves and trocars, color coded as
to sizes.

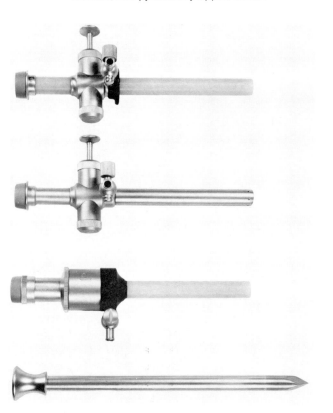

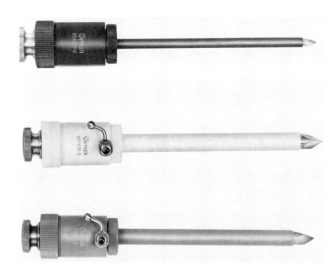

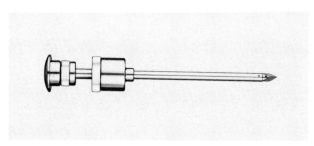

Figure 17
Secondary trocar sleeve and trocar for secondary
instruments.

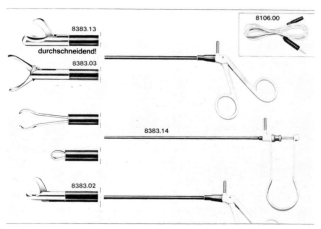

Figure 18
Secondary instruments used in operative
laparoscopy. Each instrument is designed for
specific tasks, such as aspiration, manipulation,
grasping, cutting, biopsy, coagulation, or a
combination of these functions.

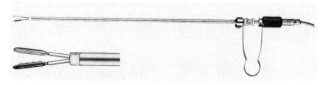

Figure 19
The bipolar instrument of Berci designed for tubal
sterilization using low-voltage electrocoagulation.

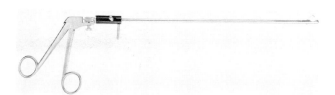

Figure 20
The bipolar instrument of Corson designed for tubal
sterilization using low-voltage electrocoagulation.

Secondary Trocar

These trocars and their sleeves are available with or without valves in 6 mm and 4 mm sizes
(Figure 17). Again, the pyramidal tip is recommended, at least for the 6 mm size. The sleeves
should be nonconducting. Rubber sealing caps are
made to fit each sleeve size, so equipment personnel must inspect and be cognizant of their inventory.

Secondary Instruments

There is a variety of diagnostic and operating secondary instruments. Many of the designs
are being changed, and new instruments are being
developed each year. Many of the secondary instruments have been redesigned for the 3 mm or 5
mm operating channel of the operating laparoscope. Figure 18 displays some of the instruments
that are most commonly chosen by laparoscopists.

In any basic set, an instrument for palpating and displacing the mobile viscera is necessary.
Some type of grasping instrument is imperative.
Insulated instruments are available for electrosurgery. The choice between specialized instruments—such as scissors versus a knife—is largely
individual and those who are enthusiastic and
knowledgeable about operative laparoscopy feel
that all the instruments, with few exceptions, have
a place in laparoscopy and should be available in
the surgical suite.

A word of caution—always read the instructions which accompany any secondary instrument. An example is the biopsy drill of Palmer:
there are several different versions and the mechanics can confuse the operator, thus raising a
potential risk for the patient.

A special comment should be made about
bipolar electrosurgical instruments (Figures 19–
22). First, they can be used only with low-voltage
coagulators. These forceps are designed primarily
for coagulation in tubal sterilization and are not
meant to be effective against any but the smallest
bleeder. Thus, unipolar systems must always be
available in the operating theater. Other specialized instruments for sterilization are discussed in
Chapter 15.

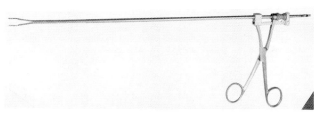

Figure 21
The bipolar instrument of Kleppinger designed for
tubal sterilization using low-voltage
electrocoagulation.

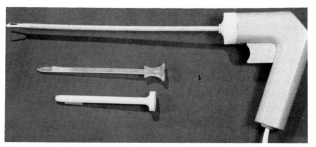

Figure 22
The bipolar instrument of Rioux designed for tubal
sterilization using low-voltage coagulation.

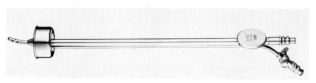

Figure 23
Semm vacuum cannula for uterine manipulation and
tubal lavage.

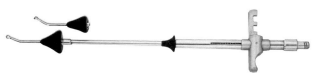

Figure 24
Cohen cannula with spring-loaded handle for uterine
manipulation and instillation of dye.

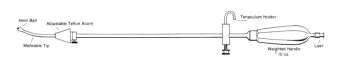

Figure 25
Corson uterine manipulator with weighted handle
and attachment for uterine insufflation.

Uterine Manipulators

A "must" in gynecologic laparoscopy is
some instrument placed into the endometrial cavity
of the uterus which will extend far enough through
the vaginal introitus to allow the operator and/or
assistant to manipulate the uterus manually during
the procedure. Many operators who wish to include
tubal insufflation in their procedure prefer the vacuum cannula of Semm with a cervical cap (Figure
23).

The acorn-tipped tubal insufflation cannula has been redesigned specifically for laparoscopy. Melvin Cohen, M.D., has introduced a
spring-loaded channel into the shaft of his cannula,
which attaches to the single-tooth tenaculum
placed on the anterior lip of the cervix so that the
cannula is self-sealing, thus preventing dye instillation leakage. This also eliminates the problem of
suction leakage with the Semm cannula (Figure
24).

Stephen Corson, M.D., has designed a
similar acorn cannula, with the addition of a
weighted handle, which is helpful in displacing the
uterus anteriorly away from the small bowel, which
might be contained in the pelvic cavity. It is particularly advantageous during tubal sterilization procedures using electrosurgery (Figure 25).

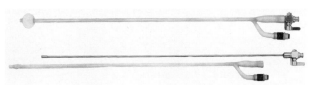

Figure 26
Hasson balloon cannula for uterine insufflation and manipulation.

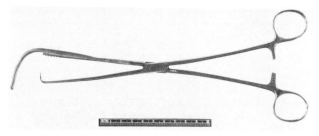

Figure 27
Tenaculum-type uterine manipulator.

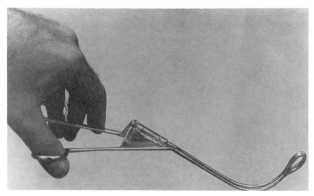

Figure 28
Hulka uterine manipulator for postabortal tubal sterilization.

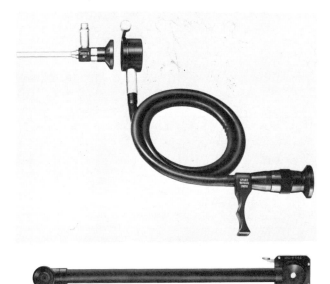

Figure 29
Flexible and rigid teaching attachments for dual vision through the endoscope.

Because uterine perforation occurs occasionally with rigid uterine manipulators, H. Hasson, M.D., has designed a balloon catheter for placement in the endometrial cavity. A semirigid metal tube inside the lumen of the catheter gives sufficient rigidity for uterine manipulation and allows the instillation of dye for tubal insufflation. The distended balloon prevents dye leakage (Figure 26).

For cases which do not require tubal patency studies, I prefer the Velsellum or tenaculum-type uterine manipulator, as illustrated in Figure 27. A special ring forceps has been redesigned by Jaraslov Hulka, M.D., as a uterine manipulator for the postabortion uterus in laparoscopic sterilization. It permits easier uterine manipulation and reduces possible uterine perforation (Figure 28).

Teaching Attachments

Optical systems are available to aid the student in observing the teacher and vice versa. The rigid-type system has more clarity than the flexible type, but the flexible teaching sidearm is more comfortable to use and is preferred by those who do a significant amount of endoscopy training. Complications during the training phase of laparoscopy can be reduced markedly with the use of a teaching sidearm (Figure 29).

Summary

In general, all kinds of laparoscopes perform their tasks well. Some can now be autoclaved—a debatable advantage since it has been shown after thousands of laparoscopies that gas sterilization every 24 hours, with cold sterilization (i.e., Cidex) between cases, is quite safe (Figure 30). As is true with any other fine optical instrument, proper maintenance is mandatory (Figure 31), and if possible, special personnel should be assigned to the care of laparoscopic equipment.

Unfortunately many parts—i.e., trocars and additional instruments—are not interchangeable from one company to another, so a hospital operating theater may be forced to use only one manufacturer's instrument and accessories. The laparoscopist must define his needs and goals, examine all instruments in coordination with his surgical personnel, and finally review his existing equipment before making a purchase decision.

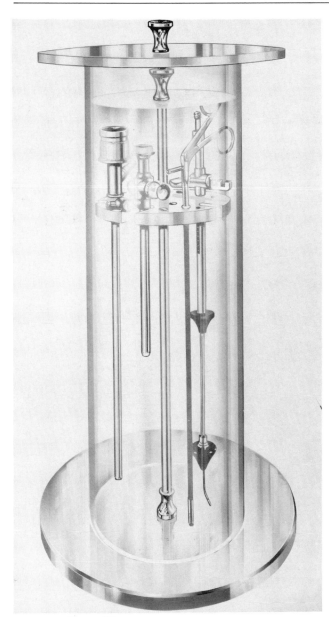

Figure 30
Soaking container for cold sterilization.

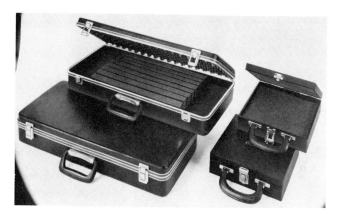

Figure 31
Storage container for the protection of laparoscopy
equipment.

Editorial Comments

Dr. Soderstrom was charged with the difficult task of covering an amoeboid-like topic. A
thorough description of laparoscopic instruments,
which does not read like a catalog, is the happy
result of his efforts. Laparoscopists tend to be
gadget-oriented, and few operating suites have
budgets which will satisfy completely the desires of
every laparoscopic surgeon.

Light sources and insufflators should be
chosen with respect to price, service after the sale,
durability, versatility and compatibility with equipment from other manufacturers. The article by
Rioux and Yuzpe[1] on generators will serve as a
consumer's guide for years to come.

It may be necessary to purchase more
than one type of laparoscope. I favor a 5 mm scope
for routine pelvic laparoscopy. Upper abdominal
cancer detection, biopsy procedures and photographic and teaching ventures all require greater
illumination and magnification, which are provided
by the 10 mm telescope. The lens angle should be
that most comfortable for the individual.

Recommended ancillary instruments include those necessary to perform sterilization
(preferably bipolar) and a blunt, calibrated probe
for manipulation of pelvic organs. An intrauterine
instrument allowing for tubal lavage and uterine
mobilization is a prerequisite for successful laparoscopy.

On the next level, one might wish to have
instruments with which to perform more involved
procedures. Among the items necessary are elec-
trified scissors, grasping and biopsy tongs, a suction probe with coagulation capability and aspiration biopsy needles. If I had to choose one all-
purpose instrument to have, it would be the Cohen-
Eder modification of the Palmer tonged-drill biopsy
tool. With it one can manipulate, sterilize, biopsy
and remove foreign objects from the abdomen.

S.L.C.

Reference

1. Rioux J-E, Yuzpe AA: Know thy generator. Contemp Obstet
   Gynecol 6:15, 1975

Chapter 6

Instrument Maintenance and Personnel Training

Tibor Engel, M.D.

Laparoscopic equipment is, at best, fragile; at worst, poorly constructed. The ruggedness and durability which seem to characterize broncoscopic and/or urological endoscopic equipment have not been passed onto the realm of peritoneoscopy. Sharp edges dull quickly, forceps lose proper occlusion, electrosurgical equipment insulation fails and optics become less clear. It is seldom that all four sets of the instruments in our hospital (from two manufacturers) are completely functional. Often two or three at a time are back at the factory for repair.

Given the premise that the tools are delicate, the hallmark of maintenance must be gentleness. Careful handling in washing and wrapping, during sterilization and while in use will greatly prolong the life of these instruments.

Preoperative Sterilization

The safest and most effective method for sterilizing endoscopic equipment is that of the gas autoclave. This method is effective for all bacteria and spore-forming organisms. The entire instrument package, including the telescope and all accessories, may be sterilized by this method. Instruments with component parts, such as the Veress needle and the trocars, may be sterilized while completely assembled so that small, individual pieces are not misplaced or lost. This package concept also allows mobility when the surgeon uses a single set of instruments in more than one hospital.

The sterilization procedure is carried out at 140 F and takes only 115 minutes plus an extended time span for the gas to dissipate.* This time is necessary because rubber and teflon retain ethylene oxide, a very caustic gas which may burn skin or intraabdominal organs. Shelf aeration alone requires seven days, but with a vacuum exhaust system the time may be shortened to 12 hours (using a low vacuum) or eight hours with a high-vacuum system.

---

* The figures for time and temperature vary for each manufacturer. The figures in this chapter refer to the Steri-Vac Model 400 Gas Autoclave, manufactured by the 3M Company, St. Paul, Minnesota.

To most laparoscopists this time period is unacceptable. Many have several instruments available so that once a week, in rotation, the gas method may be used to assure total sterility, whereas the more rapid methods are used at other times. The most commonly used technique involves soaking the instruments in a solution of activated dialdehyde† for an appropriate length of time. This solution will eliminate all organisms except spores after 10 minutes. Many operating rooms (OR) require 20 minutes as a safety margin. Spores are eliminated in 10 to 20 hours. Theoretically, soaking must be done in a plastic container because dissimilar metals will ionize and create a plating process. However, most laparoscopy instruments employ surgical grade stainless steel or chromium-plated surfaces. The instruments must be completely disassembled while soaking to assure complete contact with the solution. Also, they must be completely rinsed with sterile water because the activated dialdehyde is also caustic and harmful to intraabdominal organs. While this method is fast and allows the use of the instruments throughout the day in a busy operating room, the obvious drawback of incomplete sterilization must be considered. However, it is safe in the vast majority of instances. In grossly contaminated cases, such as pelvic inflammatory disease, the instruments should be gas sterilized as a precaution against infection. The soaking of instruments in a solution for any length of time obviously will have an effect upon the seals of the optical equipment as well as coating the fiber optic surfaces. While manufacturers do not readily acknowledge this problem, its occurrence has been documented by our operating room personnel. Droplets of water will occasionally seep through the eyepieces or more commonly through the end of the telescope, thus requiring lengthy waits during factory repair of the instrument. Bearing this in mind, the soaking of instruments for one to two hours does not increase sterility but does hasten the possibility of dissolving the glue of the lens system in the telescope. An autoclavable telescope is manufactured, but the fiber optic light cord is not autoclavable. Previous experience shows that this telescope is not as durable as the nonautoclavable scopes.

Steam autoclaving the stainless steel instruments, such as trocars, is fast and certainly adequate. Care must be taken so that the fiber optic, fiberglass and rubber materials are not steam autoclaved. This procedure reduces the life span of all these instruments by half.

Some hospitals will use only a single method, such as gas autoclaving or soaking, for the entire instrument package, so the more sensitive components may not be accidently steam autoclaved. Rigid sidearm teaching devices must never be immersed in a solution, let alone autoclaved.

Preoperative Inspection and Care

Once sterilized, the equipment is ready to use. The operator should inspect the instruments prior to beginning a case to assure that they are complete. This is particularly true when they have been disassembled for soaking. They must then be tried for mobility of the forceps and trapdoors and for proper lubrication of the valves. A drop of sterile mineral oil or silicone spray will provide adequate lubrication. All the insulation must be inspected, the electrical connections checked and the light source and cable tried out. Finally, the operator should look through the telescope to check the lens system. It has been the practice in some operating rooms to soak the telescope in hot saline prior to insertion into the abdomen to prevent fogging of the lens. This is not good practice because the hot saline ultimately will dissolve the glue at the end of the telescope and allow moisture to seep inside the lens system. Holding the end of the telescope to bring it to body temperature will suffice. The operating room should stock sterile spare parts such as bulbs, gaskets and electric cords in case the need for them develops during an operation.

---

† Cidex, Arbrook, Inc., Arlington, Texas.

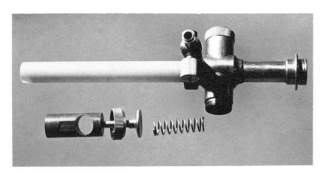

Figure 1
Component parts of trocar

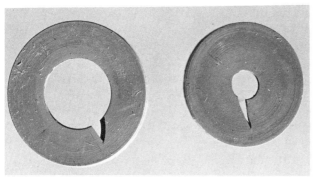

Figure 2
Damaged rubber gasket

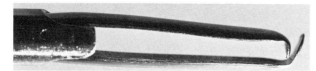

Figure 3
Forceps with bent tong

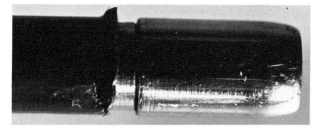

Figure 4
Frayed insulation on Palmer forceps

Postoperative Maintenance

Once the operation is completed, the instruments must be washed and made ready for future use. Care must be taken to gently place all instruments into a receptacle with "green soap"‡ and water. Powdered soap should not be used because undissolved particles can remain inside the equipment. They should not be treated casually but with finesse, as previously mentioned. The instruments should be disassembled completely so that all the blood can be easily washed away. The inner sleeves of the trocar can be cleaned with fine, long brushes and the smaller diameters with pipe cleaners and compressed air. The stainless steel trocars should not be left in saline for long periods because prolonged soaking will pit the steel. Instruments can be cleaned ultrasonically after the major debris is removed. The advantage of this method of cleaning is that it cleans hard-to-get places. The drawbacks are that the lubrication is gradually removed, which shortens the life of the instruments when used excessively, and the fiber optic cord shatters in this process. Some operating rooms have elected to use this method at the end of each day rather than between each case.

Once the equipment is cleaned, a routine inspection may be conducted. All component parts must be accounted for (Figure 1). This may be done using autoclavable color-coding tape. Edges should be inspected for sharpness. A simple carpenter's metal file will remove burrs and nicks. Fiberglass trocar sleeves have edges which fray easily, possibly from the trauma of the operation or from too much heat during a sterilization procedure. The telescope should be checked for water droplets in the lens system and for scratches and blurring of the lens. Rubber gaskets will lose their elasticity or tear as they wear out (Figure 2). Forceps jaws could lose their perfect approximation, and a hemostat can usually straighten out this kind of problem (Figure 3). Jaws and tongs should be closed for storage. The insulation along the shaft of an instrument can peel off and be deposited within the abdomen (Figure 4). The instruments are then dried and stored or made ready for another procedure. Several manufacturers have mobile carts with drawers on which rest the light source and CO_2 delivery systems and which can be used for storage of telescopic equipment. It is recommended that these carts be kept away from the busy operating room traffic (Figure 5).

---

‡ Super Edisonite, Edison Products Division, Colgate-Palmolive Company, New York, New York.

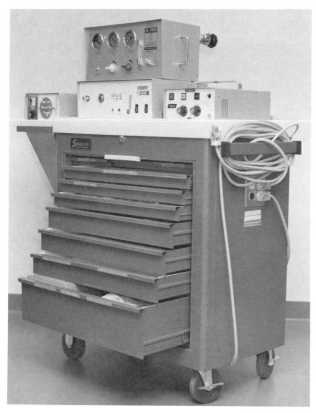

Figure 5
Mobile storage cart

It is especially important to reinforce the concept of gentleness to the OR personnel who clean the equipment postoperatively and soak the instruments in the activated dialdehyde. This is the time when many accidents may happen; instruments sometimes slip out of the hands; gaskets, washers and springs can be misplaced; the telescope may be inadvertently knocked against a pan or another instrument. If the fiber optic cable is bent in two, it results in the breakage of individual fine glass filaments and a break in the continuity of light transmission, which is indicated by black spots at the end of the cable when the light is turned on. The nurses or instrument aides must be taught to be especially careful here.

The fiber optic light source and CO_2 delivery systems need only minimal care as long as they are not abused. Prior to burning out, the light spectrum shifts toward yellow, which affects photography. The diaphragm in the CO_2 source may dry out, and the rate of flow may decrease. Light bulbs obviously burn out and valves get stuck, but major repairs are seldom needed as long as the instruments are not dropped or otherwise mishandled.

Operating Room Responsibility

In the hope of prolonging the life span of the laparoscope and ancillary instruments, various suggestions have been offered. Ideally, each laparoscopist would own one or two sets and have his or her own scrub nurse who would clean and sterilize them after each use. However, this plan is usually unrealistic, and it remains for each operating room to handle and maintain equipment for a number of surgeons. It has proven helpful to have one interested OR nurse responsible for laparoscopic equipment. Thus, all inquiries, complaints and repairs are handled efficiently by this person. Obviously, this plan is not a complete answer to the problem. One person cannot scrub on every laparoscopic case; often two or three rooms may have concurrent laparoscopic procedures; one person cannot wash and wrap every piece of equipment after every procedure; one person cannot be on continuous call for unscheduled cases. The alternative is to have one person "in charge" but to make sure that all OR nurses, scrub technicians and instrument aides are familiar with the technique and with the equipment. To this end, new nurses and scrub technicians must first learn the equipment. The purpose and operation of each instrument must be explained. The Veress needle, trocars and tubal ligation forceps should be disassembled and put back together until the process can be done by rote. The CO_2 delivery system also must be learned. The connections between the CO_2 tank, delivery system and patient require some experience to assemble. The gauges may be confusing until understood. These steps are not difficult but require time and experience to master.

Special attention must be paid to the electrosurgical equipment. In the entire procedure of laparoscopy there is no more important an area of consideration. The most dangerous complications arise from the misuse of high frequency current. The laparoscopist himself or herself should set the dials on the generator. An attempt to use the same generator is helpful in avoiding instrument variation. While the physician should check for competence of insulation and proper grounding and connections, the OR nurse can prevent many problems by being familiar with the system and checking it before each procedure. Thus, with a mastery of the instruments and with the experience of observation during the actual operative procedure, the nurse is ready to assume the responsibility for instrument maintenance. This "on the job" experience should be supplemented with frequent in-service refresher seminars—perhaps as often as every three months. They can be conducted by physicians or by other nurses well schooled in laparoscopy. There is available a cassette tape recording for OR personnel which addresses itself to the maintenance and care of instruments.§

Many operating rooms have formulated a check list which is carefully learned and applied prior to each procedure. It begins with checking the CO_2 system and light source. Next, the instruments are accounted for and the trocars, valves and springs checked for competency. The telescope is examined for optical integrity and the electrical connections and ground verified. A check list of this kind will assure that all steps have been taken to give the laparoscopist a procedure free of problems created by faulty instrumentation.

Conclusion

It must be stressed again that the hallmark of maintenance is gentleness. Careful, gentle handling of the laparoscopic equipment will easily double its life span. To accomplish this, OR teams need to know how the instruments function, need to see them in operation and must be able to dismantle and put together every item. Only with frequent exposure, both practical and didactic, will the OR personnel keep these tools functional.

Acknowledgment

The author is grateful to Valerie Voelker, R.N., Operating Room Supervisor, General Rose Memorial Hospital, Denver, Colorado for her assistance in composing this chapter.

---

§ Available from Dr. Richard Soderstrom, Mason Clinic, Seattle, Washington.

Section 3

Preparation

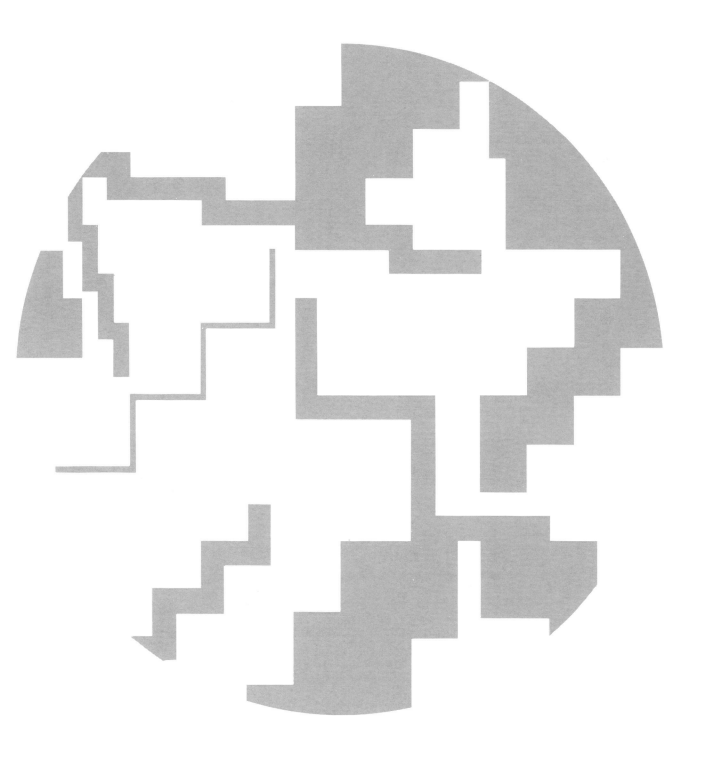

Chapter 7

Indications and Contraindications

Philip G. Brooks, M.D.
John Marlow, M.D.

General

There has been an almost meteoric rise in enthusiasm for gynecologic laparoscopy in the past few years. The primary reason is that this procedure has been found to have a wide application to diagnosis and/or treatment of gynecologic problems with reasonable safety, and it avoids expensive, hazardous and less efficient procedures. Diagnostic laparoscopy provides the physician with direct, visual access to the inner pelvic anatomy and a temporary window in the abdominal wall. A better understanding of pelvic disease and its response to treatment is available through its use.

In general, laparoscopy is useful in improving the accuracy of diagnosis when surgical intervention is undesirable but when observation or empirical therapy is ineffective or too conservative. Unnecessary laparotomies can be avoided in many of the conditions below, thus shortening hospitalizations and minimizing surgical risks and complications.

Indications

Categorizing indications for laparoscopy (Table 1) into diagnostic and therapeutic groups is very useful but difficult because of frequent overlapping. It is more appropriate to describe the application of laparoscopy according to the types of problems encountered.

Infertility

Laparoscopy has become an indispensable aid in the evaluation and treatment of the infertile woman.[4, 7] An investigation and evaluation of the factors in infertility may require several months to complete. If a rapid workup is desired, laparoscopy allows the evaluation of uterine, tubal and ovarian factors with a single visual inspection. Frequently, a more exact diagnosis can be made and specific therapy determined.

Undetectable peritubal adhesions which severely interfere with tubal mobility or obstruct ovum pickup and/or transfer can be diagnosed and frequently lysed during a laparoscopic examination. These peritubal adhesions frequently are not visualized by salpingography. The entire length of the fallopian tube can be visualized through the laparoscope; by inserting ancillary trocar sleeves into the lower abdomen, one may manipulate the tubes for a complete examination.

Table 1

I. Indications for Laparoscopy

A. Infertility:

    1. Diagnostic:
       a. Examination for tubal patency, adhesions, phimosis
       b. Assessment of type of tuboplasty to be done
       c. Assessment of ovarian function, genetic structure (karyotyping)

    2. Therapeutic:
       a. Lysis of adhesions
       b. Dilation of phimotic fimbriae
       c. Fulguration of endometriosis
       d. Removal of splints or hoods
       e. Uterine suspension

B. Endometriosis:

    1. Diagnosis.

    2. Aspiration of cysts

    3. Fulguration of implants, adhesions

    4. Assessment of adequacy of hormonal therapy

C. Pelvic pain

D. Pelvic mass

E. Hemoperitoneum

F. Endocrine disorders

    1. Primary Amenorrhea

    2. Secondary amenorrhea

    3. Intersexuality

G. Pelvic malignancy

    1. Staging

    2. "Second look" to assess therapy, to detect early recurrence

H. Sterilization

I. Miscellaneous

    1. Removal of ectopic pregnancy

    2. Removal of ectopic IUD, splints, other foreign bodies

    3. Uterine perforation evaluation

    4. Trauma

    5. Peritoneal fluid aspiration for spermatozoa, cytology, chemical analysis

    6. Ovarian wedge resection

    7. Diagnosis of unknown primary source of metastatic malignancy

    8. Oocyte recovery

J. Education

K. Research

II. Contraindications

A. "Absolute" contraindications

    1. Known acute pelvic infection

    2. Generalized peritonitis

    3. Bowel obstruction, severe ileus

    4. Abdominal, hiatal herniae

    5. Patients with severe cardiorespiratory disease

    6. Tuberculous peritonitis

B. "Relative" contraindications

    1. Extreme obesity

    2. History of previous anesthetic complications

    3. Large intraabdominal masses

    4. Extensive abdominal scars

    5. Advanced pregnancy

Retrograde tubal lavage, usually with an indigo carmine solution, affords far greater accuracy in assessing tubal patency than does hysterosalpingography or tubal insufflation (Rubin's test). This solution, of dye and normal saline injected under pressure, has therapeutic as well as diagnostic value. Fine intratubal adhesions may be released by this procedure. The location and extent of tubal obstruction may be noted. The rigidity of the wall during lavage may reflect evidence of chronic inflammatory disease of the tube. The motility and access of the fimbriae to the ovarian cortex are important information derived from the inspection. Partial tubal obstruction may not be appreciated by hysterosalpingography; however, the laparoscopist may compare the flow rate of the dye escaping from each fimbrial opening.

Tubal anomalies, Morgagnian cysts, phimosis, fimbrial adhesions, parovarian cysts and periovarian adhesions may best be evaluated by laparoscopy.

Prior to performing a tuboplastic procedure, laparoscopic examination allows for an accurate assessment of which type of procedure is indicated or whether tuboplasty is indicated at all.

When laparoscopy is performed at the luteal peak (ovulation plus eight days), the corpus luteum in the ovulating woman is seen easily. (On rare occasions, the extrusions of the ovum and its surrounding cumulus mass have been observed. This extruded mass may be seen through the laparoscope, and future observations of this phenomenon may provide a better understanding of the mechanism of tubal pickup of the ovum in humans.)

Experienced operators have reported large numbers of infertile patients for whom laparoscopic surgery has been very successful in evaluating and correcting the cause of reproductive dysfunction.[6, 9] These procedures include aspiration of peritoneal fluid and ovarian cysts, cauterization of endometrial implants, dilation of phimotic tubal ostia, uterine suspension and ovarian biopsy with preparation of the tissue for karyotyping for verification of genetic defects as a cause of the reproductive abnormality. After tuboplasty has been performed, and if fimbrial hoods or tubal splints were used, laparoscopic removal of these devices has been reported,[1, 3] thus eliminating a second laparotomy.

Other diagnostic uses of the laparoscope in infertility include an extended postcoital test to determine the presence of spermatozoa in the cul-de-sac or fallopian tube. The patient with a presumptive diagnosis of recurrent salpingitis is usually treated with antibiotic therapy and, on occasion, may require hospitalization. Early endometriosis may be mistaken for this condition and the patient subjected to repeated antibiotic exposure. Laparoscopy provides the diagnosis and, when salpingitis is discovered, more appropriate therapy. Laparoscopy provides an opportunity to obtain a direct culture from the intratubal lumen.

Endometriosis

Especially in cases where conservation of reproductive organs is desirable, the laparoscope can be invaluable in the diagnosis of endometriosis, in its treatment by way of fulguration of implants or aspiration of endometrial cysts and in the follow-up assessment of the adequacy of hormonal therapy. Of great importance is the elimination of the erroneous, presumptive diagnosis of endometriosis based on symptoms only.

The early stages of endometriosis are the most opportune for hormonal treatment but unfortunately, are also the most difficult to diagnose by pelvic examination. In the past, this stage of the disease was diagnosed at the time of exploratory laparotomy for some other, unrelated problem. With the increased use of laparoscopy, the diagnosis is being made in the early stage. Very small foci of endometriosis can be seen through the magnified view; the laparoscope can be manipulated throughout the pelvic basin for a detailed inspection of the peritoneal surfaces, thus providing a thorough examination.

The decision to treat a patient with hormone suppression for a period of six months to a year can be made more confidently following laparoscopy. The patient's response to treatment can be evaluated and, if pregnancy is desired, a more accurate timing can be provided for attempts to conceive. New drugs for the treatment of endometriosis can be evaluated objectively by the physician's noting the response of the implants to therapy. Collaborative laparoscopic studies of endometriosis may define genetic and other epidemiologic factors.

Pelvic Pain

The use of the laparoscope in unexplained acute or chronic pelvic pain offers a great opportunity to make a precise diagnosis or to rule out organic disease safely and without delays or prolonged hospitalization.

Acute salpingitis in the early stage may be confused with early appendicitis. The former disease is treated medically, and surgery is avoided; the latter is treated surgically, with morbidity related to the time from onset to intervention. The importance of early diagnosis underscores the value of laparoscopy, especially in the young woman, whose fertility may be affected. The location of the appendix may vary. It is sometimes found in the pelvis and associated with a redundant cecum. Rarely, it may be found transposed to the left lower quadrant. Locating the appendix through the laparoscope may also assist the surgeon in selecting the site for the abdominal incision.

A common and frequently perplexing problem in gynecology is the management of lower abdominal or pelvic pain. (A complete discussion of this topic is provided in Chapter 11.) Adhesions which produce traction between pelvic structures, peritoneum, bowel or omentum can be identified visually. Encapsulation of the ovary may cause pain with the swelling of ovulation. Peritoneal hyperemia or congestion may be seen. Pelvic varicosities may be associated with pain, and endoscopic inspection provides the only currently available means of defining this condition. Torsion of adnexal structures, such as pedunculated cysts or leiomyomata, old lacerations of the supporting structures of the uterus (the Allan-Masters syndrome) and small inguinal hernias may be associated with pain and may be seen through the laparoscope. (Endometriosis as a cause of pelvic pain is discussed in Chapter 11.)

In addition, laparoscopic surgical procedures, such as lysis of adhesions or fulguration of endometrial implants, can be performed to resolve the problem. Laparoscopic transection of the uterosacral ligaments to alleviate pelvic pain has been reported[4] but is not practiced widely.

Pelvic Mass

Laparoscopy is very useful in the diagnosis of pelvic masses. Uterine pathology or anomalies are distinguished easily from ovarian or tubal disease.

Laparoscopy is a rapid diagnostic tool for the patient suspected of having an ectopic pregnancy. The hospital stay during the diagnostic phase may be reduced, and the percentage of unruptured ectopic pregnancies diagnosed may be increased. The relative inaccuracy of other diagnostic methods, such as the pregnancy test, the sonogram and culdocentesis, (coupled with the fact that deaths may occur from delayed diagnosis) emphasizes the importance of the use of the laparoscope in this problem. (If an intrauterine pregnancy is suspected, the uterine cannula should not be inserted.) The differentiation between a ruptured corpus luteum and ectopic pregnancy is made easily by inspection. Likewise, the chronic ectopic pregnancy, which may be difficult to diagnose, can be identified through the laparoscope.

Patients who are overweight or who may be difficult to examine because of an inability to relax pose a problem in diagnosis when a solid or small adnexal mass is suspected. A similar problem may exist in infants or adolescents. A palpable postmenopausal ovary is worthy of attention but may be difficult to evaluate. Diagnostic laparoscopy can be used in each of these situations to rule out pelvic pathology, to confirm the presence of a benign disease such as leiomyomata or to prompt further appropriate therapy.

Puncture aspiration of ovarian cysts and hydrosalpinges has been reported as highly effective in reducing these masses.[4, 6]

Hemoperitoneum

When hemoperitoneum occurs with minimal evidence of acute blood loss, laparoscopy is useful for discerning whether the bleeding is from a ruptured tubal pregnancy or from other sources. A ruptured small ovarian cyst or corpus luteum, for example, would generally require conservative management, thus avoiding an unneccessary laparotomy.

Endocrine Disorders

Especially in primary amenorrhea, laparoscopy with or without ovarian biopsy is of great benefit in documenting genetic or congenital defects of the uterus or ovaries. In addition to assessing the extent of atresia or hypoplasia of the uterus, visual ovarian examination and biopsies can define precisely the anomaly and/or the ovulatory capacity of the ovary.

Equally important is the determination of the patient's prognosis for future fertility. Planning for the proper treatment, which may include estrogen and/or gonadotrophins, will depend upon the findings.

Stein-Leventhal ovaries, functioning ovarian neoplasms and hilar or adrenal rest tumors possibly associated with secondary amenorrhea are some of the conditions that may be detected through the laparoscope.

Laparoscopy may be performed to visualize the internal genitalia of infants born with ambiguous external genitalia. Determination of the internal reproductive organs may aid in selecting the mode of therapy. True and pseudohermaphroditism may be seen.

Uterine anomalies present a variety of appearances. The history may reveal a background of amenorrhea, infertility, repeated fetal loss or malpresentation of the fetus. Hysterosalpingography with simultaneous hysteroscopy and laparoscopy provides the most complete description of the anomaly. Thin, partial uterine septa may be resected through the hysteroscope with laparoscopic control. If metroplasty is indicated, a laparoscopic examination aids in the selection of the particular type of procedure.

Pelvic Malignancy

Laparoscopy has been utilized successfully in the evaluation and treatment of pelvic malignancy.[8] Its use in primary staging and in the so-called "second look" in order to evaluate the efficacy of chemo- or radiotherapy and to assess early "recurrences" can avoid inaccuracies or unnecessary delays.

The value of the laparoscope in the evaluation and management of pelvic malignancy was first appreciated in patients with ascites and widespread intraperitoneal metastasis. Histologic confirmation of the diagnosis was made possible and major surgery avoided. The "second look" surgery to detect response to therapy or to diagnose recurrence has also been accomplished through the laparoscope. Staging of pelvic cancer may be assisted by visual inspection. Liver, peritoneal and diaphragm metastasis may be confirmed by directed biopsy. Peritoneal fluid can be aspirated following irrigation, and cytologic evaluation can be used to assist in decisions about chemotherapy. By early investigation of adnexal masses, it may be possible to detect ovarian cancer at a more treatable stage.

Sterilization

The widest use of gynecologic laparoscopy at the present time is for tubal sterilization. This procedure, whether done by coagulation, tubal transection, resection of a tubal segment for microscopic documentation or "banding" or "clipping," is being performed very frequently because of its ease and relative safety, with a minimal hospital stay and expense (Chapter 15).

Miscellaneous Indications

In addition to the above applications of laparoscopy, several other uses have been reported, some with extensive use, others with only occasional use.

Removal of ectopic intrauterine devices eliminates the need for a laparotomy and prevents the anxiety which results from leaving the device intraabdominally.[2, 5] Other foreign bodies, such as fimbrial hoods and polyethylene tubal splints, have been removed similarly via the laparoscope. Considerable adhesions may be encountered when one attempts to remove these foreign bodies, and the surgeon should be prepared to perform exploratory surgery.

Aspiration of peritoneal fluid for spermatozoa, chemical content and/or cytology has been reported as useful in studies in reproduction and cancer therapy.

In oligoovulatory women, in whom a diagnosis of polycystic ovary syndrome has been made, several investigators have reported successfully removing a wedge of ovarian tissue via the laparoscope. It is done by grasping the ovary through one accessory cannula and using electrocoagulation to incise the ovary through another accessory cannula.

There have been several reports of removal of early ectopic gestation by laparoscopy. While extrusion of an occasional fimbrial implantation may be done via the laparoscope, the risk of extensive bleeding may be great; therefore, this indication should be reserved for rare cases and for very experienced laparoscopists.

Perforations or lacerations of the uterine wall may occur during a diagnostic D & C or elective abortion or with uterine sounding. Many of these patients will require no further treatment beyond observation. Laparoscopy frequently can be performed immediately following the uterine perforation to evaluate any significant hemorrhage at the perforation site. Should the hemorrhage require suturing or other surgery, the blood loss and subsequent need for transfusion (with the attendant risks) can be reduced.

Elsewhere in this book (Chapter 14) there is a discussion of uterine suspension via the laparoscope. While this procedure is a relatively simple one, the indications are rare, and it is most often done during laparotomy that is done for other reasons (infertility, pelvic pain, endometriosis, etc.).

The gynecologist occasionally may be called on to assist in the workup for a patient with a suspicion or frank evidence of metastatic malignancy with an undetected primary source. Certainly, laparoscopy done by an experienced laparoscopist can aid in the intraabdominal exploration (and biopsy, if needed) which is less of a surgical risk than an open surgical exploration.

Patients who have undergone trauma of the abdominal or pelvic region may be evaluated for intraabdominal hemorrhage by means of the laparoscope. Evidence of the hemorrhage may be slow to develop but deserves priority evaluation.

Education

The increasing use of laparoscopy has provided the physician with access to pelvic anatomy from a vantage point not previously available. Through the laparoscope the gynecologist can demonstrate to the student the living anatomy and pathologic variations encountered in gynecology. Television transmission has made this image available to a much larger audience simultaneously with the surgery. By means of videotape the view can be replayed for study. The findings may be documented on film or videotape for future reference. (Visual records are superior in detail to those available through the written word alone.) Electronic transmission of the images allows for consultation and educational exchanges from operating room to classroom or lecture hall or potentially to any location in the world.

Research

As a research tool, diagnostic laparoscopy allows physicians to study chronic or slowly progressive pelvic diseases, tubal and ovarian physiology, pelvic vascularity and the effects of various drugs on the pelvis. The successful use of laparoscopy as a diagnostic and surgical tool in humans has stimulated its use in research on other animal species. Multiple observations are now possible where previously only a single examination could be made.

Finally, recovery of preovulatory oocytes for reproductive studies or the *in vitro* fertilization experimentation has made the laparoscope a very useful research tool.[10]

Contraindications

While laparoscopy is a relatively safe procedure, there are times when its use is extremely hazardous.

In the presence of known, acute pelvic infection or acute, generalized peritonitis from any cause, performing a laparoscopy may spread the infection or interfere with the body's attempt at localizing the infection. In addition, when such an infection or any other intraabdominal disturbance results in distention of the intestines, laparoscopy is contraindicated because of the very high risk of lacerating or perforating the bowel.

Patients with known abdominal or diaphragmatic herniae should also be considered dangerous risks for a laparoscopic procedure because of the hazard of herniation of intraabdominal contents which results from the markedly increased intraabdominal pressures following pneumoperitoneum. Similarly, this procedure is more hazardous in patients with compromised cardiorespiratory function because the pneumoperitoneum results in decreased diaphragmatic mobility and may severely alter the blood-gas balance.

Tuberculous peritonitis, while rarely encountered in cultures with modern health measures, does occur in some parts of the world and may also contraindicate laparoscopic manipulations.

Those contraindications above are usually considered to be "absolute" ones. Other conditions which make laparoscopy more hazardous but not definitely contraindicated are considered "relative" contraindications and are related to the skill and training of the operator. Greater skill and experience are necessary in performing a laparoscopy in the extremely obese patient because of the difficulty in using trocars and needles, because of greater intraabdominal pressures required to perform pneumoperitoneum and because of greater anesthetic problems.

Patients with a history of previous anesthetic problems will warrant special precautions or alternate surgical approaches which do not require general anesthesia and endotracheal intubation.

The presence of large intraabdominal masses, advanced pregnancy or scars from multiple, previous surgeries requires great caution in the performance of laparoscopic procedures for fear of inadvertent damage to adjacent or adherent structures.

In conclusion, it must be emphasized that the risks in laparoscopy are potentially great, but that these risks can be minimized by increasing the skill and training of laparoscopists. Furthermore, it is necessary for laparoscopists to understand fully all of the effects and ramifications of the procedures. Only then can any medical or surgical problem in the patient be considered a potential contraindication.

References

1. Bagley GP: Mulligan hood removed through the laparoscope. Obstet Gynecol 40:225, 1972

2. Brooks, PG, Berci G, Lawrence A: Removal of intraabdominal intrauterine contraceptive devices through peritonescope with the use of intraoperative fluoroscopy to aid localization. Am J Obstet Gynecol 113:104, 1972

3. Esposito J: Removal of polyethylene catheters under laparoscopic supervision. J Reprod Med 14:174, 1975

4. Frangenheim H: *Laparoscopy and Culdoscopy in Gynecology*. G. Thieme, Stuttgart, 1972

5. Levinson CJ: Laparoscopic removal of perforated IUDs. J Reprod Med 10:169, 1973

6. Rioux JE: Operative laparoscopy. J Reprod Med 10:249, 1973

7. Roland M, Leisten D, Kane R: Fertility studies by means of laparoscopy. J Reprod Med 10:233, 1973

8. Rosenoff SH, Young RC, Anderson T, Bagley C, Chabner B, Schein PS, Hubbard S, DeVita VT: Peritoneoscopy: a valuable tool for the initial staging and "second look" in ovarian carcinoma. Ann Int Med (In press)

9. Siegler AM, Garret M: Ancillary techniques with laparoscopy. Fertil Steril 21:763, 1970

10. Steptoe P: Gynecological laparoscopy. J Reprod Med 10:211, 1973

Editorial Comments

The authors, Brooks and Marlow, are to be commended for their approach to the subject of indications and contraindications. They have chosen to discuss the indications in terms of symptom complexes and clinical entities; in so doing, they have avoided the stereotype of a didactic discussion. Because of the nature of their material, much of it is necessarily controversial.

I concur with the authors' suggestions for using laparoscopy for evaluation prior to tuboplasty, assessment of ovarian genetic nature, staging and "second look" evaluation of pelvic malignancy, and numerous operative procedures. However, a word of caution is in order with respect to surgery in the pelvis via the laparoscope: it requires particularly skilled hands and much experience and is not to be performed by the novice. Even when these procedures are done by an experienced surgeon, I doubt the wisdom of attempting to aspirate endometrial cysts, doing ovarian wedge resection and performing tubal plastic surgery through the laparoscope. These procedures require consummate skill, attention to detail, superior hemostasis, careful suturing and the avoidance of future adhesions. It seems unlikely to me that all this can be accomplished via the laparoscope.

C.J.L.

Chapter 8

Informing and Counseling of Patients

Edwin S. Bronstein, M.D., M.P.H.

Although all patients who are prepared for the laparoscopic procedure need to be counseled carefully, obviously the individual or the couple who seeks laparoscopy for purposes of sterilization must be counseled more carefully since the procedure provides an irreversible method of contraception. Laparoscopic sterilization, since it is an elective procedure, involves a more personal decision than a laparoscopic procedure done for diagnostic or therapeutic purposes. The patient and her husband should be counseled about the consequences of their decision. The counselor must evaluate the patient's emotional status and motivation for sterilization. After describing the alternative methods of temporary and permanent birth control, the counselor helps the patient with a mature choice of a sterilization procedure. It is also important to allay any fears of surgery or anesthesia and, above all, to answer to the patient's satisfaction any questions about a chosen procedure. Last, the counselor must see that arrangements for the procedure, whether inpatient or outpatient, are taken care of so that no additional barriers are created for the patient.

In order to carry out the above, the counselor needs to recognize the importance of the content of counseling for a sterilization procedure. He or she must have knowledge of the various types of sterilization procedures and be aware of the emotional factors in patients regarding sterilization. The approach which the counselor must take in order to be successful should foster trust and communication between patient and counselor. Brochures, audio tapes and special counseling forms, such as the one devised by the Georgia Regional Laparoscopic Program at the Medical College of Georgia[1] and another developed by Dr. James Shelton of the Maternal Health Division of the Georgia Department of Human Resources, can be used to describe the operation thoroughly.

When the couple arrives for counseling, the counselor should record the family history information and talk comfortably with the patient and her husband. During this period the counselor should observe the couple's interaction to see if both are in agreement about the need for sterilization.

The counselor atttempts to define the couple's motivation for sterilization. In assessing the strength of their decision, the counselor questions the couple about their earlier attempts at contraception and their effectiveness in limiting or spacing their children. It is necessary that each partner be involved in the decision for sterilization; the procedure should neither be forced on a reticent wife nor done without the spouse's approval and cooperation. The counselor, stressing the permanency of the procedure, should help the couple ascertain if sterilization will really accomplish the goal they have in mind. As with some surgical procedures, the outcome can often be more emotionally traumatic than physically beneficial.

The single or very young woman desiring permanent sterilization should be counseled in the same thorough and understanding manner. If her desire is real, the counselor should supply all the information and help needed for a reasonable decision. If the counselor believes the patient to have unrealistic motives or goals, he or she may suggest further consideration and counseling. The decision for sterilization rests with the couple (or the single patient) and the physician. The counselor must remain unmoralistic throughout the counseling experience, retaining his or her role as an advisor and provider of information with all patients.

The patient seeking sterilization will often have a specific procedure in mind. Perhaps she learned of this method through friends, public health staff, the mass media or another physician. The counselor introduces all available means of permanent sterilization: hysterectomy, laparoscopy, tubal ligation, culdoscopy and vasectomy. The counselor should answer briefly and completely any questions about the various procedures, encouraging the patient to discuss them with the physician. He or she should dispel any misconceptions or "old wives' tales" about sterilization. Ideally, the patient will then be more receptive to the physician's explanations and suggestions.

The main emotional barriers to sterilization procedures are fear of loss of one's "nature" (femininity or masculinity), fear of surgery and anesthesia and concern about the period of convalescence, including physical, family and financial problems. The counselor and the physician should be aware of these concerns and constantly reassure the patient of the relative safety and minimal discomfort of the laparoscopic procedure. She should understand that her "nature" will remain the same and that her sex life might even improve with the removal of the fear of pregnancy. The local family services organization can often be helpful in arranging family care and financial assistance for those unable to make adequate provisions. With the burden of these concerns lifted, the patient will be less apprehensive about the procedure. This will help in the postoperative adjustment.

The patient should be informed of the legal aspects of sterilization and know whether or not her husband must provide his consent.

Information to be Covered by Counseling

After a brief introduction to the patient, in which the counselor explains his or her purpose in getting to know more about the individual or the couple and their reasons for making the decision, the counselor stresses the need to make sure that this procedure will accomplish what the couple desires. He or she further stresses the need to avoid creating more problems by doing the procedure than are solved by it. And last, the counselor needs to make certain that the couple or the individual has a chance to ask all questions so that they fully understand the procedure they are considering.

1. The general information which should be available is the patient's name, date of birth, the source of referral, the head of the household and the address.

2. *Why does the patient want the sterilization procedure?*

It may be because of family problems such as alcoholism, infidelity, chronic illness, mental illness, another child making a bad situation worse, wanting no more children, not being able to afford more children, future pregnancies endangering the patient's health, inability to find any effective method of birth control, the patient's husband's wanting no more children and her not wanting to lose him, and the involvement of genetic problems.

3. *Has the individual or the couple used methods of contraception on a temporary basis and, if so, what has been their experience?*

It is important to discuss the current contraceptive practices of the patient and to know what information the patient has about the intrauterine device, the foam and condom, the pill or whatever method the patient has used. It is particularly important to have an understanding of the success or failure the patient has had with these methods of contraception and why she is now selecting a permanent method of contraception.

4. *What method of sterilization does the patient desire?*

Laparoscopy, tubal ligation, hysterectomy. It is important to document the patient's statements about these particular methods. For example, with laparoscopy it might be less painful, take less time in the hospital and be a more certain procedure or cost less. The individual may have personal reasons: for example, she might know of another person who has undergone the procedure and had no scar.

For tubal ligation the response might be that the patient is not familiar with laparoscopy, another family member or friend had the procedure, she desires it after a child is born or she may want to be put to sleep.

For vaginal hysterectomy the patient may want the most certain method, she may not want to have her periods anymore, as long as she is receiving surgery she may want to make certain she will not get cancer, a friend has had it and recommended it, the patient has been bothered by severe cramps throughout her lifetime.

The couple may select vasectomy for the male partner because it is an easier operation; the husband may prefer it and the wife may prefer that he have the operation.

5. *With whom has the patient discussed her decision for sterilization?*

How will she plan on handling any disapproving person? Will she ignore them? Does she feel that this will not pose a problem? Will she tell them that it is her decision and leave it at that? Does she need help with her problem? Has she discussed it with her husband, her mother, her father, her in-laws, sisters, brothers, friends? Who has been involved in this personal decision?

6. *What was the couple's desire in terms of family size?*

How many children does the patient have? How many did she want when she first started her family? Did she change her mind since that time? What caused her to change her mind? How does she cope with the children she presently has? What would happen if she knew that she could no longer have any more children? Would she deny that anything could happen to her present children? Would she want to have her tubes put back together? Would she adopt other children? Would she feel that no new child could replace one that was already born? Would she say that she does not want another pregnancy no matter what? These are all considerations and information which the counselor needs to discuss and share with the patient.

7. *What about the marital relationship?*

If the husband should die or the marital relationship break up, would the patient remarry? Would she know how to handle this? Is it too farfetched for the patient to think about, or would she say that her new husband would not need to know of her sterilization? Or that the new husband would have to accept her and her present children as they are? Possibly the patient might feel that she would never remarry.

8. *How does the patient feel about sterilization in general?*

Does she show any undue anxiety and seem to feel that she would be different after the procedure; or has the patient shown some concern that she may have some difficulty in accepting herself sterilized? Does the patient have any concern about the practical arrangements such as the bill, child care, etc? How was the patient's appearance, who came with the patient, how skillful was the patient's communication and how well thought out were her plans? Is the patient articulate? Does she have any difficulty in communicating? Was she afraid to say how she felt? Were they just random thoughts or was there a logical thought pattern? Did she listen well? All of this should be discerned by the counselor during the counseling process.

After all this has been discussed, the counselor should have an idea of which method of sterilization the patient wants. The patient then needs help with her plans for hospitalization.

If the patient's procedure is paid for out of federal funds, the counselor will have to be knowledgeable about the Federal Guidelines of April 1974.

DHEW Guidelines (April 18, 1974)

Involuntary Sterilization

There is at present a moratorium on all involuntary sterilizations for mentally retarded people or minors in programs or projects which receive federal funds.

Voluntary Sterilization

The regulations of April 18, 1974, apply principally to voluntary sterilization.

Nontherapeutic Sterilizations

Nontherapeutic sterilization is defined as any procedure or operation the purpose of which is to render an individual permanently incapable of reproducing and which is not either (a) a necessary part of the treatment of an existing illness or injury, or (b) medically indicated as an accompaniment of an operation on the female genitourinary tract. For purposes of this regulation mental incapacity is not considered an illness or injury.

Informed Consent

The voluntary, knowing assent from the individual on whom any sterilization is to be performed after she or he has been given (as evidenced by a document executed by such individual):

1. A fair explanation of the procedures to be followed,
2. A description of the attendant discomforts and risks,
3. A description of the benefits to be expected,
4. An explanation concerning appropriate alternative methods of family planning and the effect and impact of the proposed sterilization, including the fact that it must be considered an irreversible procedure,
5. An offer to answer any inquiries concerning the procedures,
6. An instruction that the individual is free to withhold or withdraw his or her consent for the procedure at any time prior to the sterilization without prejudicing his or her future care and without loss of other project or program benefits to which the patient might otherwise be entitled.

Documentation

Documentation shall be provided by one of the following methods:

1. Provision of a written consent document detailing all of the basic elements of informed consent.
2. Provision of a short-form, written, consent document indicating that the basic elements of informed consent have been presented orally to the patient. The short-form document must be supplemented by a written summary of the oral presentation. The short-form document must be signed by the counselor, the patient and by an auditor-witness to the oral presentation. The written summary shall be signed by the person obtaining the consent and by the auditor-witness. The auditor-witness shall be designated by the patient.
3. Each consent document shall display the following legend printed prominently at the top:
   Notice: Your decision at any time not to be sterilized will not result in the withdrawal or withholding of any benefits provided by programs or projects.

In addition to any other requirements of this subpart, programs or projects to which this subpart applies shall not perform or arrange for the performance of any nonemergency sterilization unless:

1. Such sterilization is performed pursuant to a voluntary request for such services made by the person on whom the sterilization is to be performed.

2. Such person is advised at the outset and prior to the solicitation or receipt of his or her consent to such sterilization that no benefits provided by programs or projects may be withdrawn or withheld by reason of his or her decision not to be sterilized.

A program or project to which this subpart applies shall not perform or arrange for the performance of a nontherapeutic sterilization *sooner than 72 hours following the giving of informed consent.*

In addition to other reports required by the Department of Health, Education and Welfare, the program or project shall report to the Secretary at least annually the number and nature of the sterilizations subject to the procedures set forth in this subpart and such other relevant information regarding such procedures as the Secretary may request.

In order to comply with the federal regulations, the Georgia Department of Human Resources developed the following document. It is presently being used on all patients whose laparoscopy will be paid for out of federal funds.

Notice: Your decision at any time not to be sterilized will not result in the withdrawal or withholding of any benefits provided by programs or projects receiving federal funds.

Explanation of Laparoscopic Sterilization Procedure
Ask Questions
If there is anything that you do not understand or that you are concerned about, be sure to **ask questions at any time.**

Your Decision Will Not Affect Other Federal Benefits and Must Be Voluntary
There is no penalty if you decide you do not want this operation. You can say "no" *at any time* and still be able to get benefits from programs or projects that get federal money, including getting a sterilization later on. Your decision to be sterilized must be voluntary. In other words, it must be of your own free will. No one has the right to force you to have the operation.

What the Sterilization Operation Does
A sterilization is an operation to make you unable to have children. You should choose to have the operation only if you are sure you *never* want to have any more children. It is occasionally possible to undo the operation, but this cannot be guaranteed, so you should consider the operation permanent. One advantage of sterilization is that you would not have to use a temporary method of birth control again (such as "the pill") and would avoid the risks of such methods. In addition, you would not need to worry about getting pregnant again. That brings peace of mind to many people.

Some Things You Need to Do
If you are married, your husband or wife must agree to the operation. However, if you are separated and he or she cannot be found, you may receive the operation without his or her signature. You must be 21 years of age or older to receive a sterilization in this program. You must wait 72 hours (3 days) after giving your consent to sterilization before the operation can be done.

Some Things You Need to Know about the Operation
The operation you would have to sterilize you is called a "laparoscopic tubal sterilization." In this operation the doctor separates or blocks each fallopian tube (which connects the womb and the ovary) so that the egg cannot travel from your ovary to your womb. Blocking the tubes makes pregnancy impossible.

How the Operation is Done

Each doctor may do the operation procedure slightly differently, but your doctor's procedure will follow this description very closely.

First, you are given an anesthetic (medicine to reduce pain). You will receive one of three types of anesthetics.

1. A "general" anesthetic, which means you are put to sleep and won't wake up until the operation is over.
2. A "local" anesthetic, which is numbing medicine (similar to what dentists use when filling cavities) injected into the skin or other tissues. Other pain-relieving drugs will probably be used along with a local.
3. A "regional" anesthetic, which is medicine injected into your back with a needle.

Local anesthesia is generally considered safer than regional, which is generally considered safer than general anesthesia.

The doctor will then put some gas into your abdomen through a needle. The abdomen is the hollow area inside your belly. Your "tubes" lie inside the abdomen. The gas is either carbon dioxide or nitrous oxide. Carbon dioxide is the same gas you breathe out of your lungs in normal breathing. The gas is put in so that the doctor can see your tubes better and make room for the operating tools.

The doctor then makes a small cut near your navel. Through this cut he or she puts a metal tube called a "laparoscope." The doctor can look down this tube to see your internal organs. The cut is so small it can be covered with a small bandage about the size of a Band aid. The scar is very small.

Sometimes the whole operation is done through this small cut, but many doctors make a second small cut lower down for a second operating tool.

The next step is to block your tubes. Your tubes will be blocked in one of these ways.

1. The doctor may pass electricity through the tubes: the heat from the electricity seals and divides each tube in half. A portion of the tube may actually be removed.
2. The tubes may be sealed with metal clips.
3. The tubes may be blocked with little rings similar to small rubber bands.

The "metal clips" and "rings" methods are newer than the "electricity" method. You would be getting the (insert name of exact procedure) type of operation.

The operation usually takes 30 minutes, and a woman can usually leave the hospital or clinic in less than 24 hours. With "local" anesthesia you may be able to leave the hospital within several hours after your operation.

Discomfort

There is usually little pain. You should expect slight, brief, pin-prick-type pain when needles are first inserted. Another slight pain may occur at the moment the tubes are blocked (similar to menstrual cramps) if a local anesthetic is used. After the operation you will probably feel some minor pain and soreness at the spot where the small cut was made. You may also feel pain in your neck and shoulders related to the gas that was in your abdomen. If you were put to sleep, you may feel some sore throat if a tube was placed in your windpipe to help you breathe during the operation. These pains usually go away within a few days. Your doctor can give you drugs to help ease any of the pains you may have.

Risks

Laparoscopic tubal sterilization is one of the safest operations a woman can have. In fact, it is probably safer than pregacy in general. However, it is associated with certain hazards and risks including death, just as any other surgery is. Serious complications do not occur often (1 to 3 in 1,000 operations). Most of the time the serious problems can be treated and cured by the doctor. If a serious problem does occur, it may mean that during the operation the doctor may have to open your abdomen and do a more major procedure (a bigger operation) than he or she had planned.

Laparoscopy   Chapter
8   Informing and Counseling
of Patients   **66**

The following problems can occur with a laparoscopic tubal ligation, although most women do not have them.

1. Bleeding from cuts made on your skin.
2. Bleeding inside your abdomen from the area where your tubes were blocked.
3. Skin burns (if electrical current was used).
4. Injury to your intestines: injury to your intestines is *rare*. When it happens, it is usually because the electrical current touches a spot on the intestine and burns it. Sometimes the doctor can tell right away if a part of the intestine is burned. If so, he or she will immediately make a larger cut into you abdomen so the burn can be repaired. Sometimes the doctor cannot tell right away if part of your intestine was burned. Infection, including a serious infection called "peritonitis," can result up to two weeks after the operation. Go back to your doctor *at once* if you get fever or severe pain in the abdomen.
5. The doctor cannot finish the operation: this could be caused by a number of problems. For instance, you might have a lot of scars around your tubes. If the doctor finds you have this scarring, he or she may have to use a larger operation to sterilize you.
6. The operation may not work: the operation cannot be 100 percent sure to make you sterile. It fails about one or two times in one thousand.
7. Anesthetic problems: the various drugs used to reduce pain can rarely cause a bad reaction, particularly if the patient is sensitive to the drug. Serious problems are (a) your heart may stop beating—**This is very rare** (b) death—**This is very rare.**

Alternatives to Sterilization

Before deciding whether or not you want to be sterilized, you should think about your other possible choices and their advantages and risks.

Pills—birth control pills are very effective. They are drugs that prevent the ovaries from releasing eggs. They must be taken every day except one week out of the month. In very rare instances the pill can cause blood clots which can result in serious problems, including death.

IUD—the "loop" or "device" is almost as effective as the pill. It must be inserted into the womb by a specially trained health professional. In extremely rare instances the IUD can cause death if the woman becomes pregnant and develops an infection during the middle of her pregnancy.

Foam, Condoms, Diaphragm—if used separately, these methods are definitely less effective than either the pills or IUD. When used together, however, such as foam and condoms together, they may be almost as effective as the IUD. A couple would need to remember to use both each time they have sexual relations. There is essentially no risk from these methods themselves, but if a woman became pregnant while using them, she would run the risks that come with pregnancy.

Rhythm and Withdrawal—these "natural" methods are much less effective than any already mentioned. There is no risk to life from the method itself.

Abstinence—you can, of course, just stop having sexual intercourse. The only risk involved in this "method" might relate to any mental stress involved.

All of the above methods are reversible. That means that after you stop using them, you *can* get pregnant.

Vasectomy—this male sterilization method is safer and cheaper than a female sterilization. It should be considered permanent.

Using No Birth Control—another alternative for you is to use no method of birth control and take the risk of getting pregnant. You should be aware that both childbirth and abortion can very rarely result in death due to bleeding, infection or other causes. The risk of death from pregnancy, in general, is probably more than for a laparoscopic sterilization.

Date _____

_____

I affirm that the above patient voluntarily requested the procedure and that he or she is not mentally incompetent to the best of my knowledge, and my explanation of the procedure agrees with the attached explanation.

Counselor's signature _____

Date _____

I affirm that the attached explanation accurately reflects my intended sterilization procedure, that the procedure is voluntarily requested and not medically contraindicated to the best of my knowledge and that the individual requesting it appears to me to be mentally able to give consent.

Physician's signature

Date

Note: State law requires that the performing physician must:

1. act in collaboration or consultation with at least one other physician in performing a sterilization.
2. give his or her own explanation of the meaning and consequences of the operation.

Questions and Answers Given

I asked the questions listed above concerning the sterilization operation.

Patient's signature

Date

I supplied the answers listed above concerning the sterilization operation.

Counselor's signature

Date

Notice: Your decision at any time not to be sterilized will not result in the withdrawal or withholding of any benefits provided by programs or projects receiving federal funds.

Family Planning Clinic

Address

City

State

Request for Referral and Consent to Sterilization

Full name of patient

Birth date

I have asked for information about sterilization and other family planning methods and the attached information was discussed fully with me by (name of counselor) of this clinic. When I first asked for the information, I was told that the decision to be sterilized was completely up to me; that I can decide not to be sterilized at any time; and that if I decide not to be sterilized I will *not* lose any help or benefits now or later which are paid for wholly or partly by the federal government. (He/she/they) explained to me the procedures that would be followed in the (insert type of sterilization) sterilization operation. (He/she/they) told me about the benefits, discomforts, risks and effects I could expect from the operation. Included was the fact that it must be considered permanent and final and cannot be reversed, although this result has not been guaranteed. (He/she/they) also told me about other possible methods of birth control, encouraged me to ask questions about the procedure, and answered them to my satisfaction.

I understand that a "sterile" woman cannot become pregnant and that a "sterile" man cannot make a woman pregnant.

I understand I can decide not to be sterilized *at any time* before the operation even after signing this consent form and I will lose no federal benefits if I do.

I further understand that the operation will not be performed sooner than 72 hours (3 days) following the signing of this consent.

I understand that in order for this consent to be valid, *I must read the explanation attached* to it and that it must agree with what the counselor told me.

I am 21 or older and legally able to consent to sterilization.

I, _____ ,

hereby voluntarily consent to having

Dr. _____ ,

and/or assistants of his/her choice, perform upon me the following sterilization operation:

Name of Procedure

and to do such other procedures as are in the physician's judgement necessary to preserve health, including giving anesthetic for the purpose of this sterilization operation.

I also consent to the release of this form and other medical records about the operation to state and federal agencies funding the operation for the purpose of seeing if appropriate laws or regulations are followed and only if my records are kept confidential.

Patient's signature

Time and date

Spouse's signature (if spouse can be located)

Date

I am separated from my husband or wife. I have made a reasonable effort to find him or her but cannot.

Patient's signature

As laparoscopy becomes a more common procedure among gynecologists and other trained physicians, and as tubal sterilization by laparoscopy becomes increasingly popular among couples deciding on a permanent method of contraception, it behooves the physician to prepare the patient for this procedure properly. Preparation must include a complete approach to counseling and informed consent, which will lead to a better understanding between the doctor and the patient and her spouse.

Reference

1. Bronstein ES: *Laparoscopy for Sterilization.* Year Book Medical Publishers, Chicago, 1975

Editorial Comments

This chapter, unfortunately, is apt to be ignored by the average gynecologist. However, it should prove to be of immense value to those interested in having informed patients and to those working in laparoscopy programs.

Dr. Bronstein stresses the need for *personal* counseling. The advising of patients requires an understanding of their motives, full comprehension of the procedure and a recognition of potential side effects. Gynecologists like to do laparoscopy, and it is the woman in a couple who visits the gynecologist's office—but that does not preclude the possibility that a vasectomy may be the appropriate mode of sterilization for the couple. Proper counseling and discussion will bring about the most appropriate decision.

Dr. Bronstein has included as part of his chapter a complete combination information sheet and consent form. In addition to supplying the needed information to the patient, such a form, routinely used, may obviate some of the difficulties of legal complications.

C.J.L.

Chapter 9

Anesthesia

John I. Fishburne, Jr., M.D.
Louis Keith, M.D.

Since the introduction of laparoscopic sterilization techniques by Palmer in 1962, surgeons have shown considerable interest in the selection of the anesthetic for this operation and in its interaction with the physiologic derangements produced by laparoscopy. Palmer's early admonition to the anesthesiologist was to avoid flammable anesthetics for general anesthesia in the event that electrocoagulation was employed.[56] Three variables are recognized presently as affecting the choice of the anesthetic agent and its management: (1) the use of pneumoperitoneum; (2) Trendelenburg position, and (3) electrocautery. In addition, the presence of gynecologic laparoscopy in an outpatient environment has required the consideration of speed of recovery from the effects of anesthesia. As a result, increased emphasis is placed upon the selection of short-acting and rapidly reversible anesthetic techniques. Regional and particularly local analgesia are most popular.

General objectives for laparoscopic anesthesia have been stated.[24] The ideal technique should:

1. Allow rapid recovery from the effects of anesthesia.

2. Maximize safety; that is, minimize the risk of aspiration of gastric contents, cardiac arrhythmias and cardiac arrest, pulmonary embolism, hypertension, hypotension, hypoxia, hypercarbia and pneumothorax.

3. Provide amnesia and adequate analgesia for anesthetic induction, surgical operation and anesthetic emergence.

4. Provide relaxation so that the operation can be performed as safely and expeditiously as possible.

5. Permit few anesthesia-related side effects.

This chapter will present the potential hazards of anesthesia and of laparoscopy as it relates to anesthesia, describe the primary anesthetic methods, discuss the management of the post-anesthetic phase and list therapeutic recommendations.

Table 1
Anesthetic and Operative Complications Related to Anesthesia

Conditions	Etiology	Diagnosis	Treatment
Cardiac arrhythmias	Hypoxia Hypercarbia Vagal stimulation Anesthetic agents such as halothane Excessive intraabdominal pressure Gas embolus Endobronchial intubation	ECG Precordial steth-oscope Pulse	100% O_2 Turn off anesthetic agent Atropine⟶ IV Lidocaine Release intraabdominal pressure Check endotracheal tube placement
Hypotension	Hemorrhage Low blood volume Bradycardia 2° to vagal stimulation Excessive anesthetic agent Aspiration of gastric contents Pneumothorax Excessive intraabdominal pressure Hypoxia Gas embolus Hypoglycemia	Systolic blood pressure by cuff <80 mm Hg	Decrease anesthetic concentration Rapid administration of IV fluids—(D5/Ringers lactate) Release intraabdominal pressure Atropine IV Listen to chest and suction endotracheal tube
Hypertension	Hypercarbia Light anesthesia History of essential hypertension Intraabdominal pressure of <20 mm Hg	Diastolic pressure by cuff >100 mm Hg	Increase ventilation Deepen anesthesia Alpha blocking agent such as droperidol or thorazine Ganglionic blocking agent or trimethaphan IV drip if severe Sodium nitroprusside IV drip
Gas embolus	Insufflation of gas into blood vessel or uterine wall	Circulatory decompensation Precordial mill wheel murmur Detection of gas with ultrasound transducer	Assume left lateral decubitus position If CO_2 embolus suspected, await absorption unless massive embolus If N_2O or air embolus, aspirate through CVP catheter Resuscitation and supportive measures Cessation of insufflation
Hypoxia	Decreased concentration of O_2 in inspired gas Equipment failure Hypoventilation Intrapulmonary shunting N_2O diffusion hypoxia Narcotic over-dosage Excessive intraabdominal pressure Trendelenburg position Endobronchial intubation	Cyanosis Decreased PaO_2	Inspired O_2 concentration—100% Assisted or controlled manual ventilation Release intraabdominal pressure Narcotic antagonist Eliminate head down tilt Check endotracheal tube to rule out endobronchial intubation
Hypercarbia	Hypoventilation CO_2 pneumoperitoneum Narcotic over-dosage Endobronchial intubation Trendelenburg position	Arrhythmia Elevated $PaCO_2$ Tachypnea	Assisted or controlled manual hyperventilation Release pneumoperitoneum (N_2O for CO_2) Check endotracheal tube for proper placement Reverse narcotic Eliminate Trendelenburg position

Table 1—*continued*
Anesthetic and Operative Complications Related to Anesthesia

Conditions	Etiology	Diagnosis	Treatment
Pneumothorax and Pneumomediastinum	Dissection of CO_2 or N_2O through anatomical opening or defect in diaphragm Rupture of pulmonary bleb Tracheal or pharyngeal injury during intubation	Subcutaneous emphysema Neck swelling Hypoventilation Increasing resistance to rebreathing bag compression Cyanosis Hypotension	Thoracentesis or thoracotomy tube Observation and supportive Rx if <20% pneumothorax
Gastric dilatation	Intubation of esophagus Energetically assisted respirations using anesthesia face mask	High index of suspicion leading to percussion of gastric gas Visible distention of the upper abdomen	Pass Levin tube
Pulmonary aspiration of gastric contents	Passive regurgitation associated with increased intraabdominal pressure Trendelenburg position lithotomy position use of muscle relaxants and atropine	Vomitus under face mask Signs of Mendelsohn's syndrome—i.e., cyanosis, copious secretions, rales, rhonchi, tachypnea	Suction trachea Methyl prednisolone 30 mg/kg IV O_2 Positive pressure ventilation

Potential Hazards of Laparoscopy as Related to Anesthesia

Cardiovascular

1. *Cardiac arrhythmias* have often been noted during anesthesia given for laparoscopy. Scott[67] observed an occurrence rate of 27 per 100 cases monitored by electrocardiography. The incidence of arrhythmias is directly related to the anesthetic technique employed[52] and to the selection of insufflation gas. Cognat[14] noted 25 cardiac arrests in an unpublished study based on 48,049 laparoscopies—a rate of one per 1,922 procedures. Nineteen of them were reversible, but six led to death—a mortality rate of one per 8,008. Most of the arrests were noted suddenly, often in association with intraperitoneal insufflation, although two occurred in association with hypotension or arrhythmia.[14]

Hypercarbia occurs under anesthesia as a result of hypoventilation or because of absorption of the insufflation gas (CO_2) from the peritoneal surface. As a result, endogenous catecholamines are released which produce arrhythmias in a myocardium already sensitized by anesthetic agents such as halothane.[7] Further evidence that intraperitoneal insufflation of CO_2 is responsible for the production of ventricular arrhythmias has been given by Lewis.[42] After noting arrhythmias in two patients during insufflation of CO_2, he treated them with sodium bicarbonate and noted prompt reversion to normal sinus rhythm. Since arrhythmias secondary to epinephrine administration failed to respond to bicarbonate injection, this seemed to offer further corroboration that insufflation of CO_2 was related to the production of cardiac arrhythmias. The most common arrhythmia noted by Scott and Julian[66] was the coupling of a ventricular extrasystole with a normal P-wave with the ectopic beat super-imposed upon the conducted beat. Bigeminy has also been observed.

Hypoxia may produce ventricular arrhythmias and has been noted in patients breathing spontaneously and receiving low concentrations of oxygen in the inspired gas.[11] Vasovagal phenomena have also been linked with the production of cardiac arrhythmias. Motew[53] and co-workers have described a dramatic vasovagal reflex associated with CO_2 insufflation which could have resulted in cardiac arrest had it not been immediately reversed by injection of atropine sulfate. Vasovagal phenomena have also been associated with manipulation of the pelvic organs. Marshall et al[46] have suggested that vagal activity may be responsible

for the rise in central venous pressure noted by himself as well as Motew and co-workers at intraabdominal pressures of less than 20 mm Hg.

2. *Hypotension* may occur as a result of cardiac arrhythmia or cardiac arrest. It may also be related to the increased intraabdominal pressure generated by the insufflating gas.[54] Motew and co-workers[53] have noted decreases in central venous pressure, systolic pressure, pulse pressure and cardiac output, all associated with intraabdominal pressures in excess of 20 mm Hg. They suggested that these phenomena indicate reduced cardiac venous return. High intraperitoneal pressures may also raise intrathoracic pressures, thus decreasing the total chest compliance and forcing the anesthetist to use higher airway pressures to ventilate the patient. This chain of events may further reduce cardiac output by diminishing venous return and by raising intrapulmonary vascular resistance.

Reduced blood volume states will increase the frequency of hypotension, as noted by Keith and co-workers,[33, 36, 37] who found a 16% incidence of hypotension in postpartum patients. They recommend that the blood volume be acutely increased in these patients by the rapid infusion of 750 ml of Ringer's lactate solution just prior to peritoneal insufflation.

Hartzell and Newberry[28] reported that the fasting state was significantly related to the degree of the hypotensive response to moderate hypoxia. This suggests that glucose-containing solutions should be used to reduce the likelihood of hypotension.

Vasovagal phenomena have been associated with hypotension, as reported by Mall and Kalischer,[45] who noted severe hypotension following irritation of the peritoneum.

Gas embolization may also produce hypotension through obstruction of blood flow through the right side of the heart.

3. Preexisting, mild, essential *hypertension* seems to be exacerbated by the light forms of general anesthesia now used most frequently for laparoscopy. The patient who is lightly anesthetized is susceptible to release of endogenous catecholamines with resultant increase in blood pressure. Similarly, tracheal intubation and surgical stimulation have both been associated with elevations in systemic blood pressure, while carbon dioxide accumulation secondary to hypoventilation or absorption from the peritoneal cavity has been associated with release of endogenous catecholamines and subsequent hypertension. Kelman et al[38] noted an increase in mean arterial pressure (93.6 to 103.6) as the intraabdominal pressure increased to 20 cm H_2O. This was associated with an increase in central venous pressure and cardiac output.

4. *Gas embolism* may occur during production of pneumoperitoneum and reportedly has produced cardiovascular collapse and occasionally death.[38, 51, 67, 84] The three gases used to produce pneumoperitoneum are carbon dioxide, nitrous oxide and air; the first is the most soluble in blood and has the least toxicity. In a comparative study of air and carbon dioxide as embolic agents Graff et al[27] discovered that air was five times as toxic as CO_2, with the toxicity correlated with solubility. Nitrous oxide, on the other hand, is only 68% as soluble as CO_2 in blood.[66] Stauffer and co-workers[74] injected carbon dioxide intravenously for angiocardiography in the dosage of 7.5 cc per kg and found this dosage well tolerated. Moore and Braselton[50] compared the effects of the injection of air and carbon dioxide into the pulmonary vein in cats and discovered that CO_2 was extremely well tolerated whereas air, in doses of 0.25 cc per kg, produced death from coronary artery obstruction. Carbon dioxide has been used diagnostically in humans, with amounts of up to 200 cc injected with no untoward results.[62]

The diagnosis of gas embolism should be suspected when sudden, profound hypotension occurs. It is confirmed by auscultation of a "mill wheel" murmur over the precordium. Ultrasonic transducers have recently proven effective in detecting gas trapped in the heart: quantities as small as 2 cc are readily identified.[48] When CO_2 is the etiologic agent, turning the patient to the left lateral decubitus position reduces obstruction to the outflow tract of the right heart until the gas has been absorbed. With air, however, absorption is slow

and the gas must be aspirated by means of a central venous pressure catheter placed in the right atrium. In order to minimize the chance of intravascular administration of the pneumoperitoneum gas, Esposito[23] recommends aspiration of the Veress needle to avoid intravascular injection. Steptoe[76] suggests that the Veress needle not be inserted with the gas tubing connected to it. Another possible source of embolism is direct injection of gas into the uterine wall with subsequent entry into the uterine venous sinuses.

Thrombus formation with possible pulmonary embolism is another potential complication of surgery and anesthesia and has been reported in conjunction with combined suction curettage and laparoscopic sterilization.[85]

Respiratory Complications

1. *Hypoxia*: This condition may arise from: (a) faulty anesthesia equipment, (b) administration of inspired gas with a low oxygen partial pressure, (c) hypoventilation, (d) intrapulmonary shunting, (e) N_2O rediffusion, (f) narcotic sedation, and (g) misplacement of endotracheal tube. Scott[67] calculates that given an intraabdominal pressure of 25 mm Hg, a pressure of 30 gm per square centimeter, or a total pressure of 50 kg, will be exerted against the diaphragm. Also, with the patient in the Trendelenburg position, pooling of blood may occur in the more dependent portions of the lungs, a factor which leads to ventilation perfusion inequalities.[11] Furthermore, with the diaphragm elevated, lung tissue is compressed and ventilation may be impaired further.

Hypoxia secondary to narcotic sedation is prevalent after general anesthesia and during local anesthesia. Brown et al[9] and Alexander and co-workers[2] measured arterial blood gases following sedation and determined that significant decreases in Pa_{O_2} appeared. On the other hand, breathing 100% oxygen or the stimulus of the surgical procedure itself both served to increase ventilation and restore a normal Pa_{O_2}.

Respiratory embarrassment has also been associated with assumption of the Trendelenburg position.[30, 75] In this position the full weight of the viscera is borne by the diaphragm, which is already elevated by the intraabdominal pressure secondary to the pneumoperitoneum. This further compromises aeration of the lower lobes and predisposes to postoperative atelectasis.

Plasma cholinesterase deficiency has also been associated with apnea during and after laparoscopy when succinylcholine was used to facilitate tracheal intubation.[41] Controlled ventilation is continued until spontaneous respirations return.

Some authors have speculated that the absorption of nitrous oxide from the peritoneal cavity might lead to diffusion hypoxia, i.e., the diffusion of nitrous oxide into the alveoli with the displacement of oxygen and the production of hypoxia. Corbett and co-workers[16] measured end-expired nitrous oxide levels after pneumoperitoneum and found this gas to be absorbed into the blood stream in very small concentrations (0.38%); however, nitrous oxide was detectable up to 13 hours following production of the pneumoperitoneum.

2. *Hypercarbia*: The partial pressure of carbon dioxide (P_{CO_2}) in the blood may rise because of two factors: (a) absorption, and (b) hypoventilation. Many authors,[3, 5, 6, 19, 21, 26, 29, 39, 43, 44, 53, 66, 69, 70] have reported an increase in $PaCO_2$ either associated with intraabdominal insufflation or following establishment of the CO_2 pneumoperitoneum. Although an elevation in Pa_{CO_2} can be accounted for entirely by hypoventilation, the fact that an increase is also seen in end-expired CO_2 concentrations[9, 68, 72] implies absorption of this gas from the peritoneal surface. The rate of CO_2 absorption is determined by the blood flow to and around the peritoneal cavity, the diffusion gradient across the peritoneum and the tissue solubility of CO_2.[6] Furthermore, blood flow to the peritoneum may also be increased because of the vasodilatory effect of CO_2.

Hypoventilation may occur for any number of reasons, e.g., use of narcotics,[2, 9] changes in the ventilation-perfusion relationship, diaphragmatic elevation secondary to excessive intraabdominal pressure, Trendelenburg position, inadequate spontaneous ventilation secondary to the use of muscle relaxants or excessive anesthesia, and inadequate mechanical ventilation. If intrapulmonary pressures increase while a pressure-operated respirator is being utilized, the tidal volume generated by the respirator will then be diminished, thus leading to hypoventilation with resultant hypercarbia. Spontaneous ventilation under anesthesia combined with CO_2 pneumoperitoneum inevitably leads to hypercarbia. Scott and Julian[66] recorded a mean Pa_{CO_2} of 60.8 mm Hg with CO_2 as the insufflation gas whereas when nitrous oxide was

used to inflate the abdomen, the mean Pa_{CO_2} was 50.5 mm Hg. As previously mentioned, the incidence of arrhythmia is considerably higher in patients who are hypercarbic. Lewis et al[43] investigated the effect of spontaneous ventilation and CO_2 pneumoperitoneum on blood gases. Although no marked changes occurred during insufflation, Pa_{CO_2} increased significantly postinsufflation. Most authors[3, 5, 6, 19, 26, 29, 39, 69, 80] prefer mechanical ventilation or manually assisted ventilation with tracheal intubation to eliminate CO_2 produced via respiration and thus to avoid hypercarbia. Fishburne and co-workers[24] have reported adequate pulmonary clearance of CO_2 by increasing ventilation to 1.5 times the basal requirement predicted by Radford et al.[63]

3. *Pneumothorax and Pneumomediastinum*: The problem of pneumothorax was reviewed in 1973 by Doctor and Hussain,[20] who added another case, the chief clinical features of which were cyanosis, hypotension, difficulty in ventilating and neck swelling. They reviewed seven cases of pneumothorax associated with laparoscopy. In the same year an additional case was reported by Smiler and Folick.[71] The most probable route of entry of the gas into the thorax is retroperitoneally via anatomical foramina or congenital defects in the diaphragm. Pneumothorax may also occur under anesthesia with positive pressure ventilation secondary to rupture of a pulmonary bleb. It is important to differentiate between these causative factors because entry of CO_2 into the chest cavity via the diaphragm should not lead to tension pneumothorax whereas a ruptured bleb can produce this problem rapidly. Thoracentesis with simultaneous expansion of the lungs or passive absorption may be used to treat the first condition. A ruptured bleb, on the other hand, must be treated with immediate insertion of a thoracotomy tube.

Gastrointestinal Complications

The major problems which confront the anesthesiologist are: (1) regurgitation of gastric contents with pulmonary aspiration, and (2) gastric dilatation with subsequent perforation by the laparoscopist.

Passive regurgitation of gastric contents is enhanced by the Trendelenburg position and in the presence of increased abdominal pressure resulting from intraperitoneal insufflation of gas. To minimize this risk the authors employ routine intubation of the trachea.

Gastric dilatation may result from enthusiastic use of the rebreathing bag to assist or control respiration in a patient who has not been intubated or esophageal placement of the endotracheal tube. Gastric perforation has been reported by Reynolds and Pauca,[64] who cited a case in which the endotracheal tube was inadvertently placed in the esophagus. Insertion of the Veress needle led to penetration of the stomach; subsequent insufflation of CO_2 produced eructations. When gas aspirated from the stomach was noted to have a CO_2 content greater than 10%, it became apparent that the Veress needle had perforated the stomach. There have been other reports of gastric perforation by the laparoscope trocar.[86] To avoid the problem of gastric dilation Soderstrom[73] and other authors have recommended that a Levin tube be passed into the stomach to ensure deflation whenever assisted ventilation is employed without tracheal intubation.

Electrical Hazards

Electrocution may occur under anesthesia with very small currents, provided that they are delivered to the vicinity of the heart. When electrocautery is being used in the presence of pacemaker electrodes or a CVP catheter, it is possible to induce small currents without a direct electrical connection. It is axiomatic that only *nonexplosive, nonflammable* anesthetic agents should be administered when electrocautery is being used. In modern anesthesia this is seldom a problem since explosive agents have been removed from most operating rooms in order to conform with stringent NFPA standards.

When patients are monitored with a direct electrocardiogram (ECG) system, the anesthetist must be alert to the possibility of a burn at the ECG grounding electrode. In the event of a disruption in the patient ground plate circuit, electrocautery current would become concentrated at the ECG grounding electrode—thus producing a significant burn.

Finally, the anesthetist should take care to avoid patient movement, which may occur with light anesthesia or inadequate muscle relaxation, during the time of electrocoagulation of the fallopian tubes.

Introduction to Anesthetic Methods

All three categories of anesthesia, i.e., general anesthesia, regional analgesia and local analgesia, are currently being used for laparoscopic procedures. The superiority of one method over others, however, has not been demonstrated. Various anesthetists and surgeons defend their favorite technique while trying to overlook its limitations. The purpose of this section is to provide general information regarding the three basic types of anesthesia for laparoscopy and to present the advantages and disadvantages of each so that the laparoscopist and anesthetist may cooperatively and objectively select the best method for a given patient. A recommended technique will be presented for each method, but the reader should understand that numerous acceptable variations exist.

General Anesthesia

General anesthesia has perhaps achieved the greatest popularity among laparoscopists. In some institutions it has been tailored to outpatient or short-stay usage as well as inpatient utilization.

Advantages of general anesthesia:

1. Excellent relaxation can be provided by means of muscle relaxants, which control voluntary and involuntary movements.
2. Ventilation can be controlled, thus enabling the anesthetist to eliminate CO_2 and prevent hypercarbia.
3. A quiet, operative field may be provided for the use of electrocautery.
4. Complete analgesia is obtained.
5. Amnesia is present.
6. Anxiety can be eliminated.

Disadvantages:

1. General anesthesia is more costly; special equipment, personnel and environments are required for its use.
2. Recovery may be prolonged, especially if inhalation agents are slowly metabolized or exhaled.
3. Additional stress may be placed on the ill patient with severe cardiac or pulmonary disease.
4. Postoperative sore throat may result from intubation.
5. Muscle fasciculations secondary to succinylcholine may cause postoperative pain.
6. Nausea and vomiting are common following general anesthesia.
7. Inappropriate use of positive pressure face mask ventilation may lead to distention of the stomach and inadvertent puncture.
8. Over-zealous assisted or controlled ventilation may produce pneumothorax, especially in patients with pulmonary blebs.

Indications for general anesthesia:

1. The anxious patient is particularly well suited for general anesthesia; she can be assured that she will be completely analgesic and amnesic during the procedure.
2. The less experienced surgeon should operate under general anesthesia until he or she can avoid sudden movements, which may provoke pain or alarm the patient.
3. Because of pain related to intraperitoneal CO_2, general anesthesia should be considered when this gas is to be used.

Contraindications to general anesthesia:

1. Severe cardiac or pulmonary disease.
2. Fear of general anesthesia.

Recommended Technique

Preanesthesia. There is some controversy as to whether or not premedication should be employed routinely. Pent and Loffer feel that the use of any premedication will prolong recovery unnecessarily.[59, 60, 61] Other authors[17, 18, 22, 31, 32, 34, 35, 38, 53, 62, 68, 69, 72, 77, 78, 81] favor the use of some premedication. The most popular premedication regimen consists of atropine, a barbiturate and/or a narcotic. Initially, one of us (JF) used diazepam extensively for premedication. The drug was given intravenously just prior to surgery, but the practice was discontinued when many of the patients complained of superficial thrombophlebitis several days postoperatively.[40] If premedication is to be used, it should be administered while the patient is in the preoperative holding area, approximately one-half hour prior to surgery.

Monitoring of the Patient. All patients under general anesthesia should be monitored extensively. The anesthetist should record the brachial blood pressure every five minutes and preferably at least every minute during the time of peritoneal insufflation in order to detect the onset of hypotension. Since hypertension is also likely to occur, it may be diagnosed early and treated appropriately. A precordial stethoscope should be used routinely so that respirations and heart beat can be monitored continuously. Diminishing breath sounds from pneumothorax may thus be appreciated and a "mill wheel" murmur due to gas embolization of the right heart may be heard and treatment rapidly instituted. Although not mandatory, it is helpful to monitor the electrocardiogram continuously during the procedure. The preferred method is to telemeter the ECG and avoid the remote possibility of burns at the ECG grounding electrode. Arrhythmias diagnosed by continuous ECG monitoring may be treated rapidly and before cardiac arrest ensues. Calverly and Jenkins[10] advise that the anesthetist monitor the intraabdominal pressure since he or she is the only member of the team who can feel the increased pressure as it is transmitted to the rebreathing bag. He or she is also in an excellent position to observe the intraabdominal pressure manometer and can readily respond by advising the surgeon to release excessive pressure.

Anesthetic Agents and Technique. All patients for whom general anesthesia is planned should breathe 100% oxygen for three to five minutes prior to anesthetic induction. This not only increases the oxygen stores but also enables the patient to remain well oxygenated for several minutes in the event of a difficult intubation.

Almost all anesthetic agents have been used for laparoscopy,[3, 6, 10, 15, 24, 32, 59] but nitrous oxide along with a short acting narcotic such as fentanyl has achieved the greatest popularity. Atropine should be utilized routinely, either administered intramuscularly with premedication or immediately prior to induction as a 0.4 mg to 0.6 mg intravenous dose. Curare 3 to 6 mg is given intravenously prior to induction in order to diminish fasciculations, which normally would be experienced with succinylcholine. When fentanyl is used, it should be administered one to two minutes prior to induction of anesthesia and given via the intravenous route.[24] Sodium thiopental, 3 to 4 mg per kg intravenously, is the most commonly used induction agent, although the other short-acting barbiturates have achieved some popularity. Following barbiturate induction, succinylcholine (1 mg/kg) is given intravenously to facilitate intubation. Intubation should be accomplished with a cuffed endotracheal tube, usually size $7^1/_2$ to 8 mm. Anesthesia is maintained with nitrous oxide and oxygen in a 2:1 mixture, respectively (66.7% N_2O and 33.7% O_2). In order to facilitate elimination of CO_2, ventilation should either be assisted or controlled. Subsequent muscle relaxation may be achieved via a continuous succinylcholine infusion of 1 mg per ml or by means of a nondepolarizing muscle relaxant such as curare in a dosage of 15 to 24 mg intravenously. If succinylcholine is used, it should be discontinued as the pneumoperitoneum is terminated. Curare may be reversed with neostigmine 2.5 mg and atropine 1.5 mg at the same time. Nitrous oxide administration is discontinued as the skin incision is closed. The patient should be extubated when she breathes and coughs spontaneously. Delayed extubation may result in the patient's remembering a feeling of suffocation as she emerges from anesthesia with the tracheal tube in place.

Regional Anesthesia

Spinal and epidural anesthesia have been employed by some laparoscopists, although regional techniques have not achieved general acceptance. Aribarg[4] reported 125 patients who had laparoscopy under epidural anesthesia. In his study excellent analgesia was obtained, and laparoscopy was well tolerated.

Advantages of regional anesthesia:
1. Since the patient is awake, she is able to give early warning of some complications such as pneumothorax, gas embolus, arrhythmias and vasovagal reflex.
2. There is a reduced need for systemic sedation and analgesia, which may have undesirable side effects and may prolong recovery.
3. There is a decreased incidence of nausea and vomiting with regional anesthesia.
4. A quiet operative field is provided for the surgeon, and good muscle relaxation is generally present.

Disadvantages:
1. Epidural anesthesia is not easy to administer; it requires a skilled technician and the ready availability of resuscitation equipment.
2. The block takes a relatively long time to administer. "Set-up" time may be as long as 20 to 30 minutes.
3. Local anesthetic agents may produce systemic toxicity; this is especially true in the event of inadvertent intravascular administration.
4. The level of the block must be high in order to block peritoneal reflexes.
5. Diaphragmatic pain may be referred to the chest and shoulders and can occur when carbon dioxide is used as the insufflating agent.
6. Recovery from the block is slower than that experienced with local anesthesia.

Indications:
1. Fear of general anesthesia.
2. Chronic pulmonary disease, provided that the block is not so high as to severely limit vital capacity through the paralysis of intercostal muscles.

Contraindications:
1. History of neurologic disease such as multiple sclerosis.
2. Infection at the site of puncture.
3. Severe hypovolemia from marked dehydration or hemorrhage.
4. History of allergic reaction to local anesthetic drugs.
5. Preexisting back disorder.

Recommended Technique

The premedication recommended by Aribarg[4] consists of morphine, 10 mg, and atropine, 0.6 mg, given intramuscularly one hour prior to operation. It is our opinion that the routine use of a narcotic or sedative for premedication is unnecessary in conjunction with regional anesthesia; these drugs should be used only if the patient appears unduly anxious. Atropine (0.4 to 0.6 mg) should be used for its vagal blocking effect, however.

The method usually employed is that described by Moore.[49] The single injection technique relies on the initial administration of an adequate quantity of local anesthetic drug. The senior author (JF) prefers to place an epidural catheter in the epidural space once the needle is positioned in order to provide flexibility in the event that the initial dose is insufficient to give suitable analgesia. Although Aribarg[4] describes the use of 1.5% lidocaine solution, we (JF) prefer to use 2-chloroprocaine (Nesacaine CE) because of its more rapid onset and shorter duration of action. Chloroprocaine is also tolerated better and is considerably less toxic than lidocaine.

Spinal anesthesia has been used effectively and is administered according to the method described by Bonica.[8] Tetracaine in dosage of 8 to 12 mg is the usual drug employed; however, lidocaine may be preferred because of its shorter duration of action.

Local Anesthesia

As laparoscopy moves from a strictly hospital-based procedure to one which can be and is being done in free-standing clinics,[57] local anesthesia is receiving greater acceptance. Many authors[1, 2, 9, 12, 13, 15, 17, 18, 57, 58, 81, 82, 83] have reported the use of local anesthesia for laparoscopy. Almost all use lidocaine for infiltration of the abdominal wall. A few use paracervical block (PCB), and others describe the use of local anesthetic solutions (lidocaine, dyclone) applied directly to the fallopian tubes. The local technique preferred by one of us (JF) is described below.

Advantages of local anesthesia:
1. Avoidance of the risks of general anesthesia.
2. Rapid recovery when little or no sedation is used.
3. Rapid induction with minimized anesthesia time.
4. Low cost.
5. Ready adaptability to the outpatient (non-operating room) setting.
6. Early awareness of complications such as arrhythmia, CO_2 embolus, pneumothorax, etc.
7. Decreased postoperative nausea and vomiting.
8. The ability to demonstrate anatomy and/or pathology directly to the patient by means of a fiber optic teaching extension.

Disadvantages:
1. Requires precise and gentle surgical technique.
2. There may be increased patient anxiety.
3. Mild to moderate patient discomfort.
4. Delayed treatment of certain complications such as organ injury or hemorrhage.
5. Necessity to talk with the patient during the procedure.
6. Increased risk of electrical burn if the patient moves during electrocautery.
7. Increased pain during manipulation of the pelvic organs. Since diagnostic laparoscopy often requires insertion of a second trocar, this procedure may produce additional patient discomfort.

Indications:
1. Nonoperating room setting.
2. Fear of general anesthesia.
3. Pulmonary disease.

Contraindications:
1. Lack of resuscitation equipment and the skill to use it.
2. Peritoneal irritation and pelvic pain.
3. An anxious patient.
4. A patient with suspected intraabdominal adhesions.

Recommended Technique

Although laparoscopy can be accomplished in selected patients under local anesthesia without benefit of premedication, most patients will require some systemic analgesia.

Although Akdamar[1] strongly advocates the use of diazepam intravenously immediately prior to surgery, our experience with superficial thrombophlebitis led to the discontinuation of administration of this drug. More recent observations indicate that most patients tolerate laparoscopy under local anesthesia with only 0.05 mg of fentanyl and 0.5 mg of atropine as premedication. Occasionally, it is necessary to use additional fentanyl, but this may be associated with decreases in Pa_{O_2} if not with the clinical appearance of hypoxia.[2, 9]

Atropine is administered when the patient is on the operating table just after initiation of the intravenous infusion. In this manner the protective effect against vagal reflexes is present before any manipulation of the uterus is begun. Because fentanyl has a short duration of action, it is best administered during the draping of the patient after the prep has been accomplished. The maximal effect is thus present when uterine manipulation is carried out for insertion of the Cohen cannula or the Hulka tenaculum. Although PCB with 1% lidocaine or other equivalent drug may be used prior to insertion of the uterine controlling instrument, the authors feel that its use does not provide sufficient relief of discomfort to justify its use and the increased risk of systemic toxicity from absorption of the local anesthetic agent. PCB will diminish pain of uterine motion and block uterine vagal mediated reflexes but has little effect on pain occasioned by tubal electrocoagulation.[25]

A local field block of the abdomen is performed using a single needle entry point in the inferior umbilical fold; the technique is illustrated in Figure 1. Approximately 5 ml of local anesthetic solution (1% lidocaine or other) is infiltrated into the skin and subcutaneous tissue in the inferior umbilical fold using a 3/4-inch, 25 gauge needle. A 1 1/2-inch, 22 gauge needle or a 3-inch spinal needle is then attached to a 10 ml syringe, and 2 ml of anesthetic is injected at each of the five positions illustrated in the diagram; 1 ml is deposited below and 1 ml above the fascia at each position. If a 5 mm operating laparoscope is being used, an 8 French Fogarty catheter with the balloon tip cut off is then inserted through the operating channel, and approximately 6 to 8 ml of 1% lidocaine solution or other agent is flowed over each fallopian tube. The authors recommend that this be done in stages since the anesthetic action is very short-lived (i.e., one tube is anesthetized and coagulated, after which the second tube is similarly anesthetized and coagulated). In this manner the patient experiences very little discomfort.

If a two-puncture technique is used, additional local anesthetic must be used at the site of the second puncture. Under such circumstances careful attention must be given so as not to exceed the maximum toxic dosage (lidocaine 5 mg per kg by infiltration).

LEFT OBLIQUE VIEW   LATERAL VIEW

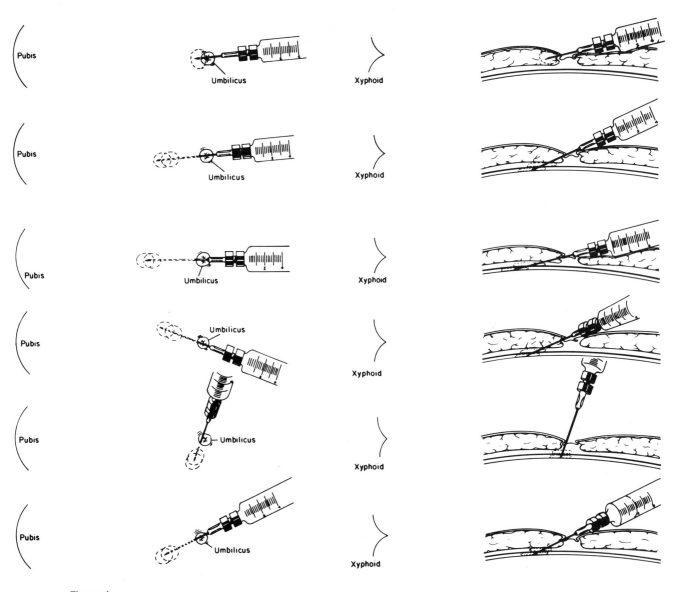

Figure 1
Technique of local anesthesia

The selection of gas for pneumoperitoneum deserves special consideration. Because of diaphragmatic and peritoneal irritation associated with CO_2 in patients under local anesthesia, most authors prefer nitrous oxide. Usage of this gas also diminishes shoulder pain in the postoperative period.

Postanesthetic Phase

Recovery From Anesthesia

Recovery from anesthesia might be delayed, although it is usually prompt. The following problems must be considered in the differential diagnosis of the causes of prolonged recovery time.

1. Excessive narcotic sedation or inadequate reversal of narcotics.
2. Barbiturate overdose.
3. Incomplete elimination of an inhalational agent.
4. Atropine overdose.
5. Chronic hypoxia.
6. Chronic hypercarbia. Since it is impossible to completely expel the pneumoperitoneum gas (CO_2), continued absorption will occur postanesthesia. In the presence of diminished CO_2 sensitivity secondary to narcotic overdose, hypercarbia may result.
7. Continued or persistent effects of muscle relaxants.

The recovery room nurse must be alert to all of these potential problems. The patient's respirations, pulse, blood pressure and general state of awareness must be monitored closely. The possibility of laryngeal edema arising from a traumatic intubation must also be considered. Since anesthesia for laparoscopy is often conducted on an outpatient basis, recovery must be prompt. When inhalation agents have been used, their elimination should be rapid. Many anesthetists prefer light halothane anesthesia in order to accomplish this. When a balanced form of anesthesia is used, such as a narcotic in combination with nitrous oxide, overdose with narcotics occasionally may occur. However, this effect may be reversed with naloxone (Narcan). The chief hazard under these circumstances is that the narcotic antagonist will be metabolized or eliminated before the narcotic itself, thus allowing the patient to become renarcotized. If the patient has been discharged from the postanesthesia recovery area prematurely, this condition may occur when the patient is unattended, and respiratory depression might ensue. If a narcotic antagonist has been employed in the operating room or shortly after the patient's entry into the recovery area, monitoring must be provided for two or three hours.

Various testing procedures have been employed to assess psychomotor recovery. The Trieger dot test[55, 79] provides a good, objective measure of patient recovery.[24] Other workers have used the Romberg test with equally good results.

Instructions for the Patient. If the patient is discharged directly from the recovery room, she must be delivered to the care of a responsible adult who will see that she is escorted home safely. The patient should not consume alcoholic beverages during the first 24 hours after her anesthetic, and she should not operate an automobile until the following day. She should also be instructed to watch for signs of laryngeal edema, which may arise as a result of traumatic intubation of the trachea.

Other Considerations

Inpatient Versus Outpatient Procedure

Almost all patients undergoing laparoscopy are potential candidates for outpatient anesthesia and surgery. However, those with a systemic illness (ASA Class II or greater) should probably be admitted to the hospital. In addition, patients who have a likelihood of experiencing a complication, obesity or a history of previous peritonitis following ruptured appendix should be admitted directly to the hospital so that a bed will be available in the event that a laparotomy becomes indicated.

Cost

Cost is a major consideration in the selection of site of surgery. Mercer et al[47] and other program directors have arranged with the hospital administration for a standard hospital admission per diem charge to cover operating room and recovery expenses. This has proven considerably less expensive than the standard charges for inpatients. When laparoscopic procedures are done in an outpatient or day surgery setting under local anesthesia, the cost can be reduced further because fewer personnel are directly involved in the care of the patient.

General Safety Measures

Because of the danger of cardiac arrhythmias, pneumothorax and major hemorrhage, resuscitation equipment should be close at hand whenever laparoscopy is performed, regardless of the method of anesthesia.

A suction source, either from a central vacuum system or a portable suction apparatus, should be near the patient's head. An oxygen source and instruments necessary for airway management should also be available (i.e., laryngoscope, endotracheal tubes, oral and nasal airways). Last, a defibrillator should be nearby. It is imperative that *all* of this equipment be checked regularly and be maintained in good working order.

Summary

In traditional surgical procedures the operating surgeon does not necessarily become involved in the problems of anesthesia. In laparoscopy, however, the interdependence of the risks and hazards existing between the operative nuances and the physiologic derangements secondary to anesthesia dictates a different approach. The surgeon and the anesthesiologist must work cooperatively to minimize the effect of the inherently unphysiologic state in which this operation is performed. Just as it is inadvisable for the untrained physician to perform laparoscopy without supervision and training, it is equally inadvisable for the anesthesiologist to disregard the necessity to gain special experience in this area and to proceed as if this were a traditional surgical procedure.

The addition of the gas system and the electrical system to the operating field adds further potential complications. This chapter has been prepared in an effort to list and categorize this aspect of laparoscopy in a manageable fashion.

References

1. Akdamar K, Lilly JO, Mary CC, Maumus L: Peritoneoscopy facilitated by premedication with diazepam. South Med J 64:891, 1971

2. Alexander GD, Goldrath M, Brown EM, Smiler BG: Outpatient laparoscopic sterilization under local anesthesia. Am J Obstet Gynecol 116:1065, 1973

3. Alexander GD, Noe FE, Brown EM: Anesthesia for pelvic laparoscopy. Anesth Anal 48:14, 1969

4. Aribarg A: Epidural analgesia for laparoscopy. J Obstet Gynecol Br Commonw 80:567, 1973

5. Baratz RA, Karis JH: Blood gas studies during laparoscopy under general anesthesia. Anesthesiology 30:463, 1969

6. Berenyi KJ, Fujita T, Siegler AM: Carbon dioxide laparoscopy. Acta Anaesthesiol Scand 14:77, 1970

7. Black GW, Linde HW, Dripps RD, Price HL: Circulatory changes accompanying respiratory acidosis during halothane (fluothane) anesthesia in man. Br J Anaesth 31:238, 1959

8. Bonica JJ: *Principles and Practice of Obstetrics, Analgesia and Anesthesia.* Davis Co, Santa Cruz, 1967, p 567

9. Brown DR, Fishburne JI, Roberson VO, Hulka JF: Ventilatory and blood gas changes during laparoscopy under local anesthesia. Am J Obstet Gynecol 124:741, 1976

10. Calverly RK, Jenkins, LC: The anaesthetic management of pelvic laparoscopy. Can Anaesth Soc J 20:679, 1973

11. Carmichael DE: Laparoscopy—Cardiac considerations. Fertil Steril 22:69, 1971

12. Chaturachinda K: Laparoscopy: A technique for a tropical setting. Am J Obstet Gynecol 112:941, 1972

13. Chaturachinda K: Laparoscopic sterilization: an outpatient procedure. Am J Obstet Gynecol 115:487, 1973

14. Cognat M, Gerald D, Vignaud A: Etude des arrets circulatoires au cours de la coelioscopie. Physiopathologie et Prophylaxie (unpublished data)

15. Cohen MR, Taylor MB, Kass MB: Interval tubal sterilization via laparoscopy. Am J Obstet Gynecol 108:458, 1970

16. Corbett TH, Peterson EP, Cornell RG, Page A, Endres J: End-expired nitrous oxide levels after pneumoperitoneum. Anesth Analg 53:527, 1974

17. Corson SL, Bolognese RJ: Laparoscopy: an overview and results of a large series. J Reprod Med 9:148, 1972

18. Corson SL, Bolognese RJ: Laparoscopic nuances. Fertil Steril 22:684, 1971

19. Desmond J, Gordon RA: Ventilation in patients anaesthetized for laparoscopy. Can Anaesth Soc J 17:378, 1970

20. Doctor NH, Hussain Z: Bilateral pneumothorax associated with laparoscopy. Anaesthesia 28:75, 1973

21. Drury WL, LaVallee DA, Vacanti CJ: Effects of laparoscopic tubal ligation on arterial blood gases. Anesth Analg 50:349, 1971

22. Edgerton WD: Experience with laparoscopy in a nonteaching hospital. Am J Obstet Gynecol 116:184, 1973

23. Esposito JM: Hematoma of the sigmoid colon as a complication of laparoscopy. Am J Obstet Gynecol 117:581, 1973

24. Fishburne JI, Fulghum MS, Hulka JF, Mercer JP: General anesthesia for outpatient laparoscopy with an objective measure of recovery. Anesth Analg 53:1, 1974

25. Fishburne JI, Omran KF, Hulka J, Mercer JP, Edelman DA: Laparoscopic tubal clip sterilization under local anesthesia. Fertil Steril 25:762, 1974

26. Gordon NLM, Smith I, Swapp GH: Letter. Cardiac arrythmias during laparoscopy. Br Med J 1:625, 1972

27. Graff TK, Arbegast NR, Phillips OC, Harris LC, Frazier TM: Gas embolism: a comparative study of air and carbon dioxide as embolic agents in the systemic venous system. Am J Obstet Gynecol 78:259, 1959

28. Hartzell WG, Newberry PD: Effect of fasting on tolerance to moderate hypoxia. Aerosp Med 43:821, 1972

29. Hodgson C, McClelland RMA, Newton JR: Some effects of the peritoneal insufflation of carbon dioxide at laparoscopy. Anaesthesia 25:382, 1970

30. Inglis JM, Brooke BN: Trendelenburg tilt—an obsolete position. Br Med J 2:343, 1956

31. Ivankovich AK, Albrecht RF, Zahed B, Bonnet RF: Cardiovascular collapse during gynecological laparoscopy. Ill Med J 145:58, 1974

32. Keith L, Stepto RC, Bozorgi N, Havdala HS, Prenzlau MS, Salvo B: Ketamine anesthesia for laparoscopy. J Reprod Med 10:256, 1973

33. Keith L, Webster A, Lash A: A comparison between puerperal and nonpuerperal laparoscopic sterilization. Int Surg 56:325, 1971

34. Keith L, Silver A, Becker M: Anesthesia for laparoscopy. J Reprod Med 12:227, 1974

35. Keith L, Silver A, Becker M: Anesthesia for laparoscopy. In *Gynecological Laparoscopy: Principles and Techniques.* (JM Phillips, L Keith, Eds.) Stratton Intercontinental Book Corp, New York, 1974, p 91

36. Keith L, Webster A, Houser K, Lash A, Barton J: Laparoscopy for puerperal sterilization. Obstet Gynecol 39:616, 1972

37. Keith L, Houser K, Webster A, Lash AF: Puerperal tubal sterilization using laparoscopic technique. J Reprod Med 6:133, 1971

38. Kelman GR, Swapp GH, Smith I, Benzie RJ, Gordon NLM: Cardiac output and arterial blood-gas tension during laparoscopy. Br J Anaesth 44:1155, 1972

39. Kunzel W, Kastendieck E, Ferneding G: Der Saure-basenstatus und die ventilation wahrend gynakologischer laparoskopien. Der Anaesthesist 21:294, 1972

40. Langdon DE, Harlan JR, Bailey L: Thrombophlebitis with diazepam used intravenously. JAMA 223:184 1973

41. Lemaire WJ, Nagel EL, Smith J: Plasma cholinesterase deficiency. Obstet Gynecol 39:552, 1972

42. Lewis GBH, Prasad K: Sodium bicarbonate treatment of ventricular arrhythmias during laparoscopy. Anesthesiology 41:416, 1974

43. Lewis DG, Ryder WT, Burn N, Wheldon JT, Tacchi D: Laparoscopy—an investigation during spontaneous ventilation. Anaesthesia 26:510, 1971

44. Lewis DG, Ryder W, Burn N, Wheldon JT, Tacchi D: Laparoscopy—an investigation during spontaneous ventilation with halothane. Br J Anaesth 44:685, 1972

45. Mall K, Kalischer F: Letter. Transient hypotension after anesthesia of peritoneum. Lancet 2:894, 1974

46. Marshall RL, Jebson PJR, Davie IT, Scott DB: Circulatory effects of carbon dioxide insufflation of the peritoneal cavity for laparoscopy. Br J Anaesth 44:680, 1972

47. Mercer JP, Lefler HT, Hulka JF, Fishburne JI: An outpatient program for laparoscopic sterilization. Obstet Gynecol 41:681, 1973

48. Michenfelder JD, Miller RH, Gronert GA: Evaluation of an ultrasonic (Doppler) for the diagnosis of venous air embolism. Anesthesiology 36:164, 1972

49. Moore DC: Regional block. In *Handbook for Use in the Clinical Practice of Medicine and Surgery.* 4th ed., CC Thomas, Springfield, 1965, p 411

50. Moore RM, Braselton CW: Injections of air and of carbon dioxide into a pulmonary vein. Ann Surg 112:212, 1940

51. Morison DH, Riggs JRA: Cardiovascular collapse in laparoscopy. Can Med Assoc J 111:433, 1974

52. Morley TR: Letter. Cardiac arrhythmias during laparoscopy. Br Med J 2:295, 1972

53. Motew M, Ivankovich AD, Bieniarz J, Albrecht RF, Zehed B, Scommegna A: Cardiovascular effects and acid-base and blood gas changes during laparoscopy. Am J Obstet Gynecol 115:1,002, 1973

54. Neely MR, Elkady AA: Modified technique of puerperal laparoscopic sterilization. J Obstet Gynecol Br Commonw 79:1025, 1972

55. Newman MG, Trieger N, Miller JC: Measuring recovery from anesthesia—a simple test. Anesth Analg 48:136, 1969

56. Palmer MR: Essais de sterilisation tubaire coelioscopique par electrocoagulation isthmique. Bulletin de la Fédération des Sociétés de Gynécologie et d'Obstetrique 14:298, 1962

57. Penfield A: Laparoscopic sterilization under local anesthesia. Am J Obstet Gynecol 119:733, 1974

58. Penfield A: Laparoscopic sterilization under local anesthesia. J Reprod Med 12:251, 1974

59. Pent D, Loffer FD: Laparoscopy at the surgicenter. J Reprod Med 10:239, 1973

60. Pent D: Laparoscopy: its role in private practice. Am J Obstet Gynecol 113:459, 1972

61. Pent D, Loffer FD: Laparoscopy as an ambulatory procedure. Clin Obstet Gynecol 17:231, 1974

62. Peterson EP: Anesthesia for laparoscopy. Fertil Steril 22:695, 1971

63. Radford EP, Ferris BG, Kriete B: Clinical use of a nomogram to estimate proper ventilation during artificial respiration. N Engl J Med 251:877, 1954

64. Reynolds RC, Pauca AL: Gastric perforation, an anesthesia-induced hazard in laparoscopy. Anesthesiology 38:84, 1974

65. Scott DB: Letter. Cardiac arrhythmias during laparoscopy. Br Med J 2:49, 1972

66. Scott DB, Julian DG: Observations on cardiac arrhythmias during laparoscopy. Br Med J 1:411, 1972

67. Scott DB: Some effects of peritoneal insufflation of carbon dioxide at laparoscopy. Anaesthesia 25:590, 1970

68. Seed RF, Shakespeare TF, Muldoon MJ: Carbon dioxide homeostasis during anesthesia for laparoscopy. Anaesthesia 25:223, 1970

69. Siegler AM: Trends in laparoscopy. Am J Obstet Gynecol 109:794, 1971

70. Siegler AM, Berenyi KJ: Laparoscopy in gynecology. Obstet Gynecol 34:572, 1969

71. Smiler BG, Falick YS: Complication during anesthesia and laparoscopy. JAMA 226:676, 1973

72. Smith I, Benzie RJ, Gordon NLM, Kelman GR, Swapp GH: Cardiovascular effects of peritoneal insufflation of carbon dioxide for laparoscopy. Br Med J 3:410, 1971

73. Soderstrom RM, Butler JC: A critical evaluation of complications in laparoscopy. J Reprod Med 10:245, 1973

74. Stauffer HM, Durant TM, Oppenheimer MJ: Gas embolism. Radiology 66:686, 1956

75. Swain J: The case for abandoning the Trendelenburg position in pelvic surgery. Med J Aust 47:536, 1960

76. Stepto P: Hazard of laparoscopy. Br Med J 3:347, 1973

77. Steptoe P, Campbell FN: Letter to the editor. Br Med J 1:625, 1972

78. Tantisira B, McKenzie R: Awareness during laparoscopy under general anesthesia: a case report. Anesth Analg 53:373, 1974

79. Trieger N, Loskota WJ, Jacobs AW, Newman MG: Nitrous oxide—a study of physiological and psychomotor effects. J Am Dent Assoc 82:142, 1971

80. Utting JE: Letter. Cardiac arrhythmias during laparoscopy. Br Med J 1:566, 1972

81. Wadhwa RK, McKenzie R, Wadhwa SR: Anesthesia for laparoscopy. Pa Med 76:69, 1973

82. Wheeless CR: Outpatient laparoscopy sterilization under local anesthesia. Obstet Gynecol 39:767, 1972

83. Wheeless CR: Anesthesia for diagnostic and operative laparoscopy. Fertil Steril 22:690, 1971

84. Wheeless CR, Penfield AJ, Israel R, Neuwirth RS: Symposium: evaluating tubal sterilization by laparoscopy. Contemp Obstet Gynecol 1:71, 1973

85. Wheeless CR, Thompson BH: Laparoscopic sterilization. Obstet Gynecol 42:751, 1973

86. Whitford JHW, Gunstone AJ: Gastric perforation: a hazard of laparoscopy under general anesthesia. Br J Anaesth 44:97, 1972

Editorial Comments

This chapter, by Fishburne and Keith, may well turn out to be the classic reference for information on anesthesia for laparoscopy. The presentation is logical and comprehensive.

The use of local anesthesia for laparoscopy is problematic. There are communities in which it is not used at all, and yet there are experienced operators who prefer local anesthesia above all other forms. As with most extremes, each view is both correct and erroneous. I did not use local anesthesia at all for the first four years of my experience but subsequently have found it to be most acceptable. Circumstances must be appropriate and include the following: the patient should not be too obese and should be placid and well-adjusted (high-strung and anxious patients do not do well). The entire counseling and operating room staff must be attuned to the procedure; any anxiety or hostility on their part is immediately communicated to the patient. The doctor must be self-assured and convey this composure to the patient. Preoperative medication is not necessary. The patient must be monitored carefully throughout the procedure by competent personnel. General anesthesia should be readily available.

The problems notwithstanding, local anesthesia has many advantages. Although the patient may complain of some discomfort during the procedure, it is usually short-lived. The effects of anesthesia are brief. The patient is alert and capable of going home within one or two hours of the procedure. There is no nausea or throat discomfort and much less general debility.

C.J.L.

Section
4

Fundamentals

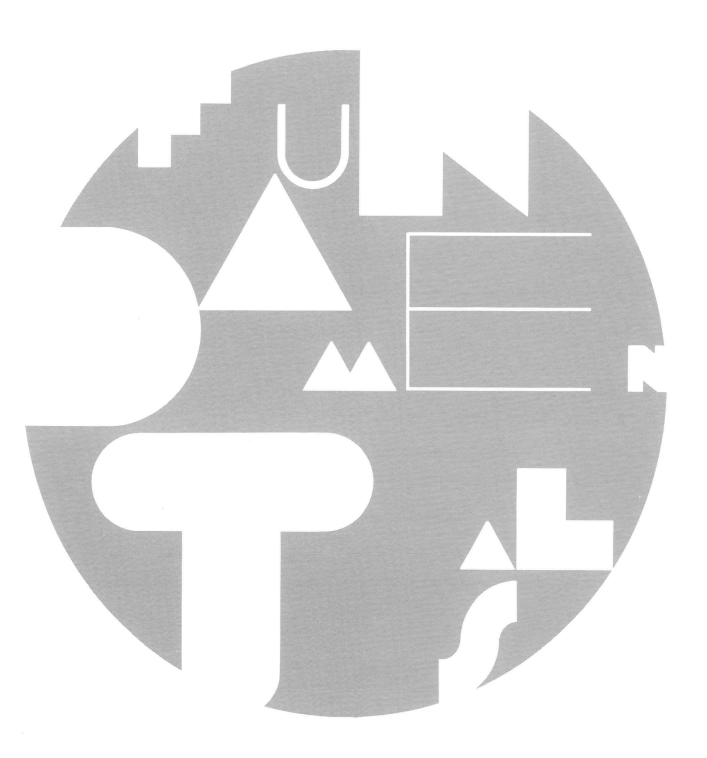

Chapter 10

Operating Room Preparation and Basic Techniques

Stephen L. Corson, M.D.

In this chapter I shall describe those maneuvers under the heading of "basic laparoscopy" which have proven helpful to me. This is done with the realization that no single technique is universally applicable. There is no claim that the method set forth here is necessarily the best or only correct approach.

As with any sophisticated procedure, the operator passes through three phases of proficiency. Phase I represents the stage of the neophyte during which patients chosen are those unlikely to represent complicated situations. Although lacking in experience, the physician should be well versed in the theoretical aspects of laparoscopy, including its anesthetic and electrosurgical correlates. During this phase procedures should be confined to diagnostic as opposed to operative ones. Experience is thus gained in recognizing variations of anatomy and in the use of the various instruments.

During Phase II confidence is acquired, and experience with wider application of laparoscopic techniques in a heterogeneous group of patients increases.

Phase III finds the skilled laparoscopist asked to consider patients whose medical condition and/or anatomy may introduce an increased degree of difficulty. Good surgical judgment is necessary to assess the expected gains versus the risks in these situations.

Any operating theater utilized for laparoscopy should have laparotomy capability. With experience and judicious patient selection, one encounters emergency laparotomy infrequently. However, laparoscopy findings may indicate concomitant laparotomy if the possibility has been discussed in advance with the patient and operating staff. This approach may be taken for diagnostic cases such as infertility, pelvic pain or mass as well as ectopic pregnancy suspects.

Therefore, the room should have the accoutrements found in a standard general operating room. A suction source, both for anesthetic and surgical use, is necessary. An electrosurgical generator should be available to control, via laparoscopy, unexpected intraabdominal bleeding sometimes encountered during nonoperative procedures. A cardiac monitor (Figure 1) should be utilized during each case, but it is no substitute for anesthetic vigilance. A sterile laparotomy set must

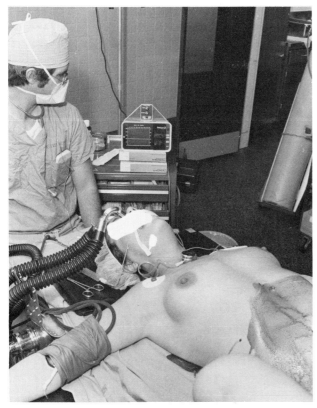

Figure 1
Cardiac monitor and chest leads. Additional lead is a carotid artery pulse monitor.

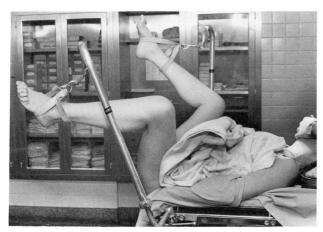

Figure 2
Drapes have been rolled back to demonstrate proper stirrup position. Near leg is correctly positioned with reduced thigh flexion to allow more room for the operator at the abdominal site.

be readily available. General anesthesia should be on hand, even if local anesthesia is employed routinely. A satisfactory intravenous drip sufficient to rapidly administer drugs or blood is a necessity. The foregoing is not inconsistent with performance of laparoscopy in a well-equipped "surgicenter" or similar, freestanding facility. It is true that in the less developed countries these conditions are rarely encountered, and laparoscopy may be performed in primitive settings.[2] It is also true that both in Europe and in North America there are a few respected and skilled laparoscopists who perform the procedure within the confines of an office.[11]

Patient preparation and instrument maintenance are detailed elsewhere, and I shall mention only those points germane to operating room care or procedure. The majority of our patients who have laparoscopic surgery are elective outpatients; therefore, they can void before entering the operating area, thus obviating catheterization, which might exacerbate a chronic cystitis. They should be given disposable, prepackaged slippers or surgical "boots" to reduce foot-borne operating room contamination.

Metal objects, such as locker keys, earrings, bracelets and rings, may act as grounding electrodes, causing skin burns as a result of high current density. They must be removed prior to surgery.

It is the responsibility of the surgeon to check the optical, mechanical and electrical components of his or her system prior to starting each case. This check includes inspecting for nonfunctioning light bulbs, frayed electrical cables, frozen valves, torn rubber seals, instrument insulation, etc.

Once suitably anesthetized, assuming general anesthesia is used, the patient is positioned in stirrups in the dorsal lithotomy position. Ankle stirrups are set slightly caudad rather than cephalad, as for a D & C, which prevents excessive flexion of the thigh on the abdomen, thus allowing more room for the laparoscopist. Figure 2 illustrates this point, with the far leg improperly positioned and the near leg showing the correct, modified position. Adjustable thigh stirrups are also suitable (Figure 3).

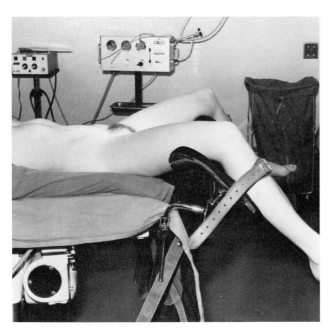

Figure 3
Thigh stirrups as an alternative method of positioning.

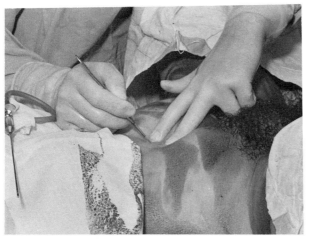

Figure 4
The initial incision is made in the infraumbilical fold, which has been everted by downward traction on the skin.

The buttocks must be at the edge of the table (at the break point) so that intrauterine instruments for D & C and manipulation can be moved freely. If the patient is too far down on the table, lumbosacral strain may be produced. In instances where there is no uterus to manipulate, i.e., prior hysterectomy or a male patient, there is little need to use this position, and a supine posture suffices. Tables with center cutouts allow one to dispense with stirrups entirely since the vaginal instruments can hang freely for manipulation.

Shoulder braces are not routinely necessary. They are reserved for very obese patients, who may slide cephalad with extreme Trendelenbeug position. If braces are used, they should be padded and comfortably adjusted with the patient awake in order to avoid nerve damage arising from direct pressure when the patient is anesthetized.

A return electrode should be positioned beneath the patient whether or not the planned procedure entails use of an electrosurgical generator. The plate should be positioned beneath the buttock so that the current has the shortest direct path through the patient. Thus, in an emergency situation electrosurgery may be employed without delay. Of course, this does not pertain to bipolar systems.

With the patient in stirrups the abdomen, from the infracostal region to the perineum and between the midaxillary lines, is cleansed with an acceptable solution such as aqueous proviodone-iodine. The prep is carried down on the thigh and posteriorly on the buttocks. Vaginal cleansing is done with the same agent. Cotton swabs may be needed to cleanse the umbilicus in some patients with chronically poor hygiene.

Various systems of draping exist utilizing linen, paper, plastic and one or multiple drapes. A small laparotomy sheet with a center hole large enough to expose the umbilical area and lower quadrant has proven convenient.

Creation of Pneumoperitoneum

The creation of the pneumoperitoneum is the first and most crucial step in the procedure. A spring-loaded needle, such as the Veress type, is preferable. The spring behind the blunt inner metal piece is designed to push away nonfixed intraabdominal structures, such as loops of bowel, to prevent inadvertent puncture by the outermost sharp needle. This construction, however, creates a narrow inner diameter for gas flow and by increasing the inherent resistance decreases the rate of gas flow.

As illustrated in Figure 4, pulling down on the skin below the umbilicus everts the infraumbilical fold, and a superficial nick is then made through the skin only with a scalpel using a No. 11 blade. This procedure ensures that the incision, later enlarged slightly to permit trocar insertion, will roll back into the umbilical depression with good cosmetic results. Incising the skin in this fashion avoids trapping a core of skin in the distal gas aperture of the needle, which would cause high pressure readings and low flow rates even if the needle were placed properly. Initial skin incision also decreases dulling and bending of the needle.

Regardless of the patient's size, the umbilicus represents the thinnest usable portion of the abdominal wall for the laparoscopist and is the site of choice. An extra long Veress needle is available and helpful for obese patients. Extremely obese patients may require use of a long spinal needle to ensure peritoneal penetration. The most popular alternate site for insertion of the pneumoperitoneum needle is 2 to 3 cm below the midpoint of the left costal margin (Figure 5). The theoretical danger of splenic perforation can be reduced greatly by palpation for an enlarged spleen under anesthesia prior to commencement of surgery. Normally, one does not find the stomach in this location, but distension as a result of general anesthesia[12, 14] may be diagnosed by a bulge in the left upper quadrant and a tympanic note to percussion. If the latter situation is present, a nasogastric tube should be passed and suction applied. A less popular site of entry is the left McBurney point; the right is avoided because of normal variation in size and position of the cecum and possible appendiceal adhesions. Laparoscopy in the face of massive liver enlargement is hazardous. The risk of bleeding, capable of causing death from liver laceration, is high. Few midline scars of previous laparotomy (or

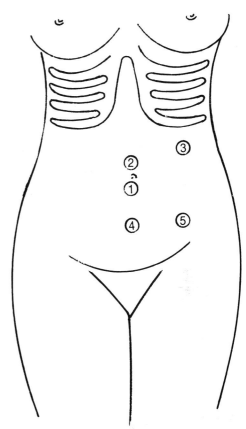

Figure 5
Usual sites for insertion of insufflating needle: (1) infraumbilical fold, (2) supraumbilical fold, (3) left costal margin, (4) midway between umbilicus and pubis, (5) left McBurney point.

laparotomies) reach the umbilicus. There is usually enough room to create the pneumoperitoneum there as usual. If dense scar tissue is encountered below the skin, the needle can be moved slightly out of the midline.

The transvaginal approach to pneumoperitoneum, especially in cases thought to present difficulties, such as obesity and prior surgery,[1, 10] does not seem to be sound.[4] One would wish to insert a trocar of 6 to 11 mm through the area previously proven to be safe by a 14 gauge needle. Puncture of a hollow viscus with the needle is usually innocuous if recognized; this is not true with the larger instrument.

I will not pass a trocar through an area which has not permitted a needle free entry to the peritoneal space. Use of the vaginal approach for gas instillation entails consideration of the contraindications for culdoscopy and exposes the patients to a "blind" puncture procedure in two distant sites. Moreover, the fat in the properitoneal space seen in obese patients extends into the cul-de-sac.

Figure 6 shows a maneuver employed by many laparoscopists.[9] Towel clips or tennaculae are used to elevate the abdominal wall, and the insufflating needle is put in the infraumbilical area at a 90° angle to the abdomen rather than at the 45° sacrally-oriented trajectory described classically.[3, 13] The proponents of this technique claim safety and easier entry into the peritoneal cavity with this method. Others raise the abdominal wall by hand (Figure 7).

The more classic 45° angle without abdominal wall elevation seems preferable (Figure 8). First, the bifurcation of the aorta is directly beneath the umbilicus in most patients. Aortic penetration has occurred with the perpendicular method, resulting in loss of 22 units of blood until bleeding was controlled, a vascular graft procedure and a large law suit. Second, I am not convinced that elevating the abdominal wall either by hand or with instruments truly raises the peritoneum in all cases. Rather, I believe that in most well-muscled patients only the skin and subcutaneous tissue are raised since the fascia is applied tightly to the underlying muscle, which resists elevation when well developed. Thus, the distance between the skin and peritoneum is increased, thus making the proper needle placement more difficult. In one particularly

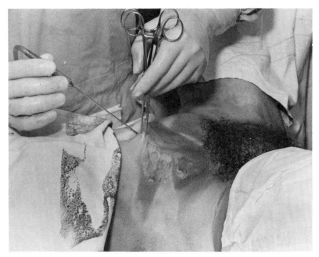

Figure 6
Elevation of abdominal wall with clamps during insufflation.

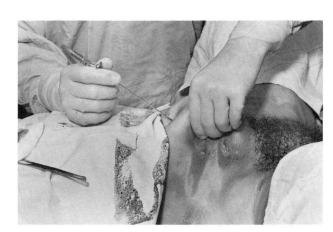

Figure 7
Manual elevation of abdominal wall during insufflation.

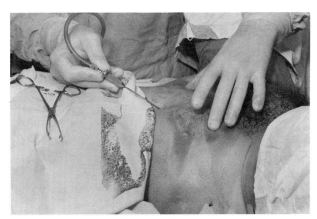

Figure 8
Classic technique of introduction of insufflating needle at 45° angle.

thin patient, use of towel clips to elevate the abdominal wall resulted in the operator's grasping the small bowel through the thin abdominal wall and eventually placing a trocar through it. Manual elevation of the abdominal wall *is* helpful in thin patients who also have lax muscles.

Directing the needle towards the sacral hollow, below the bifurcation of the great vessels, has a wide margin of safety. There are no fixed structures here normally, and bowel should move away from the blunt end of the Veress needle unless pinned between the needle and the vertebral column. The needle should be placed through the skin incision and gently advanced until the firm resistance of the fascia is encountered. The needle is then slightly withdrawn and thrust through the fascia with a quick, short stroke. A single "pop" and drop in resistance is felt and sometimes heard; a double loss of resistance suggests that the peritoneum has been traversed simultaneously. This is most common in thin patients and those with diastasis of the rectus muscles. Otherwise, the steps are repeated for peritoneal penetration. Steady, slow pressure rather than the short thrust described above will cause the peritoneum to be tented downwards before puncture, thus decreasing the intraperitoneal depth and affording less safety. Occasionally, a resistant linea alba may be encountered. Shifting the needle slightly to the left may help. Alternatively, the sharp point of the No. 11 scalpel blade may be used through the skin incision to nick the fascia. One must perform this latter maneuver carefully to avoid penetrating the peritoneum with the knife point and thereby lacerating a structure such as small intestine.

Prior to insertion of the insufflating needle, the gas system is filled with CO_2 or N_2O and is checked to ensure unobstructed flow as well as to note the pressure intrinsic to the internal resistance of the system. Improper assembly of the needle after cleaning may cause obstructed flow of gas through the distal end.

Several techniques are available for ensuring proper needle placement. If the valve has been closed during insertion, a hanging drop can be placed at the hub, as shown in Figure 9. The valve is then opened, and elevation of the abdomen or creation of first positive and then negative pressure within the abdomen by diaphragmatic excursion will cause the drop to be sucked into the needle. At this point an additional check is to connect a syringe to the needle and to attempt to aspirate blood or liquid bowel contents. Finally, 10 ml of saline may be injected via the syringe. This should pass in with no resistance and should not be retrievable.

At this point the gas line is connected and the insufflation begins. Most commercial units are calibrated for a flow rate of approximately one liter per minute at pressures between 10 to 20 mm Hg. Some insufflators have rubber diaphragms which become dry and brittle with age, thus causing a reduction of flow even at low pressures.

In patients receiving succinyl choline and a general agent, abdominal relaxation is such that insufflating pressures rarely rise over 16 mm Hg. Patients who are receiving local anesthesia may tense the abdomen and lower the diaphragm, thus causing transient pressure increases.

Percussion of the abdomen should be performed and the loss of liver dullness and generalized tympany noted. If the needle comes to rest in the infrafascial, supraperitoneal space, the pressure during insufflation will rise and only the lower part of the abdomen will distend. The abdomen may feel "doughy" rather than like the usual feel of a partially-inflated balloon. Vulvar distension and crepitus may also be observed. If the colon has been entered, a large volume of gas can be insufflated without an increase of pressure. However, the abdominal distension will be asymmetric, and the gas can be heard to escape via the anus. Placement of gas within the lumen of the stomach will produce eructation and upper abdominal distension.

Continued insufflation of gas within the layers of the abdominal wall may cause subcutaneous emphysema with an increase in diameter of the neck. This is usually harmless, if recognized, since CO_2, and to a slightly lesser extent N_2O, is rapidly absorbed. Lack of recognition causes the operator to proceed with the surgery in an unprepared peritoneal space. Bilateral pneumothorax has been described as associated with laparos-

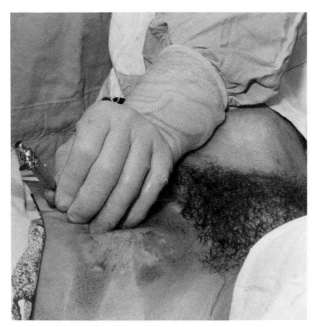

Figure 9
Hanging-drop technique may be employed during insertion of needle into peritoneal space.

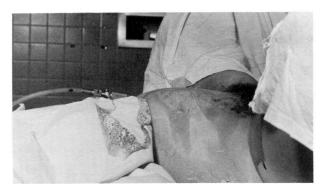

Figure 10
A symmetrical, convex, abdominal contour signifies adequate pneumoperitoneum.

copy.[6] If supraperitoneal gas is recognized, the gas line is disconnected. The valve of the needle should be opened and pressure applied to the abdomen in order to exhaust the space of as much gas as possible. A slightly steeper angle of penetration must then be employed.

The most feared complication related to gas insufflation is embolization. By extrapolation from animal studies, a 50 kg woman should be able to tolerate a flow rate of 100 ml per minute of CO_2 directly intravascularly. Embolization may occur in association with a break in the integrity of a large vessel or many small vessels, as in a placental site. A characteristic "mill wheel" cardiac murmur may be heard.

Management calls for the patient to be put in deep Trendelenburg position, left side down, to promote gas escape through the right heart into the lungs. Cardiac puncture to aspirate gas may be performed.

Cardiac arrest may occur from embolization but is commonly seen as a vagovagal reaction to anesthesia, increased abdominal pressure and hypercarbia. Prophylactic administration of 0.4 mg of atropine intramuscularly 30 minutes prior to surgery is of help in reducing cardiac irregularity. A more complete discussion is found in Chapter 9.

How much gas is sufficient for pneumoperitoneum? It depends upon the operator as well as the patient. With experience, operators tend to use less gas as their feel for the abdominal layers becomes more reliable. Large patients with lax abdominal walls may take 4$\frac{1}{2}$ liters of gas; small patients with tight abdominal walls may tense at 2 liters. A readily employed endpoint is a good degree of abdominal convexity (Figure 10) and a sensation that the abdominal wall is "bouncy." As a final check the needle may be withdrawn to the skin level and inserted at a different angle. One should be able to freely aspirate gas, seen as bubbles in saline within the syringe.

Many learned discussions have been generated by the argument over the preferred insufflating gas. Most early doyens used CO_2, and the second generation of laparoscopists in the late 1960s accepted this choice as a readily available gas whose safety factor lay in its extreme solubility in blood. That same feature of solubility which lessened embolic potential acted adversely to create hypercarbia and cardiac arrhythmia in some cases. Keith et al have recently reviewed this aspect[8] and concluded that proper techniques of hyperventilation reduce the risk of extreme hypercarbia brought about by decreased ventilation and CO_2 absorption. Use of N_2O as the distending gas avoids the metabolic derangements sometimes seen with CO_2 but substitutes a gas slightly less safe with regard to embolus formation. In contrast to CO_2, N_2O will support combustion although it will not explode. CO_2 is much more irritating to peritoneal surfaces than N_2O and causes more postoperative shoulder and rib pain.

Trocar Introduction

Where possible, the trocar should be introduced at the same site as the insufflating needle for reasons mentioned earlier in the discussion. If the primary goal is one of visualization of upper abdominal organs, the supraumbilical fold may be chosen as the entry site. The incision previously made for the needle is slightly enlarged so as to permit the trocar and surrounding sheath to be introduced.

Most operators use a slightly semilunar incision conforming to the radius of the infraumbilical fold; others prefer a vertical incision. If the incision is too long and deep, large quantities of gas will leak out during the procedure, and the wound may bleed excessively. Both of these problems are merely nuisances since the gas loss is replaced during the procedure by adjusting the flow to "manual" (fast) or "automatic" (slow) rates. A clamp can control skin bleeding until permanent hemostasis is secured at the termination of the case. If the incision is too small, however, the sheath may be impeded by the skin edge even though the narrower trocar tip has passed. This increase in frictional resistance may cause the operator to employ great force on the trocar with less ability to control the final depth of penetration. Of course, the size of the incision depends on the

diameter of the telescope utilized. The 5 mm scope requires a 6 mm outer diameter sheath and a 10 mm instrument, an 11 or 12 mm sheath. The area of the defect in the abdominal wall is, therefore, fourfold with the larger scope. Care must be taken not to incise the annular ring of the umbilicus since hernia may result. Besides the reduced chance for hernia, the smaller incision is less of a problem in coping with an outpatient population. Because of poor healing, one should suture the fascial defect in oncologic patients, obese patients and those known to have frequent coughs.

Note that the pyramidal-tipped trocars are preferred over the conical models since the former cut as well as pierce their way through the fascia and thus require less force to achieve penetration. The trocar must not be passed with a screwing motion because the sharp edges will cause excessive tissue damage. Sheaths of surgical steel glide through tissue with ease but have given way to fiberglass and plastic sheaths because of electrosurgical considerations. Trumpet-type valves or so-called automatic or clip valves allow the operator to remove the trocar or telescope from the sheath without appreciable gas loss.

The trocar and sheath are introduced through the skin incision and then run parallel to the abdominal wall just beneath the skin in the subcutaneous tissue for a distance of 2 to 3 cm (Figure 11). This prevents damage to the vulnerable fascia at the umbilicus and, on occasion, may avoid a prominent urachal remnant. The trocar is then directed at a 45° angle in the midline toward the sacrum with the patient horizontal or in mild Trendelenberg position (the "Z technique" as shown in Figure 12). The operator holds the sheath between the index and middle fingers, with the hub of the trocar against the muscles of the thenar eminence. A sharp, punching entry helps to limit depth of penetration. The other hand can be employed as a stop device by placing it between the abdominal wall and the other hand, along the length of the sheath (Figure 13). As the fascia is encountered, resistance rises and suddenly decreases as the fascia is pierced. Because the pneumoperitoneum has distended the peritoneum, it is tightly applied to the fascia, and only one "pop" is usually felt and heard.

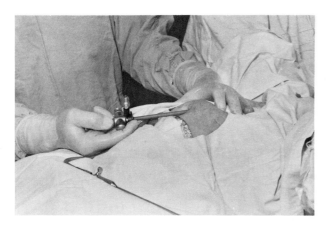

Figure 11
The trocar is first tunneled subcutaneously before
the fascia is penetrated at a greater angle.

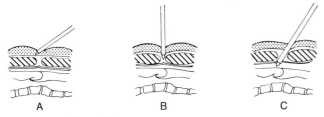

A   B   C

Figure 12
"Z" technique. Panel A shows trocar penetration of
skin. After tunneling subcutaneously, the trocar is
angled toward 45° as in "B," and the fascia is
pierced. As the peritoneum is entered, the angle is
reduced again ("C").

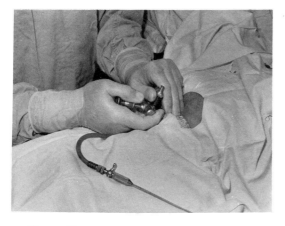

Figure 13
Limitation of trocar penetration can be
accomplished by using one hand as a stop.

As soon as the operator believes the peritoneal cavity has been entered, he or she should cease his or her efforts to advance the trocar. The sharp tip should be withdrawn into the barrel of the sheath and the sheath advanced again for a short distance to ensure that it remains within the abdominal cavity. Angular rotation of the sheath is performed to check for freedom of movement. Finally, the trocar is completely withdrawn and the valve opened manually so that the operator can listen for the hiss of escaping gas, which signifies that the sheath has entered the same anatomic space which was insufflated. Operators with hearing defects may alternatively use the side-arm gas valve of the sheath along with a syringe and saline. Withdrawal of gas into the syringe will cause bubbles. If gas is not encountered, the operator should proceed with the next step nonetheless.

As shown in Figure 14, the lighted telescope is inserted into the sheath and advanced slowly, with the surgeon observing through the lens system while the scope is within the limits of the sheath. If pelvic organs are visualized, confirmation is obtained that the peritoneal cavity has been entered although a pneumoperitoneum may not have been created. One must then carefully check for injuries to structures which may have resulted from the pneumoperitoneum needle or the trocar. If a reflecting surface or properitoneal fat is seen, one is obviously in the infrafascial space. The telescope is withdrawn and with the valve open, pressure is made against the abdominal wall. If large quantities of gas continue to escape, the original space insufflated was also supraperitoneal. But if this is not the case, one merely re-inserts the trocar and redirects the sheath slightly more perpendicularly into a properly prepared peritoneal cavity.

If the operator is unfortunate enough not to encounter either of these two views but rather a mucosal surface, he or she has inadvertently performed an intestinal endoscopic procedure or cystoscopy from above. If this is the case, *do not remove the laparoscope!* A hole made by the trocar may close because of muscular action and not leak until later. One may have to examine the entire gastrointestinal tract in order to find the site of injury. On the other hand, leaving the telescope in place may prevent excessive peritoneal soilage with liquid stomach or bowel contents. The subsequent step is to perform a laparotomy with an incision along the sheath so that the path of the trocar can be inspected and the damaged viscus identified and repaired properly. Unlike thermal-induced injuries, resection is rarely needed unless mesenteric vessel injury threatens viability; a pursestring suture and oversewing are usually sufficient. Nasogastric suction postoperatively is advised for intestinal injuries. Bladder injuries are rare with the periumbilical approach as compared with Ruddock's preferential site of pelvic entry, which was much lower on the abdominal wall.

Inexperienced laparoscopists frequently insert the telescope without viewing through the lens as it decends into the pelvis. They are greeted with a smooth, red, reflective surface and may believe that they are supraperitoneal when actually they have put the scope in too far and are touching the uterine fundus or visceral or parietal peritoneum.

If insufflation of the anterior properitoneal space has occurred, the posterior peritoneum will be lifted up and will demonstrate pockets of gas. This soon absorbs.

Assuming that all is well up to this point, the operator then attaches the gas line to the sheath. He or she may keep the valve closed and add gas intermittently as needed to sustain a good pneumoperitoneum, or he/she may deliver gas continuously at a low rate to counterbalance absorption and leakage along the sheath. Unfortunately, few insufflating units have an audible alarm system to indicate that the device needs to be refilled from the reservoir tank. Therefore, someone must observe the gauge and refill the unit when necessary. Most insufflators have either a 5 or 10 liter capacity, which is more than adequate for routine cases. Long procedures or cases with rapid gas loss may require much greater volumes.

The Telescope and Examination

The reader is referred to the sections on instruments and photography for a technical discussion of the various telescopes. As applied to general technique, the points considered here are: (1) operating telescope (single puncture technique); (2) diameter of the scope.

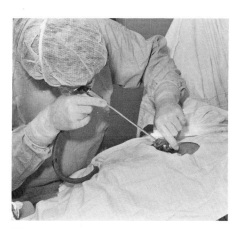

Figure 14
The telescope is inserted and advanced in the sheath under direct vision.

The passions which were generated about the merits of one- versus two-puncture techniques have simmered down, and the laparoscopic Capulets and Montagues are no longer at war. For sterilization procedures there is probably little difference between the two, and the operator should follow the method most comfortable for him/her. However, for diagnostic work, when manipulation of various structures and biopsy become necessary, the separation of optical and mechanical axes is of distinct advantage. Specific details of these procedures appear in Section VI.

For routine nonteaching pelvic use the 180° 5 mm telescope is convenient because of its small diameter and uncomplicated optics. Because the amount of light is dependent (among other things) on the number of fibers in the telescope, the smaller scope transmits less light. Thus, photography is difficult unless a photo-flash unit is used. Decreased field and light prohibits use of either a rigid or flexible teaching attachment (Figure 15). Because the smaller scope magnifies less, the novice may find it difficult to use. For patients who are having laparoscopy as a part of a cancer work-up, the operator may want all the light and magnification available. In effect then, I suggest the use of the 10 mm instrument for teaching, photography, cancer detection, and biopsy procedures.

Various films are available which may be applied to the lens of the telescope to decrease fogging. Distal fogging results from a cold lens entering a warm peritoneal cavity, and obviously can be eliminated by prewarming in warm saline or special instrument warmers. Unless the instrument is specially designed to withstand autoclaving, rinsing in hot solutions will cause minute defects in the lens sealant and actually decrease visibility by allowing moisture to collect within the instrument. Should fogging within the abdomen occur, a simple remedy is to touch the lens to the parietal peritoneum or serosal surface for temperature equilibration.

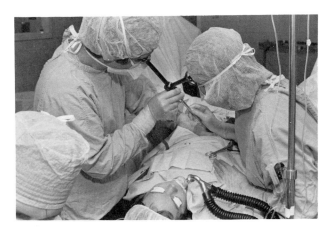

Figure 15
Rigid attachment to laparoscope, permitting simultaneous observation by the operator and an observer. A reduction in image size and illumination necessitates use of larger bore telescopes and highly efficient light systems.

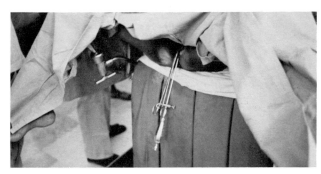

Figure 16
Weighted uterine manipulator and cannula (John Marco & Sons, Oakhurst, N.J.) in position with syringe attached. Uterus is pulled down, reducing chances of trocar damage to fundus. Uterus is rotated anteriorly to better expose adnexal structures.

If moisture within the scope is encountered and no replacement instrument is available, a temporary solution is to place the instrument in the operating room warmer to drive off the water vapor. Occasionally, blood within the sheath will leave a film over the distal lens of the scope, which can greatly hinder visualization. The solution to this problem is to remove the telescope and to run a bit of warm saline down the sheath.

Soaking the telescopes in formalin-like solutions between cases will eventually cause deposits on the lens and fiber optic linkage points. These deposits can be removed with ethanol.

Every surgeon should have a systematic approach to assessment of abdominal anatomy during laparoscopy. As soon as the telescope is in place, the uterus and then each adnexal area should be inspected. Next, the anterior and posterior cul-de-sac areas are considered. The appendix should be visualized as well if at all possible. Uterine manipulation, to expose the posterior portion of the uterus and adnexae, may be accomplished with a number of instruments. Hulka,[7] among others, has described a sturdy device. We use one of our own design,[5] as shown in Figure 16. It has no springs or valves and is weighted in order to achieve uterine anteflexion. It can be used for lavage as well. With this instrument the uterus can be moved as a piston in order to push bowel from the sacral hollow and pelvis and to elevate the ovaries for inspection and/or biopsy.

It is frequently necessary to have an accessory probe or grasping forceps within the peritoneum in order to mobilize structures. With the two-puncture technique, the abdominal wall is transilluminated (Figure 17) in order to avoid large blood vessels and a small incision is made at the level of the pubic hairline. The exact site of entry depends upon the anatomy of the patient and the preference of the surgeon. Caution must be exercised to avoid the bladder, particularly if there has been prior cesarean section. Either the 4 or 6 mm sheath is then passed at the appropriate point *under laparoscopic guidance* (Figure 18) with the operator observing the trajectory of insertion in order to avoid fixed structures and bowel. If possible, the point should be directed toward a free space in the posterior cul-de-sac. If this cannot be done the operator can aim for the fundus of the uterus, since a puncture at that point will usually bleed for a minute or so and otherwise cause no problem.

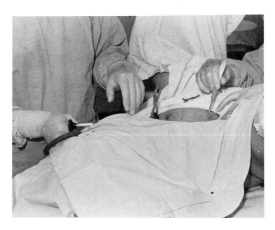

Figure 17
The laparoscope is used to transilluminate the abdominal wall in order to select a second puncture site which is not over a branch of the inferior epigastric vessels.

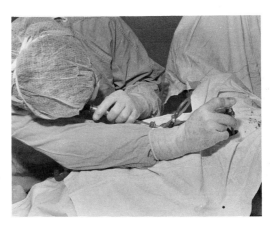

Figure 18
The second trocar is introduced under laparoscopic guidance in order to avoid pelvic structures.

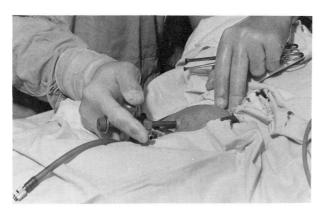

Figure 19
With the sheath valve open and with gentle abdominal pressure, the pneumoperitoneum is exhausted at the termination of the procedure.

A calibrated probe allows objective measurement of structures without distortion caused by the magnification properties inherent in the scope. Blunt 3 mm atraumatic grasping forceps are especially helpful in manipulating the tube and temporarily occluding the cornu for differential lavage studies with indigo carmine.

After pelvic inspection has been completed, the patient is returned to the horizontal position and the scope withdrawn into the sheath. By rotating the sheath cephalad and reinserting the scope, upper abdominal anatomy can be inspected. Instruments can be inserted in the upper abdomen through another sheath or percutaneously, as with certain biopsy needles, but in any case always under direct laparoscopic guidance. A blunt suction tube and attached syringe are utilized to aspirate fluid for culture, cytology and other examinations.

The information gleaned from the examination should be recorded while still fresh in the operator's mind. Best, of course, is a photographic recording. A laparoscopic reporting form as outlined in monographs by Steptoe[13] and Cohen[3] is very useful.

Termination of the Procedure

The accessory instruments should be removed first under direct vision through the scope with the jaws of the biopsy or grasping forceps in the closed position. The telescope is removed next. In cases where biopsy or cutting procedures have been performed, the degree of hemostasis should be checked.

Figure 19 demonstrates pressure applied to the abdomen with the laparoscopic sheath valve open to exhaust the pneumoperitoneum. Unless the sheath is positioned properly, the omentum will tend to follow, and adhesions or hernia may result as omentum extrudes through the peritoneal defect. Therefore, the valve on the sheath should be opened and gentle pressure made on the abdomen in order to exhaust the distending gas, after which the valve is closed. The sheath should then be rotated into a more horizontal position to raise the abdominal wall free of its peritoneal contents so that the sheath may be removed safely. If the valve remains open, respiratory efforts will suck room air into the peritoneal cavity. This air absorbs more slowly than CO_2 or N_2O and therefore causes more prolonged postoperative discomfort.

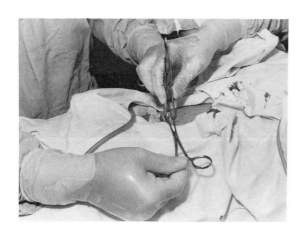

Figure 20
Application of skin clips at the operative site.

We have tried a variety of methods of skin closure. Adhesive strips do not provide enough compression of the skin edges to reliably prevent oozing. Subcutaneous or subcuticular closure with absorbable sutures may cause the wound to ooze and become inflamed. Figure 20 shows application of skin clips to the operative site. Figure 21 shows two types of clips. The type with the straight arms nicely controls skin-edge bleeding. It can be removed by the patient in 24 hours at home by pressure with the thumb and index finger. The other curved clip requires instrument removal. This point is important when dealing with outpatients.

This section has outlined one individual's approach to basic laparoscopic methods. Mastery of these elemental steps enables the laparoscopist to perform more sophistocated procedures with confidence and safety.

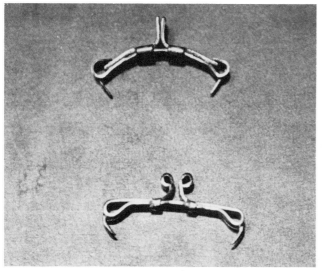

Figure 21
Straight-arm clips are removed easily by the patient at home with thumb and forefinger. Curved clips must be removed with an instrument.

References

1. Ansari AH: The cul-de-sac approach to induction of pneumoperitoneum for pelvic laparoscopy and pneumography. Fertil Steril 21:599, 1970

2. Chaturachinda K: Laparoscopy: a technique for a tropical setting. Am J Obstet Gynecol 112:941, 1972

3. Cohen MR: *Laparoscopy, Culdoscopy and Gynecology.* WB Saunders Co, Philadelphia, 1970, p 171

4. Corson SL: Letter to the editor. Obstet Gynecol 47:638, 1976

5. Corson SL: New Instruments—laparoscopic bipolar sterilizing forceps—intrauterine manipulator and lavage instrument. Am J Obstet Gynecol 124:434, 1976

6. Doctor NH, Hussain Z: Bilateral pneumothorax associated with laparoscopy. A case report of a rare hazard and review of literature. Anaesthesia 28:75, 1973

7. Hulka JF: Controlling uterine forceps for laparoscopic sterilization after abortion: a new instrument. Am J Obstet Gynecol 116:884, 1973

8. Keith L, Silver AS, Becker M: Anesthesia for laparoscopy. J Reprod Med 12:227, 1974

9. Loffer FD, Pent D: An alternate technique in penetrating the abdomen for laparoscopy. J Reprod Med 13:37, 1974

10. Neely MR, McWilliams R, Makhlouf HA: Laparoscopy: routine pneumoperitoneum via the posterior fornix. Obstet Gynecol 45:459, 1975

11. Penfield AJ: Laparoscopic sterilization under local anesthesia. J Reprod Med 12:251, 1974

12. Reynolds RC, Pauca AL: Gastric perforation, an anesthesia-induced hazard in laparoscopy. Anesthesiology 38:84, 1973

13. Steptoe PC: *Laparoscopy in Gynaecology.* ES Livingstone Ltd, Edinburgh & London, 1967, p 92

14. Whitford JHW, Gunstone AJ: Gastric perforation: a hazard of laparoscopy under general anesthesia. Br J Anaesth 44:97, 1972

Section 5

Diagnostic Procedures

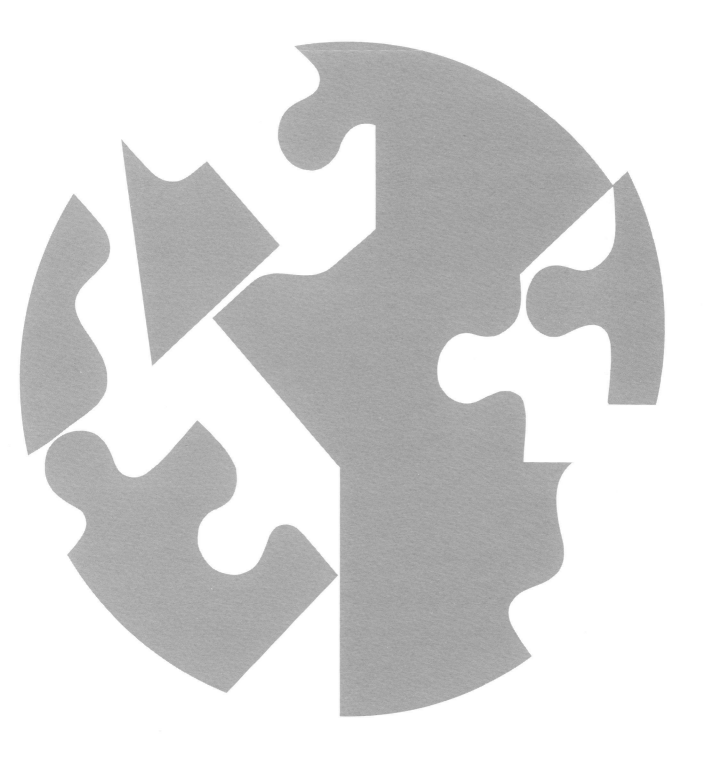

Chapter 11

Pelvic Pain

Dr. med. H. Frangenheim

Translation:
Dr. med. Walter Kleindienst

Dedicated to my dearest teacher and friend
Prof. Dr. K. J. Anselmino on his 75th birthday

Diagnostic procedures constantly evolve toward greater accuracy coupled with reduced risk to the patient. In addition, in this era of rising medical costs, economy has assumed a major role. The investigation of pelvic pain via laparoscopy fulfills these demands while affording a method of therapy at the same time.

Acute Abdominal Disease

In instances of acute abdominal pain the diagnosis often can be established because of typical clinical findings and symptoms and with the aid of laboratory data. Acute lower abdominal complaints with atypical clinical correlates may cause diagnostic difficulties. Typical diagnostic difficulties include:
1. Ectopic pregnancy
2. Acute salpingitis or ovarian abscess with accompanying peritonitis
3. Torsion of pedunculated ovarian or paraovarian cysts
4. Carcinomatous peritonitis
5. Atypical forms of intestinal obstruction
6. Rupture of ovarian cysts.

Some borderline cases between gynecology and surgery may be added:
7. Acute/chronic appendicitis
8. Perforated gastric or intestinal ulcers with atypical clinical manifestations
9. Blunt abdominal injury with suspected intraperitoneal hemorrhage in primarily or secondarily ruptured liver or spleen.

According to conventional conceptions, proper treatment consists of expectant observation or exploratory laparotomy. Today, one should not hesitate to perform laparoscopy in cases with equivocal clinical symptoms. In most of these cases "urgent laparoscopy" with readiness for major surgery will give a better diagnosis than other methods of examination. The indication for surgery can be made sooner without increasing operative risk. On the other hand, laparoscopy may help to avoid unnecessary operations. Thus, the surgeon can decide between active and conservative management.

Ectopic Pregnancy

Hardly any clinical picture can cause such a variety of symptoms as ectopic pregnancy, especially prior to rupture. Rupture of a tube will cause such dramatic clinical manifestations that, in most cases, laparoscopy will not be necessary. But the greater number of ectopic pregnancies shows no typical course. In these cases laparoscopy will clarify the situation. Thus, 25% of ectopic pregnancies are diagnosed in the intact state, thus allowing early surgical intervention, with reduced morbidity and mortality. Clinics without laparoscopic units diagnose only about 8% of the ectopic pregnancies in the intact state. The laparoscopic success is even better in suspected chronic ectopic pregnancy, which may often simulate chronic adnexitis (Color atlas, Figure 29). Mintz, Thoyer-Rozat and Frangenheim found chronic, ruptured ectopic pregnancies in the state of organization in 65% of the suspected cases.

Ruptured Corpus Luteum

The clinical manifestations of ruptured corpus luteum come very close to those of ectopic pregnancy. Puncture of the pouch of Douglas (culdocentesis) cannot give the differential diagnosis between corpus luteum hemorrhage and ruptured fallopian tube. If, at laparoscopy, the tubes are found to be intact, an attempt at conservative treatment should be made: the blood is aspirated through an accessory channel, and the ovaries are inspected carefully. In many cases one will observe that the bleeding from the site of the ruptured corpus luteum already has come to a stop, and laparotomy will not be necessary. Occasionally, major, retrograde menstruation will cause similar symptoms.

Strangulation of Pedunculated Ovarian Cysts

Depending on the degree of torsion, mild to severe acute lower abdominal pain may arise in the case of strangulation of pedunculated ovarian or paraovarian cysts (Color atlas, Figure 27). The differential diagnosis may be established by laparoscopic inspection, thus avoiding eventual emergency laparotomy. Attempts should be made to untwist the cyst. Smaller cysts can be punctured, the liquid content aspirated and the pedicle cauterized and divided. Then the empty cystic bag may be retracted through a sheath of the laparoscope. Larger cysts may be emptied and then removed through a posterior colpotomy, causing only minor discomfort to the patient as compared with laparotomy.

Acute Salpingitis Ovarian Abscess

Diagnostic laparoscopy has been recommended for a long time (Sjövall, Samuelson, Frangenheim) for all cases of acute adnexal inflammations (Color atlas, Figure 11). The recommendation is based on the concept that serous inflammatory and suppurative processes should be differentiated and treated accordingly. Acute, serous inflammations are treated with antibiotics and high doses of corticosteroids. Pyosalpinx and ovarian abscess—especially in the menopause—as well as abscesses following voluntary abortion should be operated on and extirpated. This acute approach corresponds to appendectomy in acute appendicitis and is somewhat controversial. Twenty years of experience with laparoscopic diagnosis of these entities and subsequent extirpation show excellent results as compared with conservative treatment. Postoperative complications are rare, even in the presence of accompanying peritonitis. Operative therapy prevents eventual recrudescence of an abscess after conservative treatment. Even in young women there is no sense in preserving such gravely damaged organs, which have lost reproductive capacity. Duration of hospitalization is considerably shortened by this active form of management.

Postoperative Intraperitoneal Hemorrhage

Occasionally, major intraperitoneal and retroperitoneal hemorrhage appears after vaginal or abdominal operations. The surgeon frequently agonizes over the decision to reexplore. The situation may be evaluated by laparoscopy prior to laparotomy. Sometimes, aspiration of the blood will be sufficient if inspection has shown that the bleeding blood vessels have already clotted.

Intestinal Obstruction

Occasionally, laparoscopic examination of an acute abdomen shows incomplete intestinal obstruction, manifested by an atypical course. In some cases it is possible to divide adhesions under laparoscopic visualization with careful cauterization. In most cases the intestine recovers quickly, with restoration of good peristaltic movements. Altogether, such cases are rare.

Urgent Laparoscopy in Surgery

The success of laparoscopy for the acute abdomen in gynecology has influenced surgeons to act likewise in similar situations. In the first place, there is the differential diagnosis between appendicitis and salpingitis with accompanying peritonitis. Many women actually suffering from adnexitis undergo appendectomy, with the actual disease subsiding during the postoperative phase.

Blunt abdominal injury with suspected intraperitoneal hemorrhage or suspected hemorrhage due to secondary rupture of liver and/or spleen is another indication for surgical laparoscopy (Color atlas, Figure 88).

Active laparoscopic evaluation is an alternative to conservative expectant observation in atypical forms of perforated gastric intestinal ulcer or Meckel's diverticulum with accompanying peritonitis.

These few indications from the field of surgery led to the term *urgent* or *emergency laparoscopy.* Laparoscopy was first introduced to the surgical field as an urgent procedure, as shown by the first international symposium of Prague in 1971 and subsequent national meetings.

Chronic Abdominal Disease

Laparoscopy as a diagnostic procedure for chronic lower abdominal complaints should be performed when conservative measures have failed.

Many psychosomatic and functional disturbances in women manifest in the lower abdomen, which may be called a site of predilection for neurovegetative disturbances. To the patient, psychosomatic and organic pains are qualitatively equal. There is no objective measure of the quality or severity of pain. Also, patients differ considerably in their attitudes toward pain itself.

Women with chronic lower abdominal pain consult many physicians over the years and are tagged with various diagnoses: chronic adnexitis, chronic appendicitis, fixed retroflexion of the uterus or pains due to adhesions. In the course of treatment a number of surgical interventions may have been performed without encouraging results: appendectomy, surgical revision of tubes and ovaries, hysterectomy, ventrosuspension of the uterus or division of adhesions. In some cases iatrogenic discomfort was added to complaints already present.

Neurovegetative disturbances are of a heterogeneous nature. Because of the close proximity of reproductive organs, intestine, bones and nerves, all possibilities have to be evaluated in the differential diagnosis. Complaints may be classified according to their localization or to their psychosomatic proportion. This classification will determine whether the patient should see a gynecologist, gastroenterologist, orthopedic surgeon or psychiatrist.

If chronic lower abdominal pains are manifested mainly in the back, the orthopedic surgeon should be the first to be consulted. Those pains are often due to insufficiencies of muscles, bones and ligaments in the pelvic and vertebral area.

The differential list includes conditions of a gastrointestinal nature: irritable colon, diverticulosis of the large bowel, adhesions and colitis. The differential diagnosis of chronic adnexitis and acute relapses of regional enteritis (Crohn's disease) may also play a role. Urologic disorders offer few diagnostic problems. They will be treated specifically.

If gastroenterologic, orthopedic and psychiatric consultation does not give a definite diagnosis, laparoscopy is indicated. Results of 20 years of practical experience speak for its value. The patients can be divided into three different groups:

1.   Patients with characteristic, positive, psychiatric history and unclear or almost normal findings on palpation.
2.   Patients with unremarkable psychiatric history but chronic pelvic complaints, dysmenorrhea and normal findings on palpation.
3.   Patients with uncharacteristic history and obscure or insignificant findings on palpation.

If, in the first group, a thorough psychiatric history is taken, in many cases correlations will be found between the beginning of complaints and specific emotional events.

The most frequent laparoscopic finding within this particular group is distinct local hyperemia or hyperemia of peritoneum covering the pouch of Douglas or the sacrouterine ligaments. This finding may be registered as pelvic congestion, serous inflammation of the ligaments or spastic uterosacral ligaments (Color atlas, Figure 79). The ligaments may be thickened up to the size of a thumb. The patients often manifest chronic, particularly right-sided, pelvic pain, which may have been treated under the diagnosis of chronic appendicitis.

One of the most frequent conditions is endometriosis (Color atlas, Figure 9). In about 30% of the cases it is symptomatic prior to formation of implants accessible to palpation. Nonpalpable endometriotic lesions may cause constant peritoneal irritation. Depending on the localization, the patient reports a variety of obscure, dull, pelvic pains. In the majority of cases the lesions are localized over the uterosacral ligaments. Contraction of the peritoneum diminishes the elasticity of both peritoneum and pelvic connective tissue. Mobilization of the uterus during pelvic examination or intercourse causes considerable pain. Hormonal treatment is of transitory benefit since it causes incomplete atrophy of the foci, which basically remain sensitive to the hormonal stimuli during the menstrual cycle. A more effective approach is cauterization at laparoscopy. Thus, the lesions will be destroyed completely. Sterility often goes along with the presence of endometriosis. In some cases endometriosis results in tubal occlusion; in other cases ovarian function may be impaired considerably. But in the majority of the cases the connection between neurovegetative disturbances, endometriosis and sterility remains mysterious.

In the second group of women, with chronic, left-sided pains, vast sail- or veil-like adhesions between sigmoid bowel and the peritoneum of the pelvic wall or ovaries and tubes are common findings (Color atlas, Figures 12, 13 and 14). These alterations are classified as signs of chronic perisigmoiditis or old chronic peritonitis.

Finally, in the same group of patients often marked enlargement and congestion of the ovarian plexus are found — so-called pelvic varicocele. At laparoscopy, emptying of these varicoceles can be observed in the Trendelenburg position. Therefore, attention must be paid to this eventual finding immediately after insertion of the laparoscope, while the patient is level.

Women of the third group, complaining of intermittent colicky lower abdominal pains, often show no characteristic palpatory findings. On the other hand, at laparoscopy a great variety of pathologic alterations can be seen: unpalpable endometriosis, already mentioned above; spastic uterosacral ligaments; chronic sigmoiditis; or generalized congestion. The exploration of such complaints may lead to esoteric diagnoses: incomplete strangulation of hydrosalpinx, strangulation of paraovarian cysts by fixed tubes or strangulation of the ligament of the ovary or of the tube by adhesions between the bladder and those organs. In those cases the severity of pains will depend on the filling state of the bladder. A large number of adhesions is probably a consequence of past inflammations which were never noticed by the patient herself.

Many of these patients have undergone appendectomy. Retrospectively, the patient who is actually suffering from adnexitis may have been treated for appendicitis. Surgeons therefore should do more laparoscopies in doubtful cases, especially in girls and young women.

The Allan-Masters syndrome is another disorder manifested by chronic lower abdominal pains (Color atlas, Figure 21). It is due to traumatic insufficiency of the suspensory apparatus of the uterus. Its main symptoms are dyspareunia, secondary dysmenorrhea, disturbed defecation and others. The anatomical alterations—lacerations of the broad ligaments—are seen well at laparoscopy. Defects of peritoneum and uterosacral ligaments cause mobilization of the cervix to be rather painful. The disorder often goes along with retroflexion of the uterus and pelvic variococele. Surgical intervention proves to be more beneficial than conservative treatment. The question of suture of the lacerations or hysterectomy as the treatment of choice is decided by age and physical condition of the patient. There is also a large list of other possible accidental findings: hydro- and pyosalpinx, old ectopic pregnancy and latent genital tuberculosis, particularly tubal tuberculosis. In addition, besides old or recent inflammatory processes of the intestine there are diverticulitis, perisigmoiditis, Crohn's disease or strangulation due to adhesions; ruptured paraovarian or hydatid cysts, ruptured endometriotic cysts with subsequent chronic peritonitis and perforated intrauterine devices (IUD) in various positions (Color atlas, Figures 80, 81, and 82).

Discomfort may also be due to smaller ovarian tumors—follicular cysts, fibroma or paraovarian cysts showing a tendency towards strangulation.

Table 1 shows the results of an analysis of 475 laparoscopies for pelvic neurovegetative disturbances performed during the years 1956 to 1975. Before laparoscopy all patients had a meticulous history and physical examination; the palpatory findings of the patients were minute or vague.

Table 1

Laparoscopies for Pelvic Neurovegetative Disturbances

Normal findings	7.0%
Endometriosis	27.5%
Adhesions	10.0%
Fibroids	2.5%
Ovarian tumors (dermoid, paraovarian cysts, strangulations)	11.0%
Intestinal tumors, sigmoiditis, regional ileitis, diverticulitis	3.6%
Inflammatory processes (appendicitis, adnexitis, Tbc)	9.6%
Conglomerate tumors	4.3%
Spastic, fibrotic ligaments; varicocele	12.3%
Allan-Masters syndrome	4.6%
Chronic peritonitis	1.3%
Others (perforated IUD, pregnancy and fibroid, hydrops of gallbladder)	1.3%

Therapy

The treatment of these conditions may call for the cooperative efforts of an orthopedic surgeon, gastroenterologist, psychiatrist and gynecologist.

Conservative Treatment

Beside tranquilizing agents, smaller doses of corticosteroids, given over a long period of time, proved to be of benefit in some cases. Results of hormonal treatment of endometriosis remain dubious as long as endometriotic lesions have not been totally eradicated. Repeated presacral or paralumbar anesthetic inductions give good results in appropriate cases. The value of acupuncture for these conditions is controversial.

Operative Treatment

A considerable number of surgical procedures may be done at laparoscopy: division of adhesions, resection of the uterosacral ligaments, aspiration of cysts, ventrosuspension of the uterus and others. In other cases major operations are indicated. In specific cases presacral neurectomy will give good results. For other specific cases obliteration of the pouch of Douglas or antefixation of the uterus may be taken into consideration. The indication for surgery should be set very carefully to avoid iatrogenic damage in an already apprehensive patient.

Operative Laparoscopy

The range of operative procedures performed at laparoscopy depends on the experience and the skill of the surgeon as well as his/her surgical philosophy.

Aspiration of simple serous ovarian cysts can be recommended since about 60% of the cysts will not refill. Simple aspiration of cysts is particularly recommended in cases where one ovary has already been removed earlier.

Cauterization of endometriotic lesions is preferable to hormonal treatment alone since the latter therapy causes inactivation of those lesions only as long as the medication is continued. Isolated endometriotic foci disappear completely after cauterization.

Division of solitary or larger, veil-like adhesions deserves increased attention and consideration, especially if the danger of strangulation is imminent. Division should be preceded by cauterization in order to avoid hemorrhage.

Division of the uterosacral ligaments is connected with a certain risk. Because of proximity of large blood vessels, hemorrhage must be anticipated. The procedure should only be performed — if at all — if immediate surgical intervention is possible. So far there is no extensive experience comparing cauterization with complete division of the uterosacral ligaments.

Infiltration of the uterosacral ligaments with a local anesthetic must be followed by several presacral anesthesias at two-day intervals to successfully reduce the complaints of the patient.

Ventrosuspension of the uterus is a valuable procedure in rare cases only. The round ligaments are grasped with a forceps and linked to the abdominal fascia by suture. To some authors, retroflexion is merely one variety of several different normal positions of the uterus and therefore of no pathologic significance.

Even though it is possible to correct pathologic findings in patients with chronic pelvic neuralgic pain by operative laparoscopy or by other surgical or conventional treatment, the definitive, curative effect is not as good as we may expect or wish. Many problems are deeply connected with the psychological state of the patient. But whatever one's attitude may be towards active diagnostic procedures, our experience deserves emphasis: in 80% of the patients complaining of chronic lower abdominal pains, organic disease was found at laparoscopy. Most of these alterations were not palpable. Many unexpected diagnoses were made coincidentally.

Laparoscopy enables the physician to exclude organic disease from consideration. Knowledge of normal findings may be of important immediate comfort and benefit to the patient. In some cases this definite information by itself can cure a patient from long-suffered, imagined maladies.

Additional Reading

1. Atanov IUP, Gallinger IUI: Laparoscopy in the diagnosis of several abdominal tumors. Sov Med 35:93, 1972

2. Baerlocher C: Die Notfall-Laparoskopie. Leber Magen Darm 3:11, 1973

3. Berezov IUE, Lapin M, Sotnikov V, Musabekov, T: Laparoscopy in emergency surgery. Klin Khir 10:39, 1971

4. Breuning J: Intra-abdominal adhesions diagnosed by laparoscopy. Gastroenterology 10:104, 1972

5. Brun G: Diagnosis and treatment of pelvic pain of genital origin in women. Therapeutique 49:627, 1973

6. Bullock JL, Massey FM, Gambrell RD: Symptomatic endometriosis in teen-agers: a reappraisal. Obstet Gynecol 43:986, 1974

7. Cognat M: *Coelioscopie Gynecologique.* Simep, Villeurbanne, 1972

8. Cohen, MR: *Laparoscopy, Culdoscopy and Gynecography, Technique and Atlas.* WB Saunders, Philadelphia, 1970

9. Cortesi N, Ferrari P, Romani M, Manenti A, Bruni G: Preliminary studies of the diagnostic value of laparoscopy. Minerva Chir 28:39, 1973

10. Cortesi N, Manenti A, Romani M, Gibertini G, Barberini G: Emergency laparoscopy picture in the diagnosis of acute pancreatitis. Minerva Gastroenterol 19:52, 1973

11. Diamant YZ, Aboulafia Y, Raz S: Torsion of hydrosalpinx: report of four cases. Int Surg 57:303, 1972

12. DeLas Casas Alonso P, Mesa Rivero J: Emergency laparoscopy in various acute abdominal syndromes. Rev Esp Enferm Apar Dig 43:19, 1974

13. Deschreyer M, Hubens A: Overall indications for these technics: traumatic disorders. Acta Chir Belg [suppl] 1:95, 1973

14. Duffaut M, Bec P, Suduca P, Tournut R, Ribet A: Emergency laparoscopy in the diagnosis of jaundice associated with acute kidney failure: its value apropos of 25 cases. Sem Hop Paris 49:513, 1973

15. Dufour B, Pradel G: Retroperitoneal fibrosis: surgical aspects. Rev Prat 23:3569, 1973

16. Esposito JM, Zarou DM, Zarou GS: Localized inflammation secondary to intraperitoneal IUD. J Reprod Med 8:147, 1972

17. Fahrländer H: Emergency laparoscopy: report on 248 examinations. Langenbecks Arch Chir 331:315, 1972

18. Falk V: Gonorrhea salpingitis. Lakartidningen 68:4250, 1971

19. Ferguson IL: Laparoscopy for the diagnosis of nonspecific lower abdominal pain. Br J Clin Pract 28:163, 1974

20. Foucher G, Fresnel P, Philipps O, Otteni J, Mathey B, Sibilly A: Abdominal paracentesis. Diagnostic value in multiple injuries. Nouv Presse Med 2:2323, 1973

21. Frangenheim, H: *Die Laparoskopie und Kuldoskopie in der Gynäkologie.* Thieme, Stuttgart, 1972

22. Frangenheim H: *Laparoscopy and Culdoscopy in Gynecology.* Butterworth and Co, London, 1972

23. Frangenheim H: Die Coelioskopie in der Unterbauchchirurgie. Dtsch Med Wochenschr 43:109, 1965

24. Frangenheim H: Valeur de la coelioscopie dans le diagnostic des algies pelviennes. Rev Méd Normandes 11:549, 1969

25. Frangenheim H: Die Laparoskopie bei der Diagnostik des "akuten Bauches." Endoscopy 3:121, 1971

26. Frangenheim H: *Über die Notfall-Laparoskopie bei akuten Unterbaucherkrankungen in der Gynäkologie und in der Chirurgie.* F. K. Schattauer Verlag, Stuttgart and New York, 1972

27. Frangenheim H: *Urgent Laparoscopy in Acute Abdominal Diseases in Gynaecology.* S Karger, Basel, 1972, p 241

28. Frangenheim H: Die Stellung der Laparoskopie bei gynäkologischen und chirurgischen Problemen im Kindesalter. Pädiat Fortbldk Praxis 39:71, 1974

29. Frangenheim H, Kleindienst W: Chronic pelvic disease of unknown origin. In *Gynecological Laparoscopy: Principles and Techniques.* (JM Phillips, L Keith, Eds.) Stratton Intercontinental Medical Book Corp, New York, 1974, p 43

30. Frangenheim H, Kleindienst W: Chronic pelvic disease of unknown origin. J Reprod Med 13:23, 1974

31. Fredricsson B: Laparoscopy versus culdoscopy in the investigation of infertility. Acta Obstet Gynecol Scand 53:125, 1974

32. Grosieux P, Toulemonde-Dubois MM: Le coelioscopy gynécologique dans les syndromes douloureux pelviens de la femme. A propos de 215 observations. Rev Franc Gynécol 69:165, 1974

33. Herschlein HJ, Lechner W: The diagnosis and treatment of pelvic adhesions causing recurrent pelvic pain in cases with normal findings on pelvic palpation. Geburtshilfe Frauenheilkd 34:303, 1974

34. Kaeser O: Adhesions in the lower abdominal region as a cause of recurrent pain in normal gynecological palpation findings. Comment on the article by HJ Herschlein, W Lechner. Geburtshilfe Frauenheilkd 34:303, 1974

35. Keirse M, Vandervellen R: Laparoscopy in chronic pelvic pain. Endoscopy 5:27, 1973

36. Kenney A, Greenhalt JO: Limitations of laparoscopy in diagnosis of gonococcal salpingitis. Br Med J 906:519, 1974

37. Kramer A, Wurster H: Intraperitonealer Zwischenfall mit einem Fotolaparoskop. Z Gastroenterol 12:513, 1974

38. Kruijff E: Dysmenorrhea with pain in the leg in a girl with a urogenital anomaly. Ned Tijdschr Geneeskd 118:373, 1974

39. Lagache G, Gautier P, Desmons F, Bournoville M: Value of celioscopy in pelvic infection syndromes. Rev Fr Gynecol Obstet 67:379, 1972

40. Lapin M, Sotnikov V: Evaluation of methods of diagnosing cancer of the gastric stump. Vestn Khir 103:36, 1972

41. Lieb W, Henke M, Broicher K, Mertens H, Fraling F, Weinand A: Laparoscopic findings in extrahepatic abdominal processes. Med Welt 47:871, 1971

42. Llanio R, Sotto A, Jimenez G, Quintero M, Ferret O, Manso E, Nodarse O: Emergency laparoscopy (Study of 1265 Cases). Sem Hop Paris 49:873, 1973

43. Lundberg W, Wall J, Mathers J: Laparoscopy in evaluation of pelvic pain. Obstet Gynecol 42:872, 1973

44. Magursky V: Manipulation forceps for laparoscopy. Cesk Gynekol 37:767, 1972

45. Martinek, K: Diagnostic significance of laparoscopy in patients after surgery of organs of the abdominal cavity. Vnitr Lek 19:1014, 1973

46. Nikiforov B: Clinical aspects and diagnosis of closed injuries of the abdominal organs. Sov Med 37:66, 1974

47. Paldi E, Timor-Tritsch T, Abramovici J: La culdoscopie opératoire dans les cas de stérilisation et de syndrome de l'ovaire polycystique. Rev Franc Gynécol 68:721, 1973

48. Palmer R: La coelioskopie gynecologique. EMC. Gynecologie Fascicule 71.A. 10:2, 1965

49. Pannen F, Frangenheim H: Die "chirurgische" Laparoskopie. Chirurg, 1975 (z. Zt. im Druck)

50. Poalaggi J: Emergency laparoscopy in abdominal pathology. Nouv Presse Med 2:411, 1973

51. Postivint R, Rozenberg H, Chauveinc L, Sanchez M: Plea for laparoscopy in closed abdominal injuries. J Chir 102:77, 1971

52. Potkonjak D, Filipovi Christi ČB, Elakovi CJ, Vicentijev CR, Petrovic Z, Sosic M, Micic D: Comparison of laparoscopic, surgical and histological findings in the diagnosis of malignant pancreatic tumors. Med Arh 28:195, 1974

53. Sandler B: Is your pain really necessary? Br Med J 2:550, 1973

54. Selmair H, Wildhirt E: Laparoskopie und Gezielte Leberpunktion beim Kind. Leber Magen Darm 3:20, 1973

55. Serste J, Theunis A: Use of laparoscopy in abdominal emergencies, traumatic or not. (author's transl.) Acta Chir Belg 72:387, 1973

56. Sotnikov V, Ermolov A, Litvinov V, Emellanov S, Samsonov V: Diagnosis of intra-abdominal metastases of esophageal cancer by laparoscopy. Pr Onkol 19:35, 1973

57. Steptoe PC: Laparoscopy in Gynecology. E & S Livingstone, Edinburgh, 1967

58. Stiller, H: Surgical problems in extra- and intrahepatic obstructive jaundice. Langenbecks Arch Chir 327:364, 1970

59. Thoyer-Rozat J: La Coelioscopie. Masson, Paris, 1963

60. Weinand E: Laparoskopische und histologische Klärung eines ungewöhnlichen Verlaufes kindlicher Askaridiasis. Med Welt 25:1283, 1974

61. Whitson LG, Ballard CA, Israel R: Laparoscopic tubal sterilization coincident with therapeutic abortion by suction curettage. Obstet Gynecol 41:677, 1973

62. Wurbs D: Letter: Explorative laparotomy. Dtsch Med Wochenschr 99:1512, 1974

63. Zavgorodni IL, Barilo V: Diagnostic possibilities of laparoscopy in emergency surgery. Klin Khir 9:68, 1973

64. Zielske F, Jaluvka V: Gynaecologic laparoscopy and Crohn's disease (author's transl.) Geburtshilfe Frauenheilkd 34:356, 1974

Editorial Comments

This chapter has been written by one of the world's deans of laparoscopy, a man whose personal experience has been achieved by few others. Therefore, some of the procedures advocated by him should be approached only by those who possess unusual technical skill.

Aside from considerations of manual dexterity with ancillary laparoscopic instruments, standard teaching in this country has stressed the importance of clamping the pedicle of twisted ovarian cysts prior to manipulation in order to obviate embolization. Dr. Frangenheim would rather try laparoscopic methods of untwisting and drainage for cases of acute torsion.

His discussion of laparoscopy in the management of presumed salpingitis and/or abscess parallels our experience with a large, indigent clinic population. Too often, women are treated for acute salpingitis in error when the diagnosis is made solely on clinical impression. As Swedish studies have shown, the diagnostic false positive error may be 25% to 40%. Moreover, laparoscopy does not increase the morbidity of the infectious process. Prompt surgical intervention in cases of primary acute appendicitis may have an immediate, salutary effect on morbidity and a good long-term effect on fertility. One of the worst cases of endometriosis which I have ever seen was uncovered by laparoscopy in a 19-year-old black para two who had been treated for pain, the basis of which had been assumed to be chronic pelvic inflammatory disease.

The finding of a tuboovarian abscess demands quick extirpation. Dr. Frangenheim's philosophy of active surgical management with antibiotic coverage is preferred over the tradition, which predates the antibiotic era, of waiting for the acute process to subside. This older approach often leads to worsening of the patient's condition because of poor tissue levels of antibiotics or to formation of dense adhesions which make the eventual surgical procedure more difficult and hazardous.

Even the most ardent laparoscopist would hesitate to examine a patient with intestinal obstruction. Rather, laparotomy for diagnosis and therapy is the standard form of management.

The problem of cryptic pelvic pain seems to be geographically universal and not confined to a particular class of patients. Findings of pelvic congestion and defects of the broad ligament may be noted in some cases, but causal relationship to pain needs to be scrutinized since these conditions are found also in asymptomatic women.

Dr. Frangenheim's less than enthusiastic position on hormonal therapy of endometriosis is shared by many pelvic surgeons who have operated on patients following long courses of hormonal manipulation. Dr. Siegler has aptly termed progestational treatment of endometriosis a "holding action": probably few patients are permanently cured with this approach.

Uterosacral division is a potentially dangerous procedure whose benefits are doubtful. In addition to the risk of hemorrhage, ureteral damage may ensue.

Dr. Frangenheim has supplied us with a comprehensive list of references from the European literature which is of special interest to those who may wish to pursue further particular points discussed in this chapter.

S.L.C.

Chapter 12

Blunt and Penetrating Injuries to the Abdomen

Alan B. Gazzaniga, M.D.
Robert H. Bartlett, M.D.

Laparoscopy has become popular in the diagnosis and treatment of a variety of abdominal and pelvic disorders[9] but has yet to gain wide acceptance in the diagnosis of acute abdominal injuries. The following data detail our experience at the University of California, Irvine, with use of laparoscopy in the management of acute penetrating and blunt injuries to the abdomen.

From August 1972 to January 1975, laparoscopy was performed on 37 patients selected from 132 consecutively seen patients who presented with blunt or penetrating injuries to the abdomen. Patients were selected on the basis of equivocal indications for operation, their condition and availability of equipment and personnel. Our standard method of evaluation of blunt abdominal trauma is by insertion of a peritoneal dialysis catheter with infusion of 250 to 500 cc of saline. Decisions about laparotomy depend on the content and color of the return as well as other clinical findings. Exploratory operation is performed in almost all cases of penetrating trauma except when very superficial lacerations of the abdominal wall can be documented accurately.

Laparoscopy was performed after CO_2 insufflation of the peritoneal cavity with 2,500 cc for one minute with a needle. The laparoscope was introduced 2 to 3 cm above the umbilicus in nearly all cases through a 2 cm vertical midline incision. After introduction of the laparoscope into the peritoneal cavity, additional CO_2 was added whenever necessary. The right lobe of the liver and gallbladder were visualized initially, and then the left lobe of the liver and the stomach were visualized. A nasogastric tube passed prior to laparoscopy served to deflate the stomach and to facilitate visualization of the upper abdominal organs. The patient was then turned 30° to the right, and the left upper quadrant was inspected (Figure 1). Observation of the left upper quadrant could best be accomplished with the operator in a sitting position. If omentum was present, it could be teased away from the region of the spleen with a blunt, second-puncture probe. Investigation of the bowel was carried out by direct overhead inspection with additional or maximal CO_2 insufflation (Figure 2). Initially, all patients underwent laparotomy, regardless of the findings with laparoscopy. As experience was gained and laparoscopy correlated with operative findings, patients with negative laparoscopy were not subjected to laparotomy.

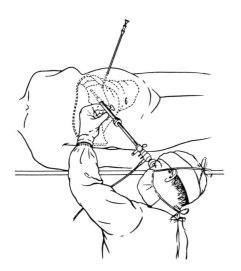

Figure 1
Inspection of left upper quadrant with patient tilted 30° to the right.

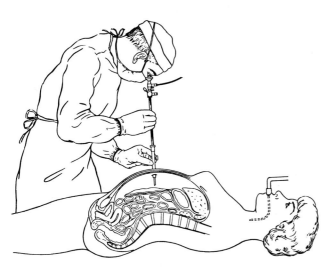

Figure 2
Inspection of small bowel; telescope perpendicular to patient and with maximum perspective.

Results were evaluated by the number of false negative and false positive findings at laparoscopy. A laparotomy was considered negative if there was no injury to the peritoneum or if there was minor intraabdominal trauma which did not require repair.

Blunt Trauma

Fifty-two patients were evaluated for blunt trauma, 14 of whom underwent laparoscopy followed by laparotomy (Figure 3). Thirteen of 14 patients had positive findings requiring surgical correction. The most common injury in this group was a ruptured spleen. Complete visualization of the spleen was not always possible. The tip of the spleen was usually identified, and if blood was superior to it or under the omentum, which had migrated to the left upper quadrant, splenic injury was always found. In no case was a normal spleen found when the preceding signs were present. The second most common injury diagnosed with the laparoscope was jejunal perforation. This diagnosis was obvious in each case by our observing small bowel contents along the lateral gutters as well as small bowel serosal inflammatory changes. These observations were best made by direct overhead visualization with maximum pneumoperitoneum (Figure 2). One patient was shown on laparoscopy to have a small liver laceration, and at laparotomy no further injuries were noted. The laceration was not bleeding and was not sutured. An additional patient had the falciform ligament torn from the liver, and it required a single suture to stop bleeding.

Ten patients sustaining blunt abdominal trauma underwent laparoscopy only; there were no false negative results in this group. Three patients had positive bloody abdominal paracentesis and at laparoscopy were found to have minor tears of the liver, falciform ligament or bleeding from a pelvic fracture with hematoma in the rectus abdominis muscle. Nine of these ten patients had possible intraabdominal damage only; their average hospital stay was two days. The other patient also had a hip fracture and required prolonged hospitalization for this reason.

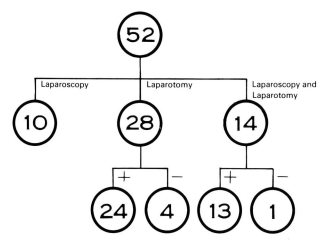

Figure 3
Treatment regimen in 52 patients presenting with blunt abdominal trauma.

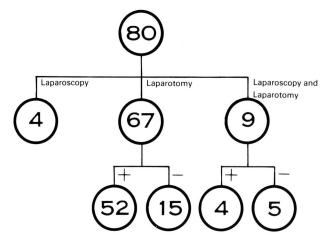

Figure 4
Treatment regimen in 80 patients presenting with penetrating abdominal trauma.

Twenty-eight patients underwent laparotomy without primary laparoscopy because indications for surgery were obvious or the attending surgeon preferred not to evaluate the patient with laparoscopy. Twenty-four of this group had definite pathology which required surgical intervention. Four patients in this group had negative findings at laparotomy. Three of these four had blood-tinged fluid on paracentesis and did not present clinical evidence of continued bleeding prior to surgical intervention. The other underwent surgery for pain only.

Penetrating Injury

Of 80 patients who were admitted with penetrating injuries, 13 underwent diagnostic laparoscopy (Figure 4). This evaluation was followed by laparotomy in nine patients. In five, laparotomy findings were negative. Four patients with penetrating injuries of the abdomen and/or chest underwent laparoscopy only. In two patients, no penetration of the parietal peritoneum was identified. In a third patient, a small nonbleeding injury to the omentum was visualized. The fourth patient represented the only possible false negative result. A 22-year-old Marine corporal was struck in the left chest with a round from an M-16 rifle. The high velocity missile entered the left seventh intercostal space, passed obliquely and exited directly posterior in the 11th intercostal space. The patient entered with a hemopneumothorax. A chest tube was inserted in the left chest, and over the ensuing two hours he developed left upper quadrant abdominal tenderness. Laparoscopy was performed, and there was no escape of CO_2 into the chest tube bottle during the procedure. The left hemidiaphragm was well visualized and was normal, without any evidence of blood in the peritoneal cavity. Four days after this procedure the patient drained feces from his chest tube, and a colopleurocutaneous fistula was documented with a gastrografin enema. The colon and diaphragmatic injury were probably due to cavitation effects. The patient was treated with a transverse colostomy and made an uneventful recovery.

Fifty-seven patients had laparotomy without laparoscopy; 52 patients had findings which required surgical intervention, and 15 patients had minimal trauma which did not require surgical repair. These last injuries included serosal stomach or bowel tears, nonbleeding superficial lacerations of the liver and minor injuries of the omentum.

In the group of patients who underwent negative laparotomy (penetrating or blunt injury), the average hospital stay was six days; in the group who had laparotomy with definite findings, the average hospital stay was 13 days.

Discussion

A Medlar search for references relating to laparoscopic diagnosis of blunt and/or penetrating trauma did not produce a single article in the English literature. In both the French and German literature, however, there are reports dealing with laparoscopy and closed abdominal trauma.[3, 6, 11] The authors of these articles are enthusiastic about its use for these problems and feel that it prevents unnecessary laparotomy and allows for a more complete evaluation of the multiply injured patient.

The use of laparoscopy in evaluating penetrating trauma was stimulated by the number of negative laparotomies at this institution prior to the use of laparoscopy as well as by reports in the literature.[10] In our series, approximately one-third of the patients had laparotomy with negative or minimal findings, i.e., avoidable laparotomy. The main limitation of laparoscopy in evaluating penetrating injuries is the inability to evaluate the entire bowel and the retroperitoneum. The use of the instrument to detect small lacerations of the liver, puncture of the parietal peritoneum and superficial lacerations of serosal injuries to the bowel has been quite good. We have not been impressed with the use of sinograms to detect whether penetrating injuries have entered the peritoneal cavity.[1] If the sinograms show penetration, then the patient may or may not undergo laparotomy, depending on clinical findings. This test does take time and usually requires transporting the patient to the radiology department. Laparoscopy can demonstrate if the peritoneum has been punctured and also give much additional information about the extent of the injury.

The use of laparoscopy in cases of blunt trauma has several advantages. If the patient has associated head, thoracic or bone injury, laparotomy evaluation of the abdomen can be difficult and pose an additional surgical insult. One patient in this series was comatose with a head injury, and laparoscopy was performed in the Intensive Care Unit, where a diagnosis of duodenal rupture was made. Abdominal paracentesis, although quite useful in evaluating the patient with blunt injury to the abdomen, can give both false negative and false positive results.[7] Accuracy of abdominal paracentesis may be improved by Gram stain and more thorough microscopic evaluation of the fluid.[8] Laparoscopy in 37 patients gave only one possible false negative result (described above). Note that laparoscopy tends to overestimate the amount of hemoperitoneum. This tendency was verified by laparoscopy in cadavers in which 50 cc increments of blood were introduced into the peritoneal cavity under direct vision. Fifty milliliters of blood appeared through the laparoscope to represent major bleeding.

In our series of 37 laparoscopies there were no complications related to the procedure. Complications can occur and have been pointed out in other reports.[2, 4] Except in one instance, the procedure was performed in the operating room under general anesthesia with endotracheal intubation and hyperventilation to prevent hypercarbia. The supraumbilical approach was used and allowed easy visualization of both lobes of the liver and access to the spleen and other upper abdominal and small bowel pathology. Hemodynamic effects of overdistension can and should be avoided in the hypotensive patient. Intraabdominal pressure of greater than 20 mm Hg can reduce cardiac output, which may be critical in the hypotensive, injured patient.[5]

Initial evaluation of the abdomen in patients with blunt trauma is best made with abdominal paracentesis. The standard method of four quadrant taps with a needle or midline needle tap has been replaced in this institution by the introduction of a peritoneal dialysis catheter into the pelvis. The bladder is first emptied with a Foley catheter and the dialysis catheter introduced below the umbilicus. If there is immediate free return of blood, the patient is considered to have a serious intraabdominal injury, indicating laparotomy. However, if the bloody return clears and the patient is hemodynamically stable after resuscitation with a crystalloid or colloid solution, laparoscopy is considered. Laparoscopy is also indicated in patients with negative paracentesis and positive physical findings or in comatose patients. Patients with penetrating injuries are considered for laparoscopy if hemodynamics are stable and the patients do not have generalized peritoneal findings.

The advantages of laparoscopy are shortened hospital stay and reduction in complications of a negative laparotomy. In patients in whom only abdominal injury was present and laparoscopy was negative, the hospital stay averaged two days. Patients who underwent laparotomy with negative findings were hospitalized for six days. In the latter group, minor complications of laparotomy, including atelectasis, ileus, etc., were noted. Long-term side effects of laparotomy, such as formation of adhesions with subsequent intestinal obstruction, may occur following negative exploration.

References

1. Cornell WP, Ebert PA, Zuidema GD: X-ray diagnosis of penetrating wounds of the abdomen. J Surg Res 5:142, 1965

2. Doctor NH, Hussain Z: Bilateral pneumothorax associated with laparoscopy. Anesthesia 28:75, 1973

3. Fahrlander H: Die notfallmabige laparoskopie. Bericht uber 248 untersuchungen. Langebecks Arch Chir 331:315, 1972

4. Keith I, Silver A, Becker M: Anesthesia for laparoscopy. J Reprod Med 12:227, 1974

5. Motew M, Ivankovich AD, Bieniarz J, Albrecht RF, Zahed B, Scommegna A: Cardiovascular effects and acid-base and blood gas changes during laparoscopy. Am J Obstet Gynecol 115:1002, 1973

6. Paolaggi JA: La laparoscopie d'urgence en pathologie abdominale. Nouv Presse Med Paris 2:411, 1973

7. Perry JF: Blunt and penetrating abdominal injuries. Curr Probl Surg, May 1970, p 1

8. Perry JF, DeMeules JE, Root HD: Diagnostic peritoneal lavage in blunt abdominal trauma. Surg Gynecol Obstet 131:742, 1970

9. Phillips J, Keith D, Keith L: Gynecological laparoscopy 1973: the state of the art. J Reprod Med 12:215, 1974

10. Ryzoff RI, Shafton GW, Herbsman H: Selective conservatism in penetrating abdominal trauma. Surgery 59:650, 1966

11. Tostivint R, Rozenberg H, Chauveinc L, Sanchez MF: Plaidoyer pour la laparoscopie dans les traumatismes abdominaux fermes. J Chir (Paris, 102:77, 1971

Editorial Comments

Those of us who have attempted to act as missionaries to our surgical colleagues are amazed at their general reluctance to accept laparoscopy as a diagnostic tool in cases of abdominal trauma.

A skilled laparoscopist can evaluate the entire peritoneal cavity and its recesses as well as or better than the surgeon who uses the usual small exploratory incision, which may be placed at a site ill-suited for the surgery eventually performed. Because of contrecoup effects, all quadrants of the abdominal cavity need to be evaluated thoroughly.

The authors have demonstrated the value of laparoscopy in this situation and have made two salient points: (1) The procedure has great value in determining the need for subsequent laparotomy: only one false negative case was noted in 37 instances; (2) The hospital stay and morbidity of patients spared laparotomy were reduced significantly. Obvious signs of hypovolemic shock or free air under the diaphragm in a scout film of the abdomen negate the need for laparoscopy prior to laparotomy just as shock and a positive cul-de-sac puncture suggest immediate laparotomy for suspected rupture of an ectopic pregnancy.

The supraumbilical approach for visualization of upper abdominal structures greatly simplifies manipulation of the laparoscope but is not a prerequisite for laparoscopy. One must keep in mind that the aorta and vena cava are more vulnerable with this approach. Reverse Trendelenburg position may be used to achieve better upper abdominal visualization.

S.L.C.

Chapter 13

Oncologic Laparoscopy

Victor Gomel, M.D.
Stephen L. Corson, M.D.

Introduction

There has been limited use of laparoscopy in diagnosing and staging intraabdominal cancer. Indeed, the bibliography of this chapter reflects Americans' reluctance to use laparoscopy as compared with their European colleagues' enthusiasm. This situation is particularly ironic when one considers the early work of Ruddock,[21] who pioneered peritoneoscopy as a diagnostic tool.

Laparoscopy may be employed in cases where the primary lesion has been determined by radiographic or other methods. Staging of intraabdominal neoplasms may determine the type of surgery to be performed or if laparotomy should be contemplated at all. A colostomy, for instance, might be substituted for a proposed en bloc abdominoperineal procedure if tumor implants are obtained via liver biopsy at laparoscopy. Laparoscopy should be considered a screening procedure prior to major surgery for extraperitoneal malignancies such as mid- and high esophogeal carcinoma and possibly for carcinoma of the breast in which a "lumpectomy" could be substituted for a radical procedure if the tumor is found in the ovaries or other peritoneal structures. Another large area for consideration is that of the "second-look" procedure after abdominal surgery for primary carcinoma. Laparoscopy can objectively assess the effect of adjunctive chemotherapy or radiation programs, thereby offering an immediate aid to the individual patient as well as to prospective multi-group study programs.

Not a few cancers have symptoms referable to the site of metastatic lesions. Laparoscopy may be helpful in identifying the primary lesion in order to establish a reasonable treatment regimen.

By now the reader might have detected our enthusiasm for the use of laparoscopy. A note of caution must be interjected at this point. First, because of the importance of accuracy in diagnosis, oncologic laparoscopy should be attempted only by the very skilled laparoscopist. We believe that laparoscopy affords a better view of the entire peritoneal cavity than the usual exploratory laparotomy incision except the "stem-to-stern" variety. Still, there are instances when visualization of a key area is less than satisfactory. The laparoscopist must recognize when an examination has not been adequate and report it as such. He or she must know how to interpret the appearance of small changes and deviations in anatomy after surgery, radiation and/or chemotherapy.

A related point is the risk factor introduced by the nature of the population in question. This kind of patient is quite different from the 32-year-old, healthy woman seen during an infertility workup or for elective sterilization. Patients are quite often in the seventh decade of life. They may have major concurrent physiologic impairments caused by pulmonary disease, cardiovascular degeneration, diabetes and the like. Prior to laparoscopy it may be necessary to remove large quantities of ascitic fluid with rapid fluid compartment shifts.

Laparoscopy following surgery and irradiation may be impossible, difficult or associated with major morbidity. Therefore, the goals and the importance of the information obtainable must be weighed against the risks. These patients must be readied for immediate laparotomy in case of laparoscopic complications.

A laparoscopic system adequate for routine use may be insufficient when utilized for this indication. A dependable, powerful light source is necessary. A xenon source or 1,000 watt mercury vapor bulb helps to illuminate dark recesses of the peritoneal cavity. A telescope of at least 7 mm is preferred because of greater light transmission and increased magnification. Laparoscopes with flexible or steerable distal tips, normally not needed for routine pelvic use, may be indispensable in these instances. A wide variety of probes and biopsy instruments must be readily available.

Superficial lesions of the peritoneum, liver and other structures may be sampled with a blunt forceps or single-toothed forceps without bleeding. Biopsies should be taken without electrosurgical techniques because of tissue distortion that might interfere with histologic evaluation. Coagulation may be employed after the biopsy has been taken. Needle-type biopsy of the liver, pancreas or retroperitoneal structures may be taken with a variety of Silverman-type needles. We have found the Travenol percutaneous disposable needle excellent here. Impressive bleeding following needle biopsy usually ceases within two minutes; a hemostatic agent such as an absorbable gelatin sponge (Gelfoam) can be placed on the site with blunt forceps. Biopsy of a suspected liver hemangioma is unwise because of uncontrollable bleeding. Metastatic disease can often be noted first in the lymphatics of the diaphragm above the dome of the liver; needle biopsy of this area is particularly helpful, but inadvertent puncture of the pleura is a risk.

Carcinoma of the Ovary

In view of the close spatial relationship of the pelvic organs, it is often difficult to establish the precise origin of a pelvic tumor by clinical means. Barium enema and sigmoidoscopy may be of limited value. Differential diagnoses include uterine myomata, ovarian tumor or a neoplasm originating from the bowel. In such cases laparoscopy may successfully replace exploratory laparotomy as a diagnostic measure to formulate a proposed regimen of therapy, which might include preoperative irradiation or chemotherapy.

In the presence of uterine fibroids whose size or symptoms do not indicate surgery, one must ascertain that no adnexal pathology exists. Laparoscopy was performed in 83 cases after a clinical diagnosis of uterine fibroids had been made. As reported by Samuelson and Sjövall, [22] leiomyomata only were found in 55 cases (66%). In ten cases (12%) there was associated adnexal pathology and in 18 (22%), adnexal pathology only. Of the 28 cases with adnexal pathology, 19 (two-thirds) were neoplastic and one was malignant.

Frangenheim and Stockhammer[10] reported 218 laparoscopies performed for pelvic mass in postmenopausal patients. In 42 of them (19.7%) a diagnosis of cancer was made; 19 were ovarian; 14, intestinal; and nine, metastatic. Aside from elucidating the diagnosis, laparoscopy answered the question of whether to operate. The authors reported that in 60.4% of the cases laparoscopy obviated the need for laparotomy, either because of the finding of benign disease or because of malignancy deemed inoperable.

Laparoscopy expedites diagnosis of small ovarian cancers. Ancillary procedures, such as biopsy, aspiration of the contents of a cyst or of the contents of the pouch of Douglas, provide material for precise histological or cytological diagnosis.[17]

Even in the most favorable groups of ovarian cancers treated with surgery and external irradiation there is a 20% mortality rate within five years. The principal route of dissemination of the disease is transcoelomic seeding. Instillation of radioactive material into the peritoneal cavity to irradiate the surfaces at risk has been an attractive idea and was tried successfully in the past.[18] The method fell into disrepute because of high morbidity, mainly due to the misplacement of the isotope.

Figure 1
Laparoscopic restaging of ovarian carcinoma*

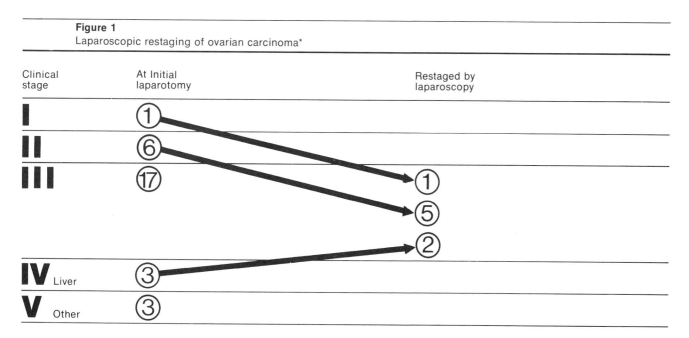

Clinical stage	At Initial laparotomy	Restaged by laparoscopy

* Data from Rosenoff et al.[20]

Intraperitoneal isotopes are presently being employed in stages I and II of ovarian carcinoma in a prospective study in British Columbia, Canada.[7] The patients are first treated with total abdominal hysterectomy and bilateral adnexectomy. Those in stage IIb also receive external cobalt irradiation to the pelvis. Later, a fine polyethylene catheter with multiple perforations is placed across the upper abdomen under laparoscopic control. Chromic phosphate P_{32} is instilled through the catheter. In this protocol, laparoscopy has proven to be a safe method for the intraperitoneal administration of radioactive isotopes. In addition, it offers the advantage of a thorough visualization of the abdominal cavity and confirmation of the extent of the disease.

DeVita's group at the National Cancer Institute has been interested in laparoscopy as related to ovarian cancer. A paper by Rosenoff and colleagues[20] describes some of their experience. Peritoneoscopy was performed in 30 patients within a month after laparotomy for ovarian carcinoma. Six of seven patients originally classified at stage I or II were reclassified at stage III because of diaphragmatic or upper abdominal metastases (Figure 1). Diaphragmatic tumor was found in 77% of all patients investigated. The authors emphasize that routine shielding of the liver during irradiation for presumed stage I/II ovarian carcinoma would program therapeutic failure for 86% of these patients. Since ovarian carcinoma is now the fifth leading cause of neoplastic death in women, these figures take on heightened significance. *True* stage I/II ovarian carcinoma has an expected five-year survival of 50% whereas later stages have rates below 10%.

Rosenoff's findings are particularly impressive considering that the technique employed Innovar and local anesthesia in a group of patients preselected for recent laparotomy.

Right hemidiaphragm involvement was found in all patients having any diaphragmatic metastases except in two, whose adhesions did not permit adequate visualization. This follows from the work of Meyers,[16] who demonstrated that intraperitoneal effusions ascend along the right gutter to the lymphatics in the right subphrenic space. The phrenicolic ligament fixes the colon to the diaphragm at the splenic flexure and retards flow up the left gutter. The thoracic duct plays a minor role in lymphatic drainage of the peritoneal space. Peritoneoscopy supplied the only objective finding of cancer recurrence in 30% of patients whose physical examination, scans and laboratory data were normal.

Figure 2
Second-look laparoscopy in ovarian carcinoma*

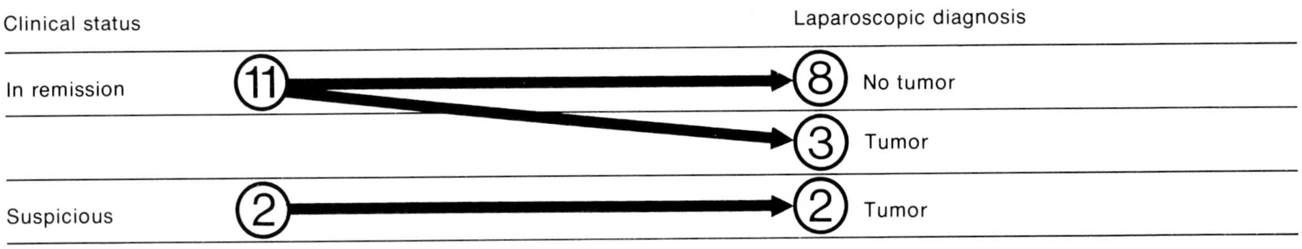

Clinical status   Laparoscopic diagnosis

In remission   ⑪   →   ⑧   No tumor

   →   ③   Tumor

Suspicious   ②   →   ②   Tumor

* Data from Rosenoff et al.[20]

Eleven patients in another group were selected for "second-look" procedures after at least one year of apparent clinical remission while they were on chemotherapy. Active disease was found in three (Figure 2). Two additional patients in whom active cancer was suspected while they were on chemotherapy had this diagnosis confirmed endoscopically (Figure 2). Relapse of two patients found negative at "second-look" laparoscopy occurred 12 and 19 months later, respectively. Rosenoff and co-workers recommend a "second-look" laparoscopy in order to more strongly document absence of tumor. This protocol confines laparotomy only to those in whom no tumor is noted during the laparoscopy—60% in their series.

Rosenoff and associates state that in a total group of 242 patients, of whom 235 had malignant disease, there were only two unsuccessful attempts at peritoneoscopy. They list five "serious" complications in this group of 242 patients: one transfusion after hypotension, one cellulitis, one pneumothrax, one brief case of respiratory distress secondary to subcutaneous emphysema, and one case of abdominal pain and transient, abnormal liver tests.

These exemplary results achieved by DeVita's group should lead toward wider use of laparoscopy in the diagnosis and management of ovarian carcinoma.

Primary and Metastatic Carcinoma of the Liver

The diagnosis of primary liver carcinoma is usually made late in the course of the disease as a result of the rarity of the lesion and its development in a voluminous organ (the larger part of which is covered by the rib cage) and because it usually develops within an already-diseased organ. The value of diagnostic biochemical tests is limited except that they occasionally find α-1 feto-protein in the blood or ascitic fluid of the patient.[11] These factors have encouraged the rise of other, more sophisticated techniques: liver scan, sonography and laparoscopy.

Etienne and associates[9] reported on 43 cases of proven primary carcinoma of the liver where laparoscopy had been performed. They found neoplastic tissue visible at the surface of the liver in 34 cases. In 28, multiple nodules were present; in six there was a single tumor. In two other patients the surface of the liver appeared raised by deeply located tumor. In seven cases the laparoscopist failed to visualize suspected neoplastic tissue. Thus, in 84% of the patients, hepatic neoplasm was directly visualized or suspected with laparoscopic inspection alone. Undirected, percutaneous liver biopsy claims only 30%[19] to 65%[1,6] positive results.

Sauer and associates[23] reported on 123 patients with primary or metastatic liver tumors, including a few benign, localized lesions. All of their patients were subjected to both liver scan and laparoscopy, and the findings were verified by biopsy, operation or autopsy. Liver scan failed to reveal the tumor in 26 cases (21%). In 88 (72%) a space-occupying lesion was recorded, and in nine (7%), suspicious findings were noted. At laparoscopy, on the basis of gross appearances alone, there were 42 (34%) false negatives. With target biopsy under direct vision this number was reduced to 24 cases (20%). By the systematic use of both liver scan and laparoscopy with directed liver biopsy Sauer and associates were able to increase the diagnostic accuracy to 93%. In 99 other cases without neoplastic involvement of the liver the scans were falsely positive in 10%. By laparoscopy there were no false positives in these 99 cases.

Figure 3
Laparoscopy in Hodgkin's disease*

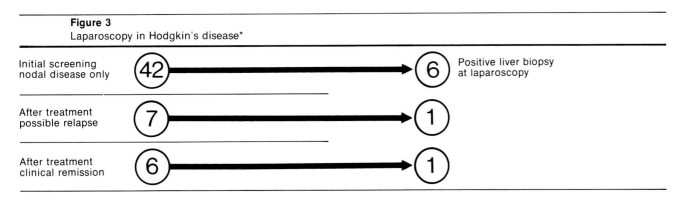

Initial screening nodal disease only	(42) ⟶ (6)	Positive liver biopsy at laparoscopy
After treatment possible relapse	(7) ⟶ (1)	
After treatment clinical remission	(6) ⟶ (1)	

* Data from Bagley *et al.*[2]

Liver scan (scintigram), although very useful, has numerous limitations, and echography has similar drawbacks:

1. Liver scan does not detect small lesions. Lesions on the surface of the liver must be at least 2 cm in diameter, and the deeply located ones must be 3 to 4 cm in diameter to be detected.
2. Liver scan does not distinguish between benign and malignant lesions.
3. The interpretation of liver scan may be misleading because of variations in the normal liver.

Laparoscopy has the following limitations:

1. The visible area of the liver is comparatively small when compared to the total volume.
2. Lesions located deep in the liver parenchyma cannot be visualized.
3. Laparoscopy is a surgical procedure but has small, associated risks and some postoperative discomfort.

Laparoscopy and scintigraphy are complementary methods. Their concomitant use markedly decreases false negative results (2.6% to 7%).[12, 24, 30] In the presence of clinically suspected, chronic, diffuse liver disease, laparoscopy with directed biopsy is a more useful and reliable tool than the scan.[25, 30]

Hodgkin's Disease

In Hodgkin's disease it is generally believed that early and wide removal of affected tissues can offer long periods of remission and sometimes clinical recovery. It is therefore important to carry out a wide range of tests to determine the extent of the disease. It is generally held that hepatic involvement occurs in the late stages of the disease. Casirola and associates[5] reported on 38 cases of early Hodgkin's disease where laparoscopy was performed routinely. In two cases (5%) unsuspected liver involvement was demonstrated. They conclude by advocating routine laparoscopy as part of the investigation in the diagnosis of Hodgkin's disease and the determination of its spread.

A study performed at the National Cancer Institute addressed the need for laparotomy versus laparoscopy as a staging procedure in Hodgkin's disease. Bagley and co-workers[2] reported on 42 patients undergoing multiple hepatic needle biopsy via peritoneoscopy as a prelude to conventional radiotherapy (Figure 3). Peritoneoscopy was performed on untreated patients whose chest and bone films, lymphangiograms, liver-bone-spleen scans and marrow biopsy had failed to demonstrate extranodal disease.

Peritoneoscopy was positive in six of the 42 patients where percutaneous "blind" liver biopsy had been negative (the sixth patient had not had a biopsy preoperatively).

An additional seven patients were evaluated who were thought to have relapsed after treatment, and one was shown to have a positive biopsy. However, of six patients thought to be in remission following chemotherapy, one had a positive biopsy at the same site prior to therapy.

Table 1
Laparoscopy in Hodgkin's Disease*

Clinical stage	Number	Laparoscopy positive biopsy		Laparotomy positive biopsy	
		Liver	Spleen	Liver	Spleen
I	19	0/19	1/15	0/19	6/19
II	21	0/21	1/17	1/21	3/21
III	11	2/11	2/11	0/8	5/8
IIIs	1	0/1	1/1	0/1	1/1
IV	13	2/13	2/10	0/10	4/10

* Modified from Spinelli et al.[29]

Comparison of the number of positive hepatic biopsies (according to stage) at peritoneoscopy with those at laparotomy in similar series led the authors to conclude that "evaluation of the liver by a sequence of percutaneous needle biopsy and needle biopsies at peritoneoscopy reveals hepatic involvement as often as does wedge biopsy at laparotomy."

The performance of peritoneoscopy as a diagnostic tool in non-Hodgkin's lymphoma was less impressive and was not advocated as a routine measure since the false negative rate was 50%, as proved at laparotomy.

We disagree with the authors' statement that one cannot see or perform biopsies on abdominal lymph nodes at the time of endoscopy. Frequently, the paraaortic nodes and the chains along the iliac vessels can be seen to bulge below the posterior peritoneal surface. Needle biopsy under vision should be performed with caution in order to avoid the ureter and great vessels.

A larger study by the group at the National Tumor Institute in Milan, Italy, compared laparotomy more directly to laparoscopy for Hodgkin's disease staging. Spinelli and associates[29] reported on a total of 91 patients first investigated with needle marrow aspiration followed by laparoscopy with hepatic and splenic biopsy. Patients with negative findings (59) went on to formal laparotomy with splenectomy and liver biopsy.

Table 1 documents the data. Of 65 untreated patients having laparoscopy, splenic biopsy was not possible in nine because of poor visualization and was unsatisfactory in two others. Hepatic biopsy was positive in four of 65 (6%) and splenic biopsy positive in seven of 54 (13%). Not shown in the table are the positive bone marrow biopsies in five cases. *Only one patient with previous negative hepatic biopsy at laparoscopy had disease in the open wedge biopsy at laparotomy (1 of 59). But splenectomy demonstrated Hodgkin's disease in 15 patients (15 of 59) previously missed at laparoscopy.* Combined laparoscopy and marrow biopsy demonstrated true stage IV disease in six of 65 (9%). Laparoscopic positive splenic biopsy with negative marrow/liver results advanced clinical staging in five patients, and negative findings reduced staging in ten for an overall change of staging in 23%.

Subsequent laparotomy worsened to stage IV only one patient (2%) with hepatic involvement missed at laparoscopy but by splenic findings worsened the staging in 8 of 59 and improved it in 9 of 59.

In 26 patients who were restaged, eventual laparotomy in 19 disclosed liver involvement in four negative at laparoscopy and splenic disease in eight originally negative at laparoscopy.

In 13 patients with Hodgkin's disease present in hepatic biopsy, ten also had splenic findings and six, positive marrow samples. Hepatic involvement was noted in 17% of those with negative liver scans.

Thus, overall, laparoscopy was successful in detecting eight cases of 13 with liver involvement prior to laparotomy. Only two patients in the laparoscopy group of 91 required laparotomy for complications related to biopsy procedures. One patient had traumatic hepatitis. This compares with the laparotomy group of 77 patients in whom 12 cases of postoperative pneumonia were noted along with one wound infection. Two patients in this group required a second laparotomy—one for hilar splenic bleeding after splenectomy and another for bowel obstruction.

The authors advocated exploratory laparotomy for staging only in those patients in whom original laparoscopy with hepatic and splenic sampling had proven negative. Their success with splenic biopsy is encouraging.

Carcinoma of the Gastrointestinal Tract

In patients with primary carcinoma of the abdominal organs (stomach, bowel, pancreas) it is essential to know whether serosal involvement and/or liver metastases are present prior to undertaking surgical treatment of the lesion. Here again, liver scan acts in concert with laparoscopy to gain more information prior to definitive therapy.

Canossi and associates[4] reported on 112 such patients subjected to liver scan and laparoscopy. In 67 patients a laparotomy followed. In 45 patients no surgical intervention was carried out, most often because of the finding of liver metastases. In the last group both the scan and laparoscopy were positive in 20 patients and negative in seven. In six cases where the scan was suspicious for metastases, laparoscopy failed to reveal liver involvement. In seven patients found suspicious at laparoscopy the scan was negative in four and positive in three. Of five cases with negative scan, laparoscopy uncovered metastatic liver lesions in all (Table 2).

Table 2

Laparoscopy and Liver Scan in Gastrointestinal Cancer*

Scan	Laparoscopy		
	Positive	**Negative**	**Suspicious**
Positive	20		3
Negative	5	7	4
Suspicious		6	

* Data from Canossi et al.[4]

Of the first group of 67 patients subjected to a subsequent laparotomy both the scan and laparoscopy were negative in 49. In two, liver metastases were found at surgery. In 14 patients with positive scans, laparoscopy failed to demonstrate liver lesions; normal liver was confirmed at laparotomy. In four patients suspicion of a lesion arose at laparoscopy. (Two of them had negative scans and two suspicious scans.) At laparotomy no liver metastases were noted (Figure 4).

Here again it is evident that liver scan and laparoscopy are complementary and must be used concomitantly. In this manner, in the above series, only 3% of the liver metastases remained undiagnosed preoperatively. Furthermore, in 45 patients (40%) a laparotomy was avoided.

At laparoscopy it is essential to do a panoramic inspection of the parietal and visceral peritoneum and to note the shape, dimension and appearance of the liver. The visualization can be enhanced by selective positioning of the operating table (Trendelenburg, Fowler, left lateral and right lateral decubitus positions) and by use of a probe.

Primary Carcinoma of the Gallbladder

The preoperative diagnosis of this lesion is often difficult. Symptoms may be lacking or, when present, may resemble those of benign biliary disease. Laparoscopy and direct visualization in the majority of cases permits an accurate and early diagnosis; in the others a suspicion of the condition is acquired.

Carcinoma of the gallbladder is often associated with cholelithiasis. The criteria for diagnosing the condition have been described by Beck.[3] Often there is a whitish, circumscribed thickening of the wall with adjoining abnormal vasculature. In other cases, associated with cholelithiasis, there is a round tumor surrounded by adhesions. Another important sign is the presence of

Figure 4
Laparoscopy in gastrointestinal cancer*

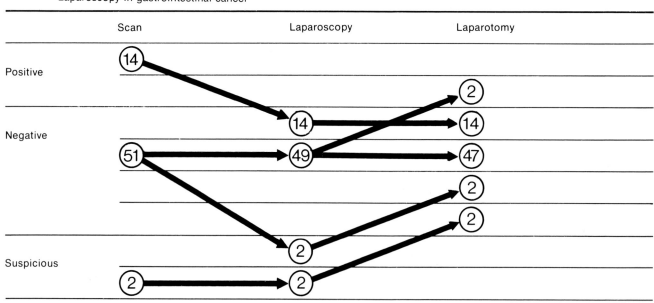

* Data from Canossi *et al.*[4]

liver metastases immediately in the proximity of the gallbladder or limited to the right lobe of the liver because the spread of the disease is either contiguous or by way of lymphatics.

DeDios Vega and associates[8] reported on 34 cases of primary carcinoma of the gallbladder diagnosed by laparoscopy. The presenting symptom in 32 was icterus; in one, right upper quadrant pain; and, in the last case, a palpable tumor in the same region.

To better visualize the region it is important to use a probe to elevate the liver and to position the operating table so that the head is elevated and the patient is in the left lateral decubitus position.

Carcinoma of the Esophagus

In esophageal cancer Sotnikov and associates[27] advocate the routine use of laparoscopy to determine whether there is intraabdominal dissemination of the disease. They reported on 65 such patients. In 16, metastases were found by laparoscopy of the liver, parietal peritoneum, lymph nodes of the lesser omentum, bowel or other organs. In cancer of the upper thoracic esophagus, intraabdominal dissemination was found in one patient

out of a total of eight. Among the 34 patients with cancer of the midthoracic esophagus, intraabdominal metastases were found in eight; of the 23 patients with lower thoracic esophageal cancer seven had intraabdominal dissemination.

Preoperative laparoscopic assessment of the peritoneal cavity in esophageal cancer permits accurate planning of the therapy. In the presence of intraabdominal dissemination, palliative surgery or conservative treatment is chosen, whereas in the absence of intraabdominal metastases, radical surgery is recommended and undertaken with greater certainty.

Carcinoma of the Rectum

Sotnikov and Aganiov[28] reported on 35 cases of carcinoma of the rectum where a routine laparoscopy was performed preoperatively. In three patients they noted liver metastasis; in four, multiple metastases were seen in the abdominal organs; in one, metastases were present in the parietal peritoneum. In the remaining 27 no metastases were noted.

The preoperative use of laparoscopy in carcinoma of the rectum permits the determination of the extent of the disease and hence the therapy to be undertaken. In cases not associated with metastasis, radical surgery was recommended.

Positioning of the operating table (Trendelenburg position) and the use of a probe to elevate the sigmoid are essential for a more accurate visualization of the pelvis.

Carcinoma of the Pancreas

Despite its location in the retroperitoneal space, the pancreas, in most cases, is accessible to laparoscopic examination and to directed biopsy. The inspection of the pancreas by laparoscopy is actually the inspection of the lesser omentum. The body of the pancreas, the lesser curvature of the stomach, the coeliac lymph nodes, etc., can be inspected successfully if the patient is not too obese.

Meyer-Burg,[13] reporting on a series of 125 laparoscopies, was able to visualize parts of the pancreatic body in 81 patients (65%). In 15 of them carcinoma of the pancreas was diagnosed, which demonstrates selection in the patients subjected to the procedure. In this series, material was obtained for histological examination in 16 patients and for cytological examination in 31. There were no associated complications. The author attaches special importance to the palpation of the pancreas during its inspection.

The technique requires elevation of the head of the operating table and the patient to be in the right decubitus position. A 130° scope is preferable. The left lobe of the liver is elevated with the rounded tip of the laparoscope or with a probe. Needle biopsies may be obtained under direct vision.[14,15] It must be stressed, however, that this technique allows the visualization of only parts of the pancreatic body.

Second-Look Procedures

The question of tumor progression following the initial phases of treatment often arises. Symptoms of bowel obstruction, pain and weight loss may arise from treatment procedures such as radiation or chemotherapy rather than from a continuing neoplastic process. In these circumstances peritoneal endoscopy is particularly helpful.

Such a case was encountered recently in a 54-year-old woman lost to follow-up for two years after radiation therapy for a stage IIa cervical carcinoma. She reappeared with left flank pain and a nonfunctioning kidney on that side. Pelvic examination could not differentiate between tumor and radiation reaction. Vaginal biopsy and cystoscopy were not positive for tumor recurrence. Laparoscopy with biopsy of retroperitoneal tumor and lymph nodes solved the issue.

Smith,[26] at the Mason Clinic, has evaluated 27 patients following initial treatment for cancer of the cervix, endometrium, ovary, tube, colon, stomach, kidney, lung and breast. In two patients a pneumoperitoneum could not be established. Recurrence was documented in 15 of the remaining 25. Cope and Gomel[7] recommend left subcostal insufflation in this group of patients.

We recently evaluated a patient who had an emergency cecostomy performed for obstruction secondary to a carcinoma at that site. Subsequent irradiation was given prior to a planned radical surgical procedure. Laparoscopic biopsy, however, demonstrated metastases to the uterine serosa and cul-de-sac, which altered the plan of management.

Laparoscopy soon after removal of stage I ovarian carcinoma may be helpful in evaluation of further treatment in asymptomatic patients. It may then be used to follow the course of patients receiving further therapy.

Conclusions

Laparoscopy has great potential in the diagnosis and staging of intraabdominal malignancy. The value of this procedure in the primary diagnosis of carcinoma of the ovary, liver, gallbladder and pancreas has been outlined. Its importance in determining the extent of the disease process in carcinoma of the esophagus and abdominal organs (stomach, bowel, rectum, etc.) and Hodgkin's disease has been demonstrated. It allows proper planning of the therapy and, in many cases, avoids unnecessary laparotomy or radical procedures which offer no hope for cure. The current consensus is that staging laparotomy should be performed only if laparoscopic inspection and biopsies are negative.

Laparoscopy is presently being tried as a therapeutic tool with a view to improving results in ovarian carcinoma. It is probable that laparoscopy will play a particularly useful role in periodic assessment of treated cancer patients. Nevertheless, much of the potential is yet to be realized. With adherence to proper technique, the procedure has a wide margin of safety. Large series demonstrating safety and accuracy would encourage a more liberal use of the procedure. Second- and third-look laparoscopies may become routine in the follow-up of intraabdominal malignancies.

References

1. Albert ME, Hutt MSR, Davidson CS: Primary hepatoma in Uganda. A prospective clinical and epidemiologic study of forty-six patients. Am J Med 46:794, 1969

2. Bagley CM, Thomas LB, Johnson RE, Chretien PB, DeVita VT: Diagnosis of liver involvement by lymphoma: results in 96 consecutive peritoneoscopies. Cancer 31:840, 1973

3. Beck K (Editor): Color Atlas of Laparoscopy. F. K. Schattauer, Berlag, 1969

4. Canossi GC, Cortesi N, Manenti A, Gibertini G, Jr.: Scintigrafia epatica e laparoscopia nella ricerca della metastasi del fetago. Minerva Chir 30:126, 1975

5. Casirola C, Ippoliti G, Marini G: Laparoscopy in Hodgkin's Disease. Acta Haematol 49:1, 1973

6. Chan KT: The management of primary liver carcinoma. Ann R Coll Surg Engl 41:253, 1967

7. Cope JL, Gomel V: Laparoscopy in the treatment of early ovarian malignancy (unpublished data)

8. De Dios Vega JF, Hita Perez J, Mura González J, Cosme Jiménez A, Miño Fugarolas G, Cano López JM: Valor de la laparoscopia en el diagnóstico del cáncer de vesícula biliar. Rev Esp Enferm Apar Dig 61:867, 1973

9. Etienne J-P, Chaput J-C, Feydy P, Gueroult N: La laparoscopie dans le cancer primitif du foie de l'adulte. Ann Gastroenterol Hepatol 9:49, 1973

10. Frangenheim J, Stockhammer, H: La laparoscopie dans le diagnostic-différentiel des tumeurs du petit bassin chez les femmes ménopausées. Gynaecologia 167:503, 1969

11. Jacobs ME: La laparoscopie dans le diagnostic du cancer primitif du foie. Arch Fr Mal App Dig 61:407, 1972

12. Lenzi G, Grillo A, Bonazzi L, Zini M, Gritti FM: Laparoscopia e scintigrafia. Minerva Gastroenterol 21:154, 1971

13. Meyer-Burg J, Ziegler U, Palme G: Zur supragastralen Pankreaskopie. Dtsch Med Wochenschr 97:1969, 1972

14. Meyer-Burg J: The inspection, palpation and biopsy of the pancreas by peritoneoscopy. Endoscopy 4:99, 1972

15. Meyer-Burg J: Inspección laparoscópica del páncreas. Rev Esp Enferm Apar Dig 38:697, 1972

16. Meyers MA: The spread and localization of acute intraperitoneal effusions. Radiology 95:547, 1970

17. Mintz M, Elmach H, Brux J: de Cancer de l'ovaire décelé par ponction d'un kyste sous coelioscopie. XXe Congr des Féd. de Gyn et Obst de langue franc, Lille, 1963 (Masson, Paris 1963)

18. Müller JH: Curative aim and results of routine intraperitoneal radiocolloid administration in the treatment of ovarian cancer. Am J Roentgenol Radium Ther Nucl Med 89:533, 1963

19. Nelson RS, de Elisalde R, Howe CD: Clinical aspect of primary carcinoma of the liver. Cancer 19:533, 1966

20. Rosenoff SH, Young RC, Anderson T, Bagley C, Chabner B, Schein PS, Hubbard S, DeVita VT: Peritoneoscopy: a valuable tool for the initial staging and "second look" in ovarian carcinoma. Ann Int Med (In press)

21. Ruddock, JC: Peritoneoscopy. Southern Surgeon 8:113, 1939

22. Samuelson S, Sjöval A: The value of laparoscopy in the differential diagnosis between uterine fibromyomata and adnexal tumours. Acta Obstet Gynecol Scand 49:175, 1970

23. Sauer R, Fahrländer H, Fridrich R: Comparison of the accuracy of liver scans and peritoneoscopy in benign and malignant primary and metastatic tumours of the liver. Scand J Gastroenterol 8:389, 1973

24. Sauer R, Müller J: Der Wert der Kolloid-und Leberzellszintigraphic sowie der Laparoskopic und Leberserologic bei der Diagnose von Lebergeschwülsten. Schweiz Med Wochenschr 104:1085, 1974

25. Sauer R, Fridich R, Fahrländer H: Zur Diagnostik chronischer Lebererkrankungen mit Hilfe der Radiokolloid-Szintigraphie. Ein Vergleich der szintigraphischen und laparoskopischen Treffsicherheit anhand von 309 simultan untersuchten Patienten. Fortschr Geb Roentgenstr nuklearmed 119:175, 1973

26. Smith M: Personal communication

27. Sotnikov VN, Enmolov AS, Litvinov VI, Emeljyanov SS, Samsonov VS: The diagnosis of intraabdominal metastases of esophageal cancer by means of laparoscopy. Vopr Onkol 19:38, 1973

28. Sotnikov VN, Agamov AG: Laparoscopic diagnosis of intraabdominal metastases in cancer of the rectum. Sov Med 10:108, 1974

29. Spinelli P, Beretta G, Bajetta E, Tancini G, Castellani R, Rilke F, Bonadonna G: Laparoscopy and laparotomy combined with bone marrow biopsy in staging Hodgkin's disease. Br Med J 4:554, 1975

30. Vido I, Hundeshagen H, Becker H, Schmidt FW: Vergleich laparoskopischer und szintigraphischer Befunde bei chronischer Hepatitis, Leberzirrhose und Lebertumoren. Dtsch Med Wochenschr 100:129, 1975

Section 6

Operative Procedures

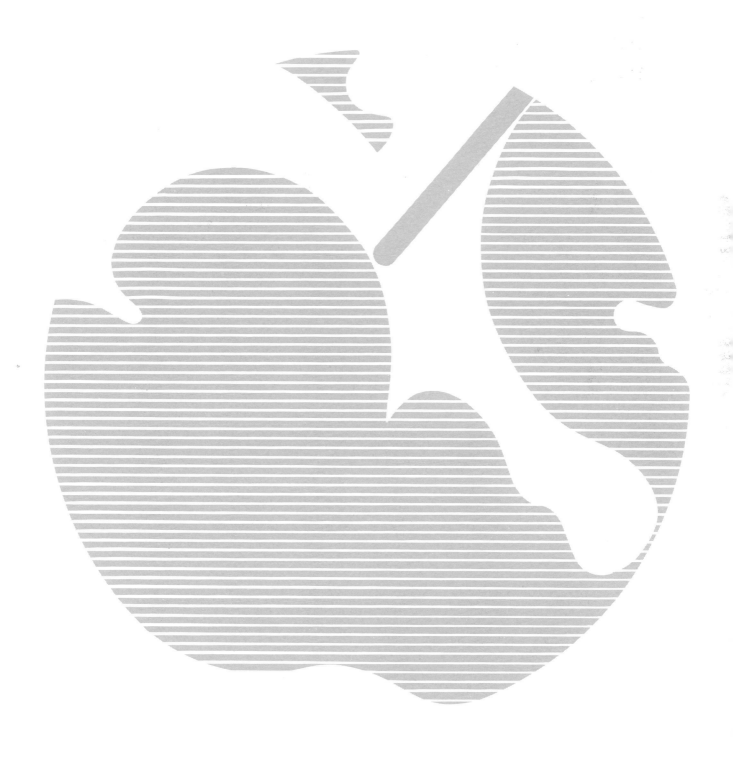

Chapter 14

Operative Laparoscopy: An Overview

Alvin M. Siegler, M.D.

Laparoscopy has become an essential component of training in gynecology because of its value in improving the accuracy in diagnosis of many pelvic diseases. In addition, specialized operative procedures such as tubal sterilization and recovery of extrauterine intrauterine devices (IUD) have become accepted extensions of its use. As the surgeons became more skillful, other minor procedures involving the uterus, tubes, ovaries and uterine ligaments were developed. Unquestionably, some of these operations are technically more difficult, increasing the risk to the patient. It is incumbent upon the physician to decide in each instance whether the hazard of operative intervention is offset by its benefits and the expected relief of the patient's preoperative complaints. The authors of the chapters in this section on operative laparoscopy have described some of these specialized techniques, and all of them agree that at least two abdominal punctures are necessary, one for the laparoscope and the other for accessory instruments.

The diagnosis of an unruptured tubal pregnancy is clinically difficult. If the rupture is accompanied by hemorrhagic shock, an immediate laparotomy is required and laparoscopy is contraindicated. The increased use of laparoscopy has improved the accuracy in early diagnosis: about 20% are discovered prior to rupture. Opportunities resulted for removal of some unruptured tubal pregnancies under laparoscopic control, and techniques were described by several authors. Esposito emphasizes that one prerequisite is a 2 to 3 cm gestational mass in a freely moveable, intact, middle or outer tubal segment. Given this gross appearance, the pathologic area can be grasped and either excised by coagulation, by the snare technique or hypothetically by a tubal ligation procedure. However, bleeding can occur from the resected area, the specimen can be too large to withdraw through the sheath used for the accessory instrument and sometimes these operative methods leave behind an appreciable residual segment of proximal tube which possibly predisposes the patient to another tubal pregnancy. Complete salpingectomy at laparotomy or, in selected instances, tubal conservation by techniques involving removal of the products of conception seems safer and more desirable.

Laparoscopy permits performance of minor operative procedures on infertile patients. Gomel describes the laparoscopic surgical treatment of pelvic endometriosis and endometriomas, polycystic ovaries, ampullary or fimbrial phimosis, clinically significant adherent tubes or ovaries and distal tubal occlusion. In all of these conditions the double- or triple-puncture technique is advocated.

Coagulation is suggested for endometriotic implants, and some ovaries which adhere to the posterior leaf of the broad ligament can be mobilized by lysis of periovarial adhesions. It is important to avoid excessive current, its prolonged application and injury to juxtaposed organs such as the fallopian tube, intestines and ureter. Gomel recommends aspiration of endometriomas. The evidence that such techniques corrected infertility is not convincing because in many patients progestins also were used postoperatively. Ovarian endometriosis, which causes adherence to the posterior leaf of the broad ligament, results from multiple, thick, relatively inaccessible adhesions which are difficult to remove under laparoscopic control. Clinically significant endometriosis in the infertile woman probably is treated best by careful, sharp dissection and excision or coagulation of implants during laparotomy.

The diagnostic value of ovarian biopsy in the management of polycystic ovaries is questionable because the gross appearance of bilateral, smooth, gray-white, enlarged ovaries with subcapsular vessels and small cysts is characteristic. Ovaries larger than 4 cm probably should be resected primarily. Ovarian wedge resection made under laparoscopic control rarely is indicated and can be dangerous. The failure to consistently induce ovulation following carefully selected doses of clomiphene citrate for a few months in the smaller polycystic ovaries or to effect a pregnancy after a trial of six to eight months in some of these patients who ostensibly ovulate is another indication for wedge resection. At laparotomy the surgeon has the opportunity to precisely resect and approximate ovarian edges. One reason for a patient's failing to conceive subsequently despite ovulation results from postoperative periovarial or peritubal adhesions. Meticulous hemostasis, imbrication of cut surfaces and precise ovarian reconstruction are not feasible by laparoscopic techniques. Although ovulation and occasionally conception may follow a unilateral ovarian biopsy in patients with polycystic ovaries, some women with this disease become pregnant without therapy.

Yuzpe describes the techniques for obtaining adequate specimens and correctly emphasizes that the biopsy site should be near the free ovarian surface rather than the mesovarium. The defects rarely require coagulation, and the risks are minimal. Laparoscopic ovarian biopsy can be helpful in the diagnosis of patients with primary amenorrhea and normal pituitary gonadotropins. If numerous primordial follicles are seen in the ovarian specimen, then stimulation with menotropins is indicated. A reliable endocrinologic assay showing a normal follicle stimulating hormone (FSH) almost always indicates a follicular apparatus whereas a high FSH means that little endogenous estrogen is available. The causes of secondary amenorrhea in women who have had a normal pelvic examination can be ascertained in most instances by their response to intramuscular progesterone and the findings from radioimmunoassay of FSH and luteinizing hormone (LH). The additional information provided by study of ovarian histology usually is not helpful in diagnosis or management of these patients. In the patient suspected of having a dysgenetic gonad, ovarian specimens are sometimes difficult to procure because of their small, linear shapes and proximity to the posterior leaf of the broad ligament. Ovarian specimens thus obtained can be submitted for karyotyping to exclude an XY pattern and possible need for gonadectomy.

In Yuzpe's series 12% of the ovarian biopsy specimens obtained by laparoscopy did not show follicular or stromal activity, and these ovaries were classified as inactive. How did the histology correlate with the clinical history and endocrinologic findings? Were these inadequate biopsies? If no follicular tissue is found, amenorrhea is persistent and unresponsive to treatment.

Unlike ovarian operations by laparoscopy to correct infertility, some types of tuboplasty seem feasible and logical. Thick pelvic adhesions involving omentum or intestine cannot be dissected safely by coagulation and lysis under laparoscopic control. Severe bleeding or thermal intestinal injuries are potential complications. Lysis of thin, avascular peritubal adhesions can free adherent tubes or fimbriae. Gomel reported that 17 of 37 women (46%) who had peritubal adhesions, some with fimbrial phimosis or periovarial adhesions, became pregnant and delivered following surgical treatment under laparoscopic observation. These results are extraordinarily good in any group of infertility patients, and other investigators should attempt to duplicate his experience. Fimbriae are very delicate and sometimes bleed easily while held with fine forceps, and thrusting blunt ones into fimbrial ostia for dilatation is only for an expert laparoscopist. Laparoscopic tubostomy of distally occluded tubes following a previously failed tuboplasty is suggested by Gomel. Although he does not advocate the operation as a primary procedure, intrauterine pregnancies followed in three of seven such patients. The results obviously are excellent, and the technique deserves an extended trial by others.

Hasson defines *open laparoscopy* as a combination of a subumbilical "mini" laparotomy with laparoscopy during which a large, blunt trocar and sleeve are inserted into the peritoneal cavity. Pneumoperitoneum is created subsequently. The additional time required to create adequate abdominal distention (4 to 20 minutes) is discounted because of the accuracy and safety claimed for this technique. Another theoretical advantage is repair of the abdominal wall in anatomical layers following removal of the trocar. In 500 patients open laparoscopy permitted adequate observation of the pelvic organs in every instance. Indications are the same as those for conventional laparoscopic procedures (56% tubal sterilization), and Hasson's incidence of 1.6% complications requiring laparotomy (8 patients) was comparable to other series of similar sizes and types of patients. Although 137 (27%) of the patients had a previous laparotomy, most investigators do not believe conventional laparoscopy is hazardous in these women. Hasson and co-workers have had the largest experience with this variation of laparoscopy. Although the method appears more complicated, open laparoscopy could be valuable in women in whom initial induction of pneumoperitoneum followed by trocar insertion was potentially more hazardous, such as the patient with proven ovarian cancer.

Suspension of a moveable but retrodisplaced uterus can be performed under laparoscopic control according to the technique described by Marik and a few other gynecologists. The risks are greater than the potential benefits. Most retrodisplaced uteri unassociated with significant pelvic pathology are asymptomatic. Correction of a retroverted uterus fixed by endometriosis, intestinal adhesions or adnexal masses requires a laparotomy to cure the principal pathology; the uterine suspension is an ancillary procedure. What are the indications for uterine suspension by laparoscopy, and were the patients' complaints relieved? Judgement combined with skill contributes to better surgical practice; based upon clinical experience, the indications for laparoscopic uterine suspension must be very infrequent. There are no contemporary data to support the use of this procedure as a primary operation.

Although the intrauterine contraceptive device (IUD) is universally accepted as a safe, reliable method of contraception, occasionally these devices are misplaced during their insertion or become displaced following an initial, partial uterine perforation. Under laparoscopic control the intraperitoneal position of IUDs can be localized and their removal accomplished with accessory instruments. Ectopic IUDs generally are free in the cul-de-sac but sometimes are covered or enmeshed with filmy adhesions. They can be freed and manipulated without difficulty in most instances. Traction can dislodge them from omentum or adhesions. The device can be grasped and removed easily by pulling it out together with the sleeve of the trocar. Israel has described preoperative methods of localization and laparoscopic techniques for removal of ectopic, intraperitoneal IUDs. Although little scientific evidence exists to support the argument for removal of all such misplaced devices, the consensus seems to be for their extraction whether they are classified as open or closed.

Ovarian Biopsy

A. Albert Yuzpe, M.D.

In many patients who have ovular dysfunction and menstrual disorders a clinical diagnosis is established by means of a thorough history, physical examination and various biochemical and endocrinological tests.

Sometimes, information about ovarian histology can aid in formulating a more precise diagnosis, prognosis and plan of management. In addition, the tissue can be karyotyped as well as analyzed biochemically. Such analyses include the biosynthesis of estrogens, progesterone and androgens as well as the effects of exogenous gonadotropins on their *in vitro* production. Pure cultures of granulosa cells may also be prepared from such specimens and studied in a similar fashion. Also, prostaglandin levels in ovarian tissue and follicular fluid may be evaluated.

The indications for performing laparoscopic ovarian biopsy are presented in order of frequency and importance (Table 1). It is essential to remember, however, that not every case in each category requires or merits biopsy. This issue will be considered further in the subsequent discussion.

Table 1
Relative Indications for Laparoscopic
Ovarian Biopsy

Amenorrhea— primary   — secondary
Infertility— primary   — secondary
Oligomenorrhea
Hirsutism
Failure to respond with ovulation to clomiphene citrate alone or combined with human chorionic gonadotropin
Assessment prior to treatment with human gonadotropins
Suspected genetic anomaly
Suspected ovarian neoplasm
Precocious puberty of ovarian or undiagnosed origin

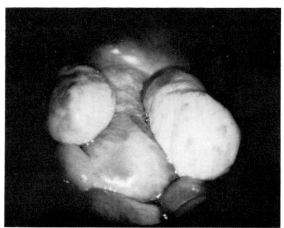

Figure 1
Ovarian position in preparation for biopsy. The uterus has been forced into retroversion, displacing the ovaries into an anterior position.

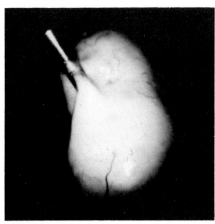

Figure 2
The ovary is grasped at its antehilar margin.

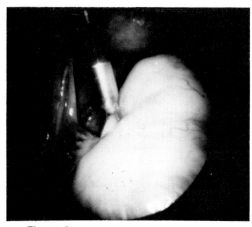

Figure 3
The biopsy forceps is turned at right angles to the ovary.

Technique of Ovarian Biopsy Under Laparoscopic Control

The procedure is performed under general anesthesia with endotracheal intubation and assisted ventilation. Since electrosurgery may be employed, a ground plate must be placed securely under the patient's buttocks.

To make the ovaries easily accessible for biopsy the uterine corpus is first retroverted or forced back into the hollow of the sacrum, using a uterine manipulator (Cohen-Eder, Corson or Semm). The fundus is then swept anteriorly along either of the pelvic sidewalls with a prying motion of the manipulator. This procedure forces the tube and ovary on the appropriate side to come to rest anterior to the fundus in full view (Figure 1). An assistant holds the instrument in position as the operator performs the biopsy; the site remains in full view throughout the procedure to facilitate inspection and possible subsequent electrocoagulation. This maneuver is extremely helpful, especially if bleeding is excessive.

Other alternatives for exposing and immobilizing the ovaries are necessary in patients in whom (1) the vagina is too narrow for insertion of the uterine cannula, (2) the uterine fundus is too small to manipulate the ovaries into the proper position, (3) the ovarian ligament is too short to permit ovarian mobilization, (4) the gonads are very small and not mobile, (5) the ovary and/or the tube are/is fixed by adhesions.

Technical variations to overcome some of the anatomical abnormalities cited are described below:

1. The operating laparoscope is used with a 3 or 5 mm channel plus an ancillary instrument inserted through a second puncture. The ovary can either be stabilized or biopsied with a second puncture instrument or with the instrument passed through the operating laparoscope

2. Through a third puncture a grasping instrument can stabilize the ovary while the biopsy is performed, if an operating laparoscope is unavailable, with the forceps inserted through the second puncture

3. Utilizing a grasping instrument to immobilize the ovary, a needle biopsy can be taken. However, this technique provides only very small specimens[3, 9]

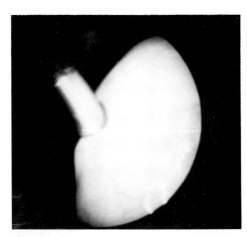

Figure 4
The knife is turned down, excising the specimen.

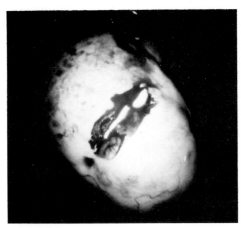

Figure 5
The biopsy site remains in full view. Bleeding is not excessive.

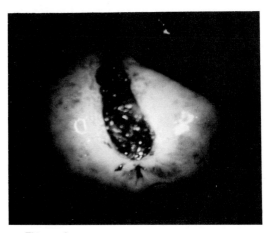

Figure 6
The ovarian biopsy site following coagulation.

4. A 3 mm punch forceps (Siegler forceps) is preferable in patients whose ovaries are small since the hilar vessels are more easily avoided. Instruments used for ovarian biopsy are listed in Table 2.

The Palmer biopsy forceps (one- or two-puncture technique), or one of its modifications, obtains the most adequate specimen in most situations.

1. The ovary is grasped at its free margin, away from the hilar vessels (Figure 2). The tissue within the jaws of the instrument eventually will be removed as the biopsy specimen

2. The forceps is turned at right angles to the ovary (Figure 3)

3. The knife or drill is rotated until the specimen has been separated cleanly from the ovary (Figure 4), and the forceps, which is still grasping the biopsy specimen in its jaws, is removed from the sheath

4. The ovarian defect is inspected (Figure 5), and if significant bleeding is present, the site is coagulated. The forceps is reinserted, and only then is the connecting cable from the electrosurgical generator attached. This avoids inadvertent injury if the foot pedal were activated accidentally during any of the previous steps. Only two or three applications of blended current are necessary for complete hemostasis (Figure 6). If the margins of the biopsy site bleed, they are grasped between the forceps jaws and coagulated. When the base of the biopsy bed bleeds, the tip of the closed forceps is applied directly to it. A spherical-, coagulating-tipped instrument may also be employed for this purpose although it is usually more convenient to utilize the same biopsy forceps.

Table 2
Instruments Used in Ovarian Biopsy*

Single Puncture Technique

Telescope— Operating Laparoscope

Biopsy Instruments— 3 mm or 5 mm instruments

Single jaw action biopsy forceps (Lancet, tapered or rounded forceps)

Single- or double-spoon-shaped jaws (for punch biopsies)

Palmer biopsy forceps—5 mm only

Double Puncture Technique

Telescope— Any Laparoscope

Biopsy Instruments— 3 mm or 5 mm instruments

Palmer biopsy forceps or its modifications— i.e., Cohen-Eder, Eder-Barton, Palmer-Neuwirth

Single jaw action— similar shapes as for single puncture

Double jaw action— Semm, single- or double-spoon jaws

* Forceps and cannulae must be insulated.

Whenever possible, both ovaries should be biopsied since similar findings in both specimens add validity to the pathologic interpretation. Furthermore, multiple biopsies, as in the case of the Stein-Leventhal syndrome, may be therapeutic.

Jaw-type forceps may require the aid of "cutting current" from an electrosurgical unit to obtain final separation of the specimen from the ovary. This is especially true when the ovarian tunica is thick, thus preventing complete closure of the jaw.

Complications

Complications specifically related to ovarian biopsy are described in the following section and also have been described in the literature.[4,5,11] In experienced hands they are rare.[13]

1. Acute or delayed hemorrhage from the biopsy site. This problem is caused by (a) too deep a cut into the ovary (especially those of small volume), thus involving medullary vessels, (b) tearing of the ovarian tissue when attempting to separate the specimen from the ovary, (c) biopsying too close to the hilar vessels, thus traumatizing one or more of them.

Excessive coagulation may act adversely in that it can cover the surface of the ovarian defect and obscure a bleeding site. As with liver biopsies, most ovaries bleed minimally after biopsy and then a clot forms, which obviates the need for electrocoagulation.

The forceps jaws also become coated with coagulum during electrocoagulation, which causes them to adhere to the biopsy site. Through another, lower abdominal puncture an irrigating cannula is inserted (a suction cannula to which a syringe containing sterile saline is attached), and the biopsy site is simultaneously irrigated and coagulated. Routine irrigation of the biopsied area following its coagulation may prevent delayed hematoma formation by identifying and coagulating remaining small bleeding points. If such a cannula is unavailable, a spinal needle attached to a syringe may be inserted transabdominally over the area of the ovary and the irrigation performed.

A suction cannula in the cul-de-sac can aspirate blood and irrigation fluid which has accumulated during the procedure. The same syringe used for irrigation may be employed for this purpose.

2. Mechanical or electrosurgical ureteral injury. Mechanical injury should never occur if the ovary is manipulated properly prior to biopsy. With

Table 3
Ovarian Biopsy—Pathologic Assessment

Name

Age   Menarche

Clinical history:

Amenorrhea	◯ Primary	◯ Secondary	Duration
Oligomenorrhea	◯ Yes	◯ No	
Hirsutism	◯ Yes	◯ No	

Other

Size

Gross appearance:

Microscopic appearance:

Capsule	◯ Thickened	◯ Normal	

Other

Follicular apparatus	◯ Normal	◯ Decreased	◯ Absent
Primary follicles	◯ Yes	◯ No	
Secondary follicles	◯ Yes	◯ No	
Tertiary follicles	◯ Yes	◯ No	
Corpus luteum	◯ Yes	◯ No	
Corpus albicans	◯ Yes	◯ No	

Other

Specialized stroma	◯ Normal	◯ Hyperplasia

Other

Supporting stroma	◯ Normal

Other

Tissue karyotype

Biochemistry

adequate pneumoperitoneum and in the Trendelenburg position the pelvis should be devoid of intestinal loops. The pelvic course of the ureter can often be identified, especially in patients with streak or hypoplastic gonads.

3. Mechanical or electrosurgical tubal injury. The uterine and ovarian manipulation procedure previously described will minimize the possibility of inadvertently grasping a portion of the tubal serosa since the tube tends to fall away laterally from the ovary.

Interpretation of Laparoscopic Ovarian Biopsies

Black and Govan,[2] and Steele and colleagues[10] suggest that biopsy specimens containing at least a 1 cm arc of ovarian circumference are representative of the entire ovary. However, Sutton disagrees with this opinion and has cited cases in which some women in whom no follicles were found on biopsy ultimately conceived. Endocrinologic evaluation, however, was also misleading in his examples. One explanation may be that the biopsy specimens in his study were not adequate enough and thus not representative of the entire ovarian substance. Sykes and Ginsburg[12] have also reported elevated gonadotropins in patients with primary amenorrhea in the presence of an apparently normal follicular apparatus.

From an ovarian biopsy specimen accurate evaluation may be made of the capsule, follicular apparatus, supporting stroma, corpora lutea and albicantia, etc. These data may be documented on a form such as that seen in Table 3.

Results

Most laparoscopic ovarian biopsies have been performed because of unexplained amenorrhea or infertility.[1, 6, 8, 12] When the basal body temperature and endometrium suggest ovulation and a good luteal phase is present, ovarian biopsy is unnecessary in the infertile patient. In instances of anovulation, hirsutism or enlarged ovaries, biopsy specimens are sometimes helpful in conjunction with endocrinologic evaluation in order to establish an accurate diagnosis and plan for treatment.

The gross and histologic appearance of the ovaries permits a more accurate classification of primary ovarian failure, according to Kinch and co-workers.[7] Follicular and afollicular forms can be distinguished, thus enabling potential candidates for gonadotropin therapy to be selected.

In a review of 454 patients who had ovarian biopsies pathology was found in 73.2%.[13] The great majority of these biopsies substantiated the preoperative clinical diagnosis. However, in 18% of cases unexpected findings resulted in an alteration of diagnosis, prognosis and subsequent management. The major unsuspected pathology was a decrease in the number of follicles. The subsequent pregnancy rate in women exhibiting such pathology regardless of therapy has been found by Sykes and Ginsburg to be decreased to 20% to 25%.

Our experience has been very similar. In such women, especially when under 25 years of age, the time available for them to conceive may be limited, and thus treatment should not be delayed. Furthermore, when no germinal tissue is present, the futility and expense of treatment can be avoided.

Conclusion

The major value of laparoscopic ovarian biopsy lies in evaluating selected cases of amenorrhea and infertility. It can be performed safely on an outpatient basis. Proper instruments and a thorough knowledge of the techniques and potential hazards of the procedure are essential prerequisites for performing the procedure.

References

1. Black WP, Govan ADT: Laparoscopy and gonadal biopsy for assessment of gonadal function in primary amenorrhea. Br Med J 1:672, 1972

2. Black WP, Govan ADT: Laparoscopy and ovarian biopsy for the assessment of secondary amenorrhea. Am J Obstet Gynecol 114:739, 1972

3. Cohen MR: Ovarian biopsy via peritoneoscopy. J Reprod Med 1:436, 1968

4. Duignan NM, Jordan JA, Coughlan BM, Logan-Edwards R: 1000 consecutive cases of diagnostic laparoscopy. J Obstet Gynecol Br Commonw 81:317, 1974

5. Esposito JM, Rubino G: Bleeding after ovarian biopsy under laparoscopic vision. Am J Obstet Gynecol 119:857, 1975

6. Khoo SK, MacKay EV: Primary amenorrhea: a study based on clinical examination, chromosomal analysis, endocrine assay and laparoscopy. Med J Aust 2:991, 1972

7. Kinch RAH, Plunkett ER, Smout MS, Carr DH: Primary ovarian failure. Am J Obstet Gynecol 91:630, 1965

8. Neuwirth RS: A method of bilateral ovarian biopsy at laparoscopy in infertility and chronic anovulation. Fertil Steril 23:361, 1972

9. Palmer R: *Les Explorations Fonctionelles Gynecologiques.* Masson et Cie, Paris, 1963, p 375

10. Steele SJ, Beilby JOW, Papadaki L: Visualization and biopsy of the ovary in the investigation of amenorrhea. Obstet Gynecol 36:899, 1970

11. Sutton C: The limitations of laparoscopic ovarian biopsy. J Obstet Gynecol Br Commonw 81:317, 1974

12. Sykes DW, Ginsburg J: The use of laparoscopic ovarian biopsy to assess gonadal function. Am J Obstet Gynecol 112:408, 1972

13. Yuzpe AA, Rioux J-E: The value of laparoscopic ovarian biopsy. J Reprod Med 15:57, 1975

Removal of Extrauterine Intrauterine Devices

Robert Israel, M.D.

Oh, do not ask, "*Where* is it?"
Let us go and make our visit.

paraphrased from
"The Love Song of J. Alfred Prufrock"
by T. S. Eliot (1917)

Although uterine perforation with an intrauterine contraceptive device (IUD) is uncommon, its occurrence requires surgical removal of the IUD. The laparoscope permits both definitive localization of the intraabdominal IUD and a route of removal.

Workup

The plan outlined in Figure 1 provides a systematic approach to the problem of attempting to locate a "lost" IUD. An initial history is taken and a physical, with pelvic, examination is performed. If the IUD is identified by the presence of its intravaginal appendage, it can either be removed or left in utero. However, if the IUD strings are *not* visualized, the uterine cavity should be probed with a sound. When the IUD is felt easily, removal should be attempted with an IUD retriever of the "crochet hook" type. Prolonged intrauterine probing must be avoided. If the position of the IUD is in question or a quick removal is not achieved, a paracervical block should be applied and the hysteroscope, if available, utilized to secure and remove the device. Even a partially embedded IUD can be grasped via direct hysteroscopic visualization, gently extracted from the myometrium and removed from the uterine cavity without undue blood loss.

If the IUD is not found in the uterus, further attempts at localization should be carried out with various x-ray techniques or ultrasound. Unless the IUD is well out of the pelvis (Figure 2), a plain flatplate of the abdomen will not diagnose it definitively as being extrauterine. Before an x-ray is obtained, one of three techniques can be employed to "mark" the uterus. Another IUD can be inserted into the endometrial cavity (Figure 3) before the routine anterior-posterior (AP) and lateral x-rays of the abdomen are obtained. Even simpler, an intrauterine sound can be inserted and held in place while the AP (Figure 4) and lateral (Figure 5) films are taken. When this technique is utilized, care should be taken to insure that the sound remains in place throughout the entire study and does not slip down into the lower uterine segment or cervix. The opposite extreme must also be avoided—perforating the uterus with the sound. Since an intrauterine sound fills only a small portion of the endometrial cavity and the surrounding myometrium can be quite variable in thickness, an IUD which is definitely extrauterine must be well away from the

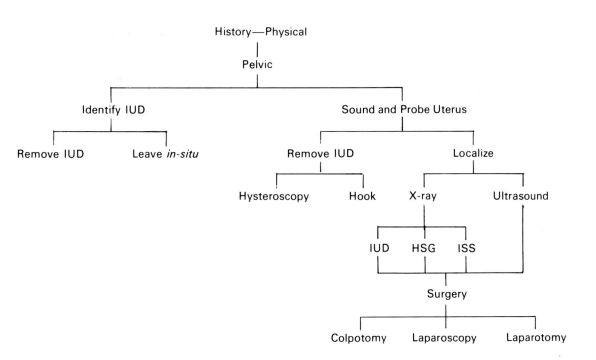

Figure 1
Diagnostic techniques for localization and removal
of extrauterine IUDs

sound and/or abnormally angulated. The most definitive x-ray technique for localizing the extrauterine IUD is the hysterosalpingogram (HSG) (Figure 6).

Once the various diagnostic techniques described above demonstrate an IUD in the abdominal cavity, surgery may be utilized to pinpoint the location of the IUD and remove it. Should the device be easily palpable in the anterior or posterior cul-de-sac, a colpotomy may be the easiest and most direct approach. However, laparoscopy will be the primary surgical technique in most cases and laparotomy reserved for the occasional failure of laparoscopic removal or for cases in which concomitant pelvic pathology is found.

Laparoscopic Techniques
Preoperatively, the patient with an intraabdominal IUD must sign an informed consent which includes the possibility of an exploratory laparotomy. Unlike laparoscopic sterilization, the removal of an extrauterine IUD might *not* be considered an outpatient procedure by some. In addition, it should only be attempted by an abdominal surgeon who is comfortable with *both* diagnostic and operative laparoscopy.

Since intraabdominal manipulation may have to be extensive in order to free up an extrauterine IUD, a general anesthetic with endotracheal intubation and relaxant medication is generally employed. For similar reasons—the need for good visualization and considerable surgical maneuvering—double-puncture laparoscopic technique is preferable. On occasion, a third puncture may be necessary in order to dissect the IUD away from investing adhesions. With the laparoscope inserted through the infraumbilical rim, lower quadrant incisions may be utilized for probes, grasping forceps and/or dissecting scissors. The previously obtained, localizing x-ray should be in the operating room for reference purposes. However, if days or weeks have passed between the x-rays and the surgery, the IUD may have continued to wander in the peritoneal cavity and be in a location other than that indicated on the films. A careful, systematic, intraabdominal search must be carried out under laparoscopic visualization with the aid of a single palpating probe placed through a lower quadrant trocar sheath. If the IUD is not located immediately, the probe can be utilized to mobilize bowel, "palpate" the omentum and compress the leaves of the

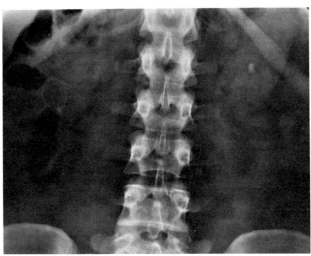

Figure 2
Abdominal x-ray showing Dalkon Shield *(right upper quadrant)*, well out of pelvis.

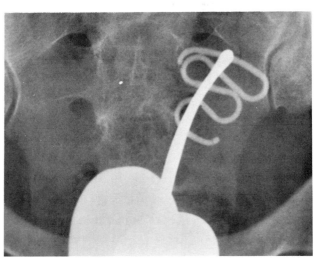

Figure 4
Intrauterine sound study (ISS). AP x-ray shows sound overlying Lippes Loop.

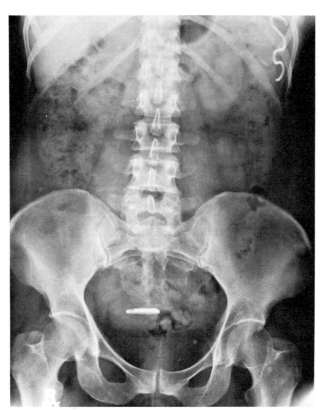

Figure 3
Abdominal x-ray showing distorted, extrauterine Lippes Loop *(left upper quadrant)* and a "marking" Lippes Loop in uterus.

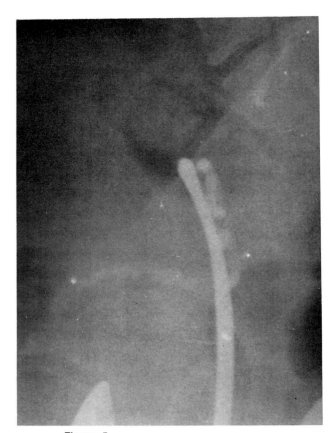

Figure 5
Intrauterine sound study (ISS). Lateral x-ray shows sound in close approximation to Lippes Loop. Together Figures 4 and 5 confirm intrauterine site for Lippes Loop.

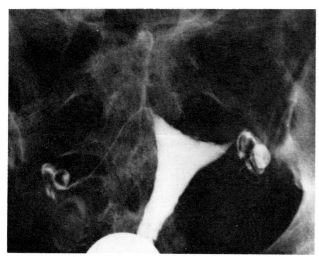

Figure 6
Hysterosalpingogram (HSG) confirms extrauterine location of Dalkon Shield seen below right fallopian tube.

broad ligament to exclude an intraligamentous perforation. In addition, the peritoneal reflection of the vesicouterine fold may be probed. With the laparoscope as a scanning eye and the accessory probe as an examining fingertip, every intraabdominal IUD should be located.

Specific kinds of IUDs can create their own particular problems. The external copper wire around the vertical arm of the copper 7 and copper T IUDs causes considerable tissue reaction. Chronic inflammatory changes and adhesions between intraperitoneal structures will occur in the presence of an extrauterine copper IUD. The controversial Dalkon Shield, although a nonmedicated plastic IUD, creates significant reactivity in the abdominal cavity. Whether this reactivity is a result of its different plastic matrix—ethyl-vinyl-acetate rather than polyethylene, or bacterial contamination from bacteria harbored in its multifilament tail,[8] the obscuring adhesions can complicate the laparoscopic detection and removal of the IUD. On the other hand, the plain polyethylene IUDs, e.g., the Lippes Loop—cause little reaction in the peritoneal cavity. However, the omentum often sweeps it out of the pelvis and incorporates it. If the device is not located on initial laparoscopic inspection, careful visualization and palpation of the omentum and upper abdomen should be carried out.

The intraabdominal IUD which is lying free in the peritoneal cavity can be grasped and brought out through the accessory sheath. Various instruments can be utilized to secure and remove the extrauterine IUD. However, the grasping forceps pictured in Chapter 5, Figure 18 has proven most reliable in firmly holding the extrauterine IUD as it is drawn out of the abdominal cavity. If the IUD is invested in surrounding adhesions, it should be grasped and elevated. This maneuver will permit many loose adhesions to fall away from the IUD and suggest to the surgeon the extent of the dissection, if any, which will be required to release the device. At this point a decision should be made about a third puncture. Often a small probe or grasping forceps placed through a third sheath in the opposite lower quadrant can be utilized to hold up the IUD. A dissecting scissors can be introduced through the accessory sheath in the other lower quadrant and the IUD freed from the adhesions. Depending upon their vascularity, the adhesions can be cut directly or coagulated and then transected. Once the IUD has been removed from the peritoneal cavity and before concluding the laparoscopy, the operative area must be scanned a final time to be certain that hemostasis has been achieved.

Complications

Complications associated with laparoscopic removal of the extrauterine IUD are no different than those which might occur with any laparoscopic procedure. Since lysis of adhesions may be a prominent feature of the surgery, bleeding from inadequately coagulated or overlooked raw surfaces or vessels must be sought out diligently. Careful inspection and use of electrosurgical equipment should reduce the frequency of inadvertent burns to adjacent structures, such as bowel. Occasionally, an exploratory laparotomy will be necessary to correct one of the above-noted complications or retrieve an intraabdominal IUD that resists laparoscopic removal. Therefore, all patients undergoing laparoscopy—for *any* reason—must sign an informed consent that includes the possibility of an exploratory laparotomy.

Conclusions

Laparoscopic identification and removal of the extrauterine IUD has been well documented in the literature.[1, 2, 3, 4, 5, 6, 7, 9, 10] Like female sterilization, the intraabdominal IUD has become a definite indication for operative laparoscopy.

References

1. Cibils LA, Moragne R: Intraabdominal Lippes Loop removed at laparoscopy: a case report. J Reprod Med 6:194, 1971

2. Koetsawang S: Laparoscopic removal of a perforated copper T IUD: a case report. Contraception 7:327, 1973

3. Kozloff SR, Engle T, Bernstein D, Silverberg S: Laparoscopic removal of ectopic intrauterine devices. Rocky Mt Med J 69:41, 1972

4. Leventhal JM, Simon LR, Shapiro SS: Laparoscopic removal of intrauterine contraceptive devices following uterine perforation. Am J Obstet Gynecol 111:102, 1971

5. Merrill LK, Burd LI, VerBurg DJ: Laparoscopic removal of intraperitoneal Dalkon Shields: a report of three cases. Am J Obstet Gynecol 118:1146, 1974

6. Smith DC: Removal of an ectopic IUD through the laparoscope. Am J Obstet Gynecol 105:285, 1969

7. Strecker, JR: Unusual uterine perforation by the copper-T intrauterine device and removal by laparoscopy. Contraception (In press)

8. Tatum HJ, Schmidt, FH, Phillips D, McCarty M, O'Leary WM: The Dalkon Shield controversy. JAMA 231:711, 1975

9. Taylor MB, White MF: Operative laparoscopy: removal of intraabdominal IUD with biopsy tongs. Obstet Gynecol 35:981, 1970

10. Whitson LG, Israel R, Bernstein GS: The extrauterine Dalkon Shield. Obstet Gynecol 44:418, 1974

Editorial Comments

The onus of removing intraabdominal IUDs seems to be falling more and more upon the laparoscopist. Lippes[1] has recently pointed out that the dangers of surgically removing any *asymptomatic,* inert, linear-shaped device (Lippes-Loop, Saf-T-Coil and Margulies spiral) are greater than the dangers posed by their ectopic location. He stressed that to his knowledge, no cases of bowel obstruction or mortality have occurred when such devices were left undisturbed. This finding is in marked contrast to the two deaths reported by Kahn and Tyler associated with removal of intraabdominal intrauterine devices.[2] In neither case, however, was the laparoscopic route of removal chosen. The closed-configuration, inert devices as well as the copper-containing ones, however, should be removed because of the potential hazards they pose.

The scheme suggested for determining the location of an intrauterine device is excellent and comprehensive.

I have never encountered an intraabdominal IUD which could not be removed via the laparoscope. The inert devices are generally found lying free in the pouch of Douglas. The copper-containing devices are almost always surrounded by, or involved in, dense adhesions; the string of the device, however, is almost always visible. Continuous, firm traction is almost always sufficient to free the device without necessitating lysis of the surrounding adhesions.

A.A.Y.

References

1. Lippes J: IUD related hospitalization and mortality. Letter to the editor. JAMA 235:1001, 1976

2. Kahn HS, Tyler CW Jr.: Mortality associated with use of IUD's. JAMA 234:57, 1975

Open Laparoscopy

H. M. Hasson, M.D.

Open laparoscopy is a surgical procedure which utilizes a small abdominal incision to carry the cannula and laparoscope into the peritoneal cavity under continuous visual control. The technique was developed to offer an alternative to the conventional method of blind abdominal puncture with the pneumoperitoneum needle and sharp trocar. The lack of certainty related to the use of these instruments has been responsible for many of the complications of laparoscopy. Significant complications reported with the use of needles include the following: laceration of blood vessels, hemorrhage and embolism; perforation and insufflation of dilated stomach, bowel and colon; emphysema and failed laparoscopy.[2, 4, 5, 6, 8, 10, 11, 12] The use of the sharp trocar has resulted in perforation of the gastrointestinal tract, laceration of abdominal organs and hemorrhage.[2, 4, 5, 6, 8, 10, 11, 12] These complications can be eliminated effectively with the use of open laparoscopy.

Equipment

The equipment utilized in open laparoscopy is standard, with the exception of the primary cannula. In addition, two sets of small Deaver retractors are used to expose the operative field. The open laparoscopy cannula* is fitted with a cone-shaped sleeve which moves freely but can be locked in any position along the cannula's shaft. The cone is sealed by a rubber cap. Two small metal hooks mounted near the proximal end of the cannula serve as suture holders. A blunt obturator replaces the sharp trocar (Figure 1). Pneumoperitoneum needles are not used in open laparoscopy.

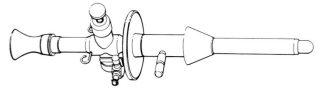

Figure 1
Open laparoscopy cannula.

* Eder Instrument Company, 5115 N. Ravenswood, Chicago, IL 60640.

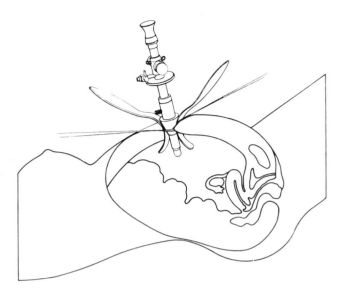

Figure 2
Cannula inserted into the peritoneal cavity, guided
by retractors.

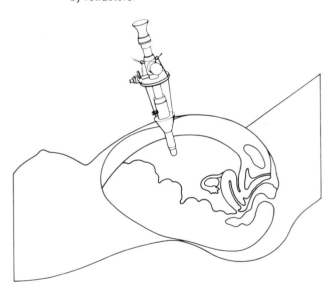

Figure 3
Fascial sutures tied to metal hooks to provide an
airtight seal and to maintain the instrument in place.

Technique

General anesthesia is administered and
endotracheal intubation is employed. A 2 cm
curved incision is made through the skin of the
anterior part of the abdominal wall, 0.5 cm below
the lower edge of the umbilical fossa. The skin
edges are retracted with two Allis clamps. The subcutaneous adipose tissues are dissected to expose
the linea alba.

The exposed deep fascia is lifted with skin
hooks or grasped with two Kocher clamps. The
fascia is held forcibly upward and incised transversely, approximately 1.1 cm, a short distance
below the aponeurotic umbilical ring. Elevation of
the fascia separates the abdominal wall from the
contents of the abdominal cavity during incision.
Two sutures are passed, one through each fascial
edge, and tagged. The fascial sutures are held upward and apart, and two small retractors are placed
laterally inside the fascial incision to expose the
properitoneal tissues.

The adipose tissue is dissected, and a
small hemostat is thrust against the peritoneum to
create an opening in the cavity. The small retractors are replaced inside the peritoneal defect and
lifted upward to increase the space between the
abdominal wall and the abdominal content. This
depth differential facilitates discrimination of
omental fat from properitoneal fat. Visualization of
small bowel and/or omentum is an essential step in
the procedure. The cone sleeve of the cannula is
then fixed in an appropriate position on the shaft to
accommodate the individual thickness of the abdominal wall, and the cannula is inserted gently
through the opening between the retractors. To
ensure clear entrance into the peritoneal cavity the
cannula must be guided by the retractors (Figure
2). The fascial sutures are then tied snugly, one to
each metal hook, pulling the fascia firmly against
the cone to provide an air-tight seal. Thus, escape
of the gas is prevented. The tied sutures also secure a sustained attachment of the cannula to the
anterior abdominal wall (Figure 3). In open laparoscopy the abdominal seal is established at the level
of the anterior rectus fascia.

Gas is insufflated through the valve of the cannula to create a pneumoperitoneum. Insufflation may be initiated while the sutures are being tied. The blunt obturator is withdrawn to permit a more rapid flow of gas. With the establishment of an adequate pneumoperitoneum the lighted laparoscope is introduced, and the procedure continues as usual. At the completion of the procedure the abdominal wall is closed in layers. It is essential to approximate the fascia well to prevent postoperative herniation. Closure of the peritoneum is less important and may be deleted if it is difficult to pursue. The present text details fine technical points which have not been reported previously.[3]

Use in Obese Patients

The incidence of obesity in our clinical sample was approximately 40%, indicating that this method is suitable for obese and markedly obese patients. Degree of obesity was based on conventional weight-height charts. Difficulties in exposure related to obesity were resolved with the use of a slightly larger incision as well as small Deaver retractors.

Use in Nulliparous Patients

The abdominal wall in most nulliparous patients was found to possess strong musculofascial supports. Three distinct fascial layers were encountered frequently: (1) posterior layer of superficial fascia or Scarpa's fascia, (2) anterior rectus sheath; and (3) posterior rectus sheath. Rectus muscle fibers occasionally extended into the umbilical fossa. The anterior rectus sheath in multiparous women is usually the only fascial layer which requires incision; however, in nulliparous women all three layers may be sufficiently developed to require incision. Rectus muscle fibers which extend into the umbilicus are separated in the midline with Deaver retractors.

Use in Patients with Previous Abdominal Surgery

Satisfactory visualization of the pelvic organs was obtained in almost all of 102 patients who had had one or more previous laparotomies. In these patients, with visual aid one is less likely to injure intraabdominal structures fixed and/or adherent to the abdominal wall or to insufflate a loculated section of the peritoneal cavity. One is more likely to enter the free peritoneal space. Open laparoscopy, however, does not guarantee pelvic visualization in patients who have had previous abdominal surgery. Dense, multilayered adhesions may render pelvic exposure impossible, which necessitates extending the procedure into a laparotomy.

It should be emphasized that although open laparoscopy is particularly indicated in obese patients and those who have had previous abdominal surgery, it should not be attempted in these types of patients until sufficient experience has been developed with the technique. One must proceed with care to avoid injury to adherent structures.

Operative Time

Open laparoscopy initially demanded an adaptive protocol while the procedure was being developed and modified. Operative time diminished readily with increased experience and presently compares favorably with the conventional method. The time required to attain entrance into the abdominal cavity and to establish an adequate pneumoperitoneum in open laparoscopy is comparable to the cumulative time required to establish the pneumoperitoneum with the needle, perform diagnostic tests to confirm proper placement of gas and puncture the abdominal wall with the sharp trocar. The time needed to establish an adequate pneumoperitoneum in open laparoscopy currently ranges from 4 to 20 minutes and averages 7 to 8 minutes. This includes operative time for insertion of the cannula as well as insufflation time.

Complications

Complications related to open laparoscopy have been limited to minor wound infections, one instance of febrile reaction of short duration and one occasion of small-bowel injury. Initially the abdominal incision was placed inside the umbilical fossa. This practice, which resulted in a wound infection in one patient, has since been abandoned. In the one potentially serious complication of bowel incision, absence of adipose tissue in the abdominal wall led to an inadvertent nick of small bowel in the process of incising the peritoneum. Current technique does not require a sharp incision in the peritoneum and thus should avoid recurrence of this more major complication. Failed laparoscopy has not occurred with the use of this technique.

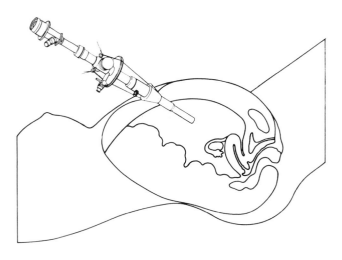

Figure 4
Open laparoscopy cannula: optimum protrusion in a thin patient.

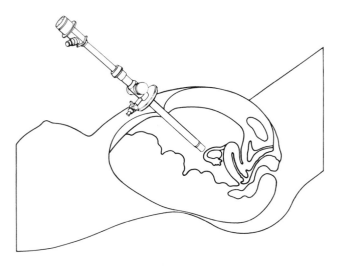

Figure 5
Standard cannula: deep insertion in a thin patient.

Advantages

Open laparoscopy offers certain advantages over the conventional method. Analysis of a series of 500 cases has revealed a virtual lack of complications related to the establishment of the pneumoperitoneum. The complications essentially were limited to minor wound infections in 1% of the patients. The fact that failed laparoscopy did not occur in any case is noteworthy. The results indicate that open laparoscopy is both safe and reliable. A more subtle advantage of the technique is the provision of optimal laparoscopic view in all patients, as illustrated in Figures 4, 5, 6 and 7. The insertion mechanics of the open laparoscopy cannula accommodates for the thickness of the abdominal wall while the standard cannula does not. The portion of the open laparoscopy cannula which protrudes beyond the fascia into the remaining portion of the abdominal wall and abdominal cavity can be adjusted to permit optimal visualization. This prevents deep cannula insertions, which limit adequate telescope mobility and view, as well as shallow insertions, which fail to traverse the abdominal wall completely.

An additional value of open laparoscopy is that it permits a more correct anatomic closure of the abdominal wall incision at the conclusion of the procedure. This closure preserves the integrity of the abdominal wall and lessens the possibility of postoperative herniation. Such a complication has been reported with the conventional method[1, 7, 9] but has not occurred in the open laparoscopy series.

Conclusion

Open laparoscopy is a safe and reliable procedure which is particularly suitable for obese patients and those with a history of previous abdominal surgery. Further, the technique allows the surgeon to have a greater degree of confidence in establishing the pneumoperitoneum as compared to other conventional methods.

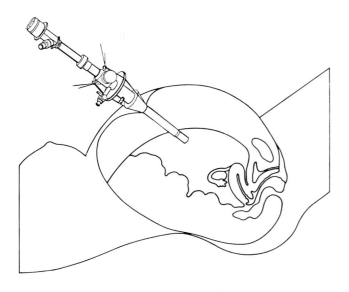

Figure 6
Open laparoscopy cannula: optimum protrusion in
an obese patient.

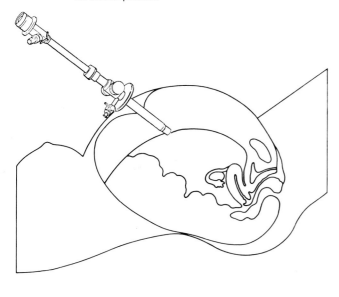

Figure 7
Standard cannula: shallow insertion in an obese
patient.

References

1. Bishop HL, Halpin TF: Dehiscence following laparoscopy: report of an unusual complication. Am J Obstet Gynecol 116:585, 1973

2. Edgerton WD: Experience with laparoscopy in a non-teaching hospital. Am J Obstet Gynecol 116:184, 1973

3. Hasson HM: Open laparoscopy: a report of 150 cases. J Reprod Med 12:234, 1974

4. Horwitz ST: Laparoscopy in gynecology. Obstet Gynecol Surv 27:1, 1972

5. Hulka JF, Corson SL, Soderstrom RM, Brooks PG: Complications Committee of the American Association of Gynecological Laparoscopists, First Annual Report. J Reprod Med, 10:301, 1973

6. Peterson EP, Behrman SJ: Laparoscopy of the infertile patient. Obstet Gynecol 36:363, 1970

7. Schiff I, Naftolin F: Small bowel incarceration after uncomplicated laparoscopy. Obstet Gynecol 43:674, 1974

8. Siegler AM: Trends in laparoscopy. Am J Obstet Gynecol 109:794, 1971

9. Smith AM: Rupture of abdominal wound after laparoscopy. Br Med J 1:159, 1974

10. Steptoe PC: Gynecological laparoscopy. J Reprod Med 10:211, 1973

11. Wadhwa RK, McKenzie R: Complications of band-aid surgery for sterilization. JAMA 222:1558, 1972

12. Whitford JH, Gunstone AJ: Gastric perforation: a hazard of laparoscopy under general anaesthesia. Br J Anaesth 44:97, 1972

Editorial Comments

In the past, lower abdominal laparotomy was considered a relative contraindication to laparoscopy. The technique described enables the procedure to be performed safely and efficiently. Although the author advocates this method for all laparoscopic procedures, in the hands of most experienced laparoscopists it does not usually seem necessary. Knowledge of the technique, however, should be a part of the repertoire of all laparoscopists.

A.A.Y.

Laparoscopic Uterine Suspension

Jaroslav J. Marik, M.D.

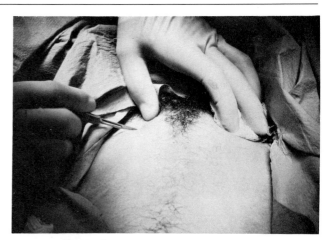

Figure 1

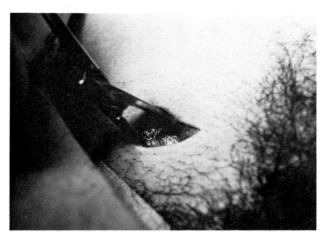

Figure 2

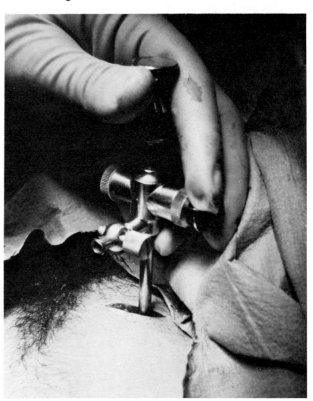

Figure 3

Among the available operative laparoscopic procedures is suspension of a retroverted uterus. The normal anteverted position of the uterus is maintained by three pairs of ligaments: round, uterosacral and cardinal. The precise role of these three ligamentous supports is not definitely agreed upon. The causes of retroversion have been discussed by others.[4, 16] The symptoms of retroversion include backaches, dysmenorrhea and dyspareunia. Retroversion is also associated with lower fertility, an increased rate of spontaneous abortions, endometriosis, a "bearing down" sensation, etc.[4, 5, 16, 17] This chapter is not meant to discuss these subjects or to set forth the indications for suspension of the uterus but to provide a technical description of the method employed to change the position of the uterus from retroverted and retroflexed to anteverted and anteflexed.

In the past, the correction of the position of the uterus was attempted by two basic approaches: the insertion of vaginal pessaries of numerous types and designs, and surgical procedures. Gynecologic surgeons approached the task by three basic routes. One was shortening the round ligament through the inguinal canal, as described by Adam[1] and Alexander.[2] Schauta[14] developed a technique of uterine suspension performed vaginally by shortening the round ligaments. Numerous surgeons preferred to do the uterine suspension via laparotomy. In general, the surgeons tried to change the position of the uterus by manipulating the round ligaments.[3, 6, 8, 9, 13] In the procedure several of them also included manipulation of the uterosacral ligaments.[10, 12, 18]

Donaldson and associates,[7] in 1942, described a technique of uterine suspension using the peritoneoscope. Steptoe[15] and Marik[11] have commented further on this procedure. The basic laparoscopic procedure is performed in the usual manner, and mobility of the uterus is a prerequisite for uterine suspension. Two skin incisions, each of 2 to 3 cm, are made in the lower abdomen 1 cm above the symphysis pubis (Figure 1). The subcutaneous tissue is separated down toward the fascia of the recti muscles. The fascia should definitely be visualized and identified (Figure 2). A 5 mm trocar and trocar sleeve are introduced through the remaining structures of the abdominal wall (Figure 3). A grasping forceps is passed through the trocar sleeve (Figures 4 and 5) and the round ligament grasped (Figure 6). The trocar sleeve is then pulled back out of the abdominal wall towards the handle

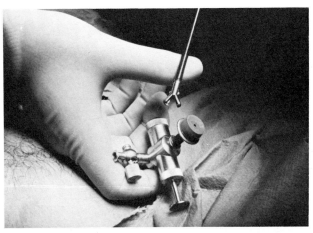

Figure 4

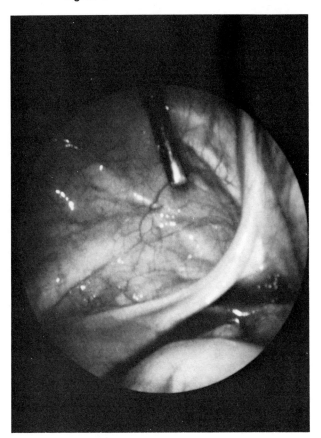

Figure 5

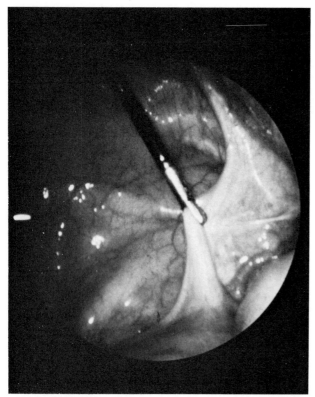

Figure 6

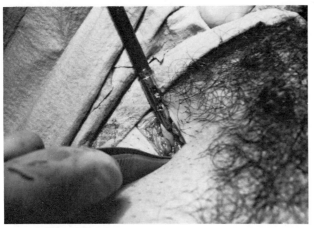

Figure 7

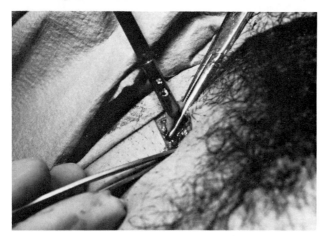

Figure 8

of the grasping instrument. A knuckle of the round ligament is delivered into the incision by drawing the forceps out of the abdomen (Figure 7). The loop of round ligament is secured with a surgical clamp (Figure 8). The identical procedure is done on the contralateral side. The position of the uterus is verified through the laparoscope (Figures 9 and 10). If it is adequately anteverted, the knuckle of the round ligament is sewn firmly to the fascia with a nonabsorbable suture (Figure 11). The skin is closed with two or three simple sutures of 000 plain catgut.

Several steps in the procedure deserve more detailed discussion. The Semm biopsy forceps, shown in Figure 4, has been found to be the most satisfactory instrument for delivering the round ligament through the abdominal wall. This instrument permits a firm grasp of the ligament because of the presence of a small tooth in each biopsy jaw which prevents the tissue from slipping out of the jaws.

It is very important that the fascia of the recti muscles be well exposed during the procedure. The subcutaneous fatty tissue should not be included in the suture when attaching the knuckle of the round ligament to the fascia. Inability to visualize the loop of round ligament after tying the stitch may well indicate that the suture was placed improperly or that only subcutaneous tissue, rather than fascia, was sutured. The round ligament thus may have slipped back into the abdominal cavity.

The ideal site at which the round ligament is initially grasped is 2 cm lateral to the incisions in the lower abdomen. The incisions through the fascia are usually made 4 to 5 cm from the midline vertical axis. If, on inspection, the new position of the uterus is not deemed satisfactory, the round ligament may be regrasped at an appropriate site to correct this.

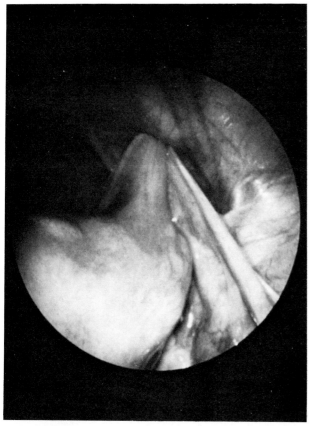

Figure 9

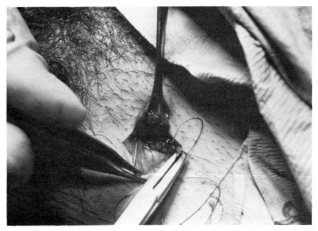

Figure 11

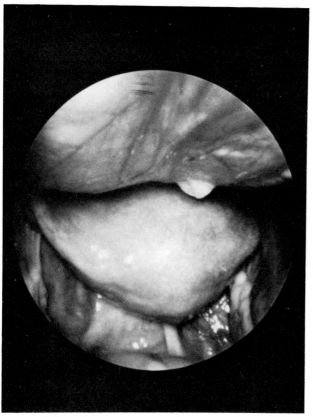

Figure 10

It is very important to release the pneumoperitoneum prior to suturing the segment of round ligament into the fascia since the new position of the uterus may vary depending upon the amount of gas remaining in the peritoneal cavity. Furthermore, the tension on the round ligament is significantly less if the pneumoperitoneum is released.

Attention should be paid to a possible space between the lateral portion of the round ligament and the abdominal wall. Although it has not caused problems in the past,[4, 5, 6] theoretically it might be a site of bowel strangulation. To prevent bowel strangulation, the two lower abdominal incisions are made very close to the pubic bone and lateral enough so that no aperture exists inside the abdomen.[15]

For an experienced laparoscopist this technique is not difficult. Uterine suspension can be performed via laparoscopy with minimal patient morbidity, hospitalization and cost.

References

1. Adams, cited by Graves WP: In *Gynecology*, W. P. Saunders Co, Philadelphia and London, 1916, p 589

2. Alexander W: A new method of treating inveterate and troublesome displacements of the uterus. Med Times Gazette 1:327, 1882

3. Baldy JM: The surgical treatment of retroversion of uterus. Surg Gynec Obstet 20:614, 1915

4. Behrman SJ, Gosling JRG: Uterine displacements and relaxations. *Fundamentals of Gynecology*. Oxford University Press, New York, 1966, p 46

5. Brewer JI: Uterine displacements. In *Textbook of Gynecology*. Williams & Wilkins Co, Baltimore, 1961, p 665

6. Coffey RC: Surgical treatment of displacements of uterus. Denver Med Times 24:339, 1904

7. Donaldson JK, Sanderlin JH, Harrell WB: A method of suspending the uterus without open abdominal incision. Am J Surg 55:537, 1942

8. Gilliam DT: Round ligament ventrosuspension of the uterus. Am J Obstet Dis Women Children 41:299, 1900

9. Graves WP: Olshausen's operation for suspension of the uterus. Surg Gynecol Obstet 52:1028, 1931

10. Javert CT: Combined procedure for anteversion of retroverted uteri. Am J Obstet Gynecol 52:865, 1946

11. Marik JJ: Report to the Annual Meeting of the American Association of Gynecologic Laparoscopists, Anaheim, California, 1974

12. McCall ML, Schumann EA: The subperitoneal Baldy-Webster uterine suspension. Am J Obstet Gynecol 51:125, 1946

13. Olshausen R: Uber ventrale Operation bei Prolapsus und retroversio Uteri. Zentralbl Gynaekol 10:698, 1886

14. Schauta R: Retrovesio, retroflexio uteri. In *Klinicka Gynekologie*. (A Ostricil, Ed) F Rivnac, Prague, 1933, p 310

15. Steptoe PC: *Laparoscopy in Gynecology*. E & S Livingston Ltd, Edinburgh and London, 1967, p 78

16. Taylor SG: Uterine retroversion. In *Essentials of Gynecology*. Lea & Febiger, Philadelphia, 1969, p 353

17. TeLinde RW, Mattingly RF: Malpositions of the uterus, cervical stump and vagina. In *Operative Gynecology*. J B Lippincott Co, Philadelphia, Montreal, 1970, p 469

18. Webster JC: A satisfactory operation of certain cases of retroversion of the uterus. JAMA 37:913, 1901

Editorial Comments

The majority of uterine suspensions being performed today appear to be done in association with several other procedures during conservative surgery for endometriosis. Laparotomy is obviously necessary in these cases. Laparoscopic uterine suspension for symptomatic uterine retroversion seems to be only a relative indication for the procedure. Many feel that laparoscopic uterine suspension is merely an exercise in "surgical gymnastics."

In the rare instance, however, when uterine suspension is the only indicated procedure, laparoscopy does offer an effective method of achieving the desired results. However, it should only be attempted by the most skilled laparoscopists.

A.A.Y.

Ectopic Pregnancy Management

John M. Esposito, M.D.

Laparoscopy has become an accepted technique in the diagnostic and therapeutic armamentarium of the gynecologist. As a result, the early diagnosis and management of ectopic pregnancy has now become a reality.[1,2,3,4,5] The early intervention which is thus possible has resulted in an increased number of patients operated upon prior to rupture of the gestational sac. It is in such cases that excision of the gestional sac under laparoscopic control may be possible and desirable.

The management of tubal eccyesis via laparoscopy decreases the length of hospital stay for the patient and therefore improves the utilization of hospital beds. Postoperative morbidity is also markedly reduced when compared to the other standard surgical approaches to the problem.

There are three techniques for accomplishing this task:

1.   Electrocoagulation and excision.
2.   Electrocoagulation of the sac without excision.
3.   The snare technique.

A fourth possibility to be considered is the procedure described by Frangenheim[2] for tubal ligation employing a loop of "self-tying" Prolene. This technique might very well lend itself to the removal of a tubal pregnancy.

When removing an ectopic gestation under laparoscopic vision the following criteria should be followed:

1.   The operator should have experience with other forms of operative laparoscopy and instrumentation.
2.   The ectopic gestation must be in a segment of the fallopian tube in which there is minimal vascularity. Excision should not be performed if the gestation is implanted in the isthmic portion of the tube immediately adjacent to the uterus, because of its proximity to the major vascular anastamosis between the uterine and ovarian arteries.
3.   The gestational sac should not exceed 3 cm in diameter.
4.   The pelvis should be relatively free of adhesions and the tube fully mobile.
5.   Under no circumstances should laparoscopy be performed on a patient in shock or should laparoscopic removal be attempted if more than 100 cc of blood is present in the peritoneal cavity.

The patient's desire for further childbearing must be taken into consideration prior to initiating the procedure and the various possible alternatives discussed with her. The very cases which are amenable to excision and removal under laparoscopic vision are those in which salpingostomy with preservation of the tube and childbearing capacity is also possible. In those who desire further pregnancy laparotomy would be the preferred method of approaching the problem.

Techniques

The two-hole approach is preferred because it provides a complete view while still permitting extensive operative manipulation.

1.   *Electrocoagulation followed by excision*

Shapiro[4] was the first to describe this procedure. Goldrath[3] described ten successful operations utilizing this technique.

The gestational sac is localized and the area distal and lateral to it is coagulated to blanching. This provides hemostasis in the branches of the uterine and ovarian artery supplying the tubal mucosa. The sac is then grasped and coagulating current applied until blanching extends well beyond it. When hemostasis is considered to be adequate, the tubal pregnancy is excised in total or by morsalization, depending on its size.

After removal is complete, free blood is aspirated from the pelvic cavity and a lavage with saline is performed. Careful inspection of the area is then made in order to ensure that adequate hemostasis has been achieved. Bleeding is controlled by further electrocoagulation, but if it persists, laparotomy may become necessary.

2.   *Electrocoagulation alone*

It has also been suggested that electrocoagulation of the sac is adequate. Eventual reabsorption then occurs. If this technique is to be employed, the gestational sac should not exceed 1.5 cm in diameter. The area is grasped with the forceps and coagulating current applied until the sac and a minimum of 0.5 cm of surrounding tissue are blanched. It is possible that after reabsorption of the gestational sac recanalization may occur and tubal patency may be preserved.

3.   *Snare Technique*

Soderstrom and Smith, in 1971,[6] described the snare technique for tubal sterilization. Soderstrom[7] subsequently reported the removal of five tubal pregnancies using this method. In his original description a two-hole technique with an operating laparoscope was used. However, if an operating laparoscope is not available, a three-hole technique may be employed.

Under laparoscopic control a grasping forceps is passed through the channel of the operating laparoscope and guided through the loop of an insulated electrocoagulating rectal snare inserted through a second puncture. The forceps is then used to grasp the segment of tube containing the gestational sac and draw it upwards through the open loop of the snare along with a small amount of normal tube on either side. Coagulating current is applied as the snare is slowly tightened until blanching is adequate. The snare is then closed, completely severing the segment of tube which is still held by the grasping forceps. The specimen is removed by withdrawing the operating laparoscope and grasping forceps as a single unit through the 11 mm sheath. If the specimen is too large to pass through the sheath, a minilaparotomy incision may be made suprapubically and the specimen withdrawn with a Kelly clamp. Following the removal, inspection of the excision site is essential in order to ensure that hemostasis is adequate.

Although the fourth technique has not been described specifically for the removal of ectopic pregnancies, the Prolene loop used by Frangenheim for tubal sterilization may be adopted for this purpose. A two-hole or a three-hole technique is used, depending on whether an operating laparoscope is available. The grasping forceps is passed through the loop and the ectopic gestation grasped. The Prolene loop is applied over it down to its base and secured tightly. The gestational sac is then excised leaving an adequate pedicle of healthy tissue in order to keep the suture from slipping. This technique seemingly would eliminate the attendant risks of electrosurgery.

It is essential to realize that techniques described for removal of ectopic gestations under laparoscopic control cannot be employed in all cases. In order to avoid complications, rigid criteria for case selection must be observed. Only a few cases have been reported in the literature. Therefore, at this time one cannot be assured that this method will be successful. In order to evaluate the procedure adequately more cases must be assessed critically.

Under no circumstances should the procedure be carried out on an outpatient basis. It must be performed in an area in which immediate laparotomy, if indicated, is possible. Adequate blood for replacement must be available at all times.

The laparoscopic excision of tubal pregnancies must be carried out only by physicians who are accomplished laparoscopists and abdominal surgeons. If the technique is performed successfully it improves bed utilization and decreases postoperative morbidity and length of hospitalization.

We would like to stress that the procedure should only be attempted by an experienced laparoscopist, and even in these hands it would be considered by many as operative gymnastics.

References

1. Esposito JM: The laparoscope: an aid in the diagnosis of the intact ectopic gestation. J Reprod Med 9:158, 1972.

2. Frangenheim H, Kleindienst W: Tubal sterilization under vision with the laparoscope: new techniques and instruments for tubal ligation and occlusion with tantalum clips. In *Gynecological laparoscopy: Principles and Techniques.* (J M Phillips, L Keith, Eds) Stratton Intercontinental Medical Book Corp, New York, 1974, p 213

3. Goldrath M, Platt L: The treatment of ectopic tubal pregnancies by laparoscopy. Presented at the Second International Congress of Gynecologic Endoscopy, Las Vegas, Nevada, 1975

4. Shapiro HI, Adler DH: Excision of an ectopic pregnancy through the laparoscope. Amer J Obstet Gynecol 117:290, 1973

5. Samuelsson S, Sjoval A: Laparoscopy in suspected ectopic pregnancy. Acta Obstet Gynecol Scand 51:31, 1972

6. Soderstrom RM, Smith MR: Tubal sterilization: a new laparoscopic method. Obstet Gynecol 38:152, 1971

7. Soderstrom RM: Unusual uses of laparoscopy. J Reprod Med 15:77, 1975

Editorial Comments

Laparoscopic removal of tubal pregnancies should be considered in the same category as uterine suspension, i.e., surgical gymnastics. However, laparoscopy has become invaluable in establishing the diagnosis of unruptured tubal pregnancy. In most cases the fetus will not be amenable to laparoscopic removal due to its size, presence of adhesions, lack of adequate instruments, desire to maintain a functional fallopian tube or inexperience on the part of the surgeon. When there is any doubt about the surgeon's ability to perform the procedure laparoscopically, it is much more prudent to use minilaparotomy or colpotomy. Minilaparotomy is generally quite easily performed through a small, one-inch to two-inch suprapubic incision over the fundus of the uterus. The uterine manipulator should be left in place during this procedure to facilitate mobilizing the uterus against the anterior abdominal wall. The gestational sac is first excised and then the tube repaired. Minilaparotomy is certainly the procedure of choice when it is desirable to conserve tubal integrity: laparoscopic removal of an ectopic pregnancy renders that tube functionless.

A.A.Y.

Chapter 15

Operative Sterilization: An Overview

Richard M. Soderstrom, M.D.

In the United States today, laparoscopic sterilization is the most common laparoscopic procedure, as well as the most common method of sterilization for women. Complications are rare when an experienced operator performs the procedure, and gives careful attention to electrocoagulation techniques.

Because laparoscopy permits direct visualization and manipulation of the abdominal and pelvic organs with an insignificant abdominal incision, it offers a number of advantages over other sterilization techniques. Hospitalization is seldom required, for most patients return home within a few hours, and 50% of patients return to full activity within 24 hours. Discomfort is minimal and incision scars are barely visible. Vaginal drainage associated with culdoscopy and colpotomy does not occur. The patient's sexual activity need not be restricted, and, as mentioned, the surgeon has an opportunity to view the abdominal viscera. Cost to the patient is lower than for more extensive sterilization procedures, such as abdominal laparotomy or vaginal colpotomy.

The disadvantages of laparoscopic sterilization are few. General anesthesia usually is required. The surgeon must have special training beyond that required for diagnostic laparoscopy. Also, cost to the patient is greater than for vasectomy, which may be the preferable sterilization procedure for some couples.

Until the late 1960s, voluntary sterilization was not available for women unless their age, times the number of children, equaled or exceeded 120.[5] In May, 1969, however, the ACOG released the bonds of restriction for women seeking voluntary sterilization and officially stated that a decision regarding voluntary sterilization is to be made by physician and patient. Only in cases of therapeutic sterilization is consultation required.[6]

This change in policy was probably the most important event in modern laparoscopy. Not only did it alert obstetricians and gynecologists to their responsibility to provide permanent contraception, but it emphasized the need to develop methods comparable to vasectomy in simplicity, recovery time and expense. Just six years later laparoscopic sterilization comprised 60% of all laparoscopic procedures performed in the United States.

Prior to laparoscopy, female sterilization was usually accomplished by mechanical means, such as a suture ligature (with or without transection) and resection, whereas operative laparoscopy equipment was oriented toward the use of electrocoagulation techniques. Thus, early reports of laparoscopic sterilization dealt with the methods and success or failure of tubal occlusion and/or transection using electrocoagulation. Though most reports were promising, it became evident that electrocoagulation is not without hazard, particularly in the hands of the inexperienced. A flurry of research began. Some investigators directed their studies toward improvement and refinements in electrosurgical units, while others reviewed and developed mechanical methods to eliminate the potential hazards of any electrosurgical procedure.

Laparoscopic sterilization may be achieved by one of three methods: (1) occlusion of the fallopian tubes by electrocoagulation or mechanical means, (2) occlusion and transection with electrocoagulation, and (3) occlusion and partial resection, combining electrocoagulation and the use of biopsy instruments. All three approaches have been performed using the operating laparoscope alone, or the diagnostic laparoscope with secondary trocar instruments, or the operating laparoscope and secondary puncture equipment. Patient acceptance and recovery are approximately the same with all methods.

A retrospective study showed that complications from laparoscopic sterilization are attributed primarily to inexperienced operators in electrocoagulation accidents, as a result of defective coagulation equipment or of inadvertent fulguration of hidden viscera. An "experienced operator" was defined as one who had participated in a postgraduate education course in laparoscopy and who had performed at least ten operative laparoscopies. In a subsequent prospective study, the complication rate was reduced tenfold by establishing a consistent operating protocol and an intensive education program for all operating room personnel, particularly with respect to diathermy principles and techniques.[11]

Before attempting voluntary laparoscopic sterilization procedures, the novice should gain experience by practicing sterilization techniques on informed, consenting patients who are undergoing benign laparotomy, such as hysterectomy. Once a level of confidence is obtained, the surgeon should build competency first with coagulation or mechanical occlusion alone, then with transection, and finally, if desired, with coagulation and resection. Occlusion combined with resection is a complicated operative procedure and should be performed only by a surgeon experienced in operative laparoscopy.

Electrocoagulation accidents can be reduced by (1) proper equipment maintenance, (2) use of low-voltage, high frequency coagulation units, preferably with isolated ground circuitry, rather than high-voltage spark gap units, and (3) visualization of the entire operative field before connecting and applying the electric current for coagulation.

It is my intent to describe each basic technique of laparoscopic sterilization and to explore those specific ingredients, precautions, and "tricks of the trade" suggested by those experts in each technique. Acknowledgment is gratefully given to Drs. Stephen Corson, H. M. Hasson, Jaroslav Hulka, Louis Keith, Richard Kleppinger, John Marlow, A. Jefferson Penfield, David Pent, Jacques Rioux, Alvin Siegler, Donald C. Smith, Clifford R. Wheeless, InBae Yoon, and A. Albert Yuzpe. Their advice and contributions to this chapter have been invaluable.

Electrosurgical Methods

All electrical methods have one principle in common—tubal occlusion as a result of tissue heat created by electrical energy. In applying this energy, the surgeon wishes to create as little tissue damage as possible while permanently obstructing ovum transportation. The more electrical energy required, both in amount and in duration, the greater the risks inherent in electrosurgery. Thus, a working knowledge of electrosurgical principles is imperative in analyzing the advantages and disadvantages of any electrosurgical method of sterilization.

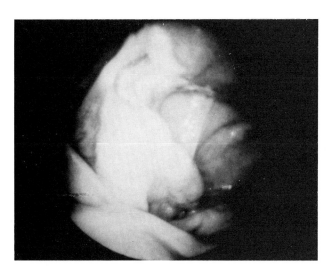

Figure 1
Adequate coagulation using the burn only technique of laparoscopic sterilization. (Figure courtesy of A. Albert Yuzpe, M.D.)

Coagulation Alone

Single-point coagulation does not destroy enough of the fallopian tube to guarantee adequate occlusion. Most authorities feel that continuous, multiple-point coagulation of the tube, destroying a minimum of 3 cm of tubal length, is the preferred method (Figure 1). This technique may be accomplished by using any appropriate coagulation forceps, introduced through the operating laparoscope or through secondary trocar sleeves. The following suggestions and comments have been taken from publications and communications from the leading authorities of this technique, Loffer, Pent, Rioux, and Yuzpe.[17]

Loffer and Pent prefer to stay 1 to 2 cm from the cornu of the uterus, whereas Rioux and Yuzpe coagulate up to and include the cornu of the uterus. Apparently, both techniques are equally successful. Identification of the tube from cornu to fimbria is considered important, as this prevents incorrect coagulation of other structures because of misidentification and alerts the operator to possible adherent viscera, which could lead to accidental burns through electrical transfer down adhesive bands. They stress the importance of adequate displacement of the small bowel from the pelvic cavity prior to electrocoagulation. The complete coagulation process is characterized by blanching, swelling, and finally collapse and dehydration of the fallopian tube. They have found that the duration of coagulation time is related to the size of the tube, the smaller diameter requiring less time. Also, since current density is increased by a decreasing size in grasping forceps, coagulation time is reduced as one reduces the surface area of the grasping forceps. Because of the discrete coagulation area found with bipolar forceps (Chapter 4), more applications of the grasping forceps are needed than with the unipolar systems.

These four authorities performed a collaborative study in 1975 that revealed a failure rate of 0.35 per 1,000, or 0.035%, in 2,100 patients followed for 18 months. No method of female sterilization yet designed can declare a higher success rate. These authorities use and recommend low-voltage, high frequency coagulation units with isolated ground circuitry. Bowel burns did not occur in their series.[17]

Coagulation and Transection

Steptoe and Wheeless popularized this approach in the late 1960s and early 1970s.[13,14,15,16] Though their instruments differ, they found two basic principles to be important. First, complete transection through the tube and into a small portion of the mesosalpinx must take place and second, generous coagulation of the transected ends of the tube decreases the chance of reanastomosis and failure. Steptoe prefers the two-hole technique and recommends a 70° lens system. He feels that the operative field can be more adequately scanned with this type of laparoscope, thus reducing the risk of inadvertent electrocoagulation of hidden viscera. Wheeless, on the other hand, has utilized the operating laparoscope (one-hole technique) and feels that the "blind spot" created by the grasping forceps placed through the operating channel is not a hazard when the surgeon adheres to the principles of operative laparoscopy. It is considered advisable to transect the tube 1.5 to 2 cm from the uterine cornu to avoid bleeding injury to the uteroovarian artery anastomoses. Some operators advise multiple transections, but there is no evidence that this approach is an improvement over an adequate single-transection technique. The 1975 AAGL survey confirms that using transection in tubal sterilization introduces the potential risk of mesosalpinx tears and bleeding.[7]

Coagulation and Resection

In a review of 29,500 tubal sterilizations by Garb, the Pomeroy partial salpingectomy method of tubal sterilization was touted as the most successful, according to the world literature.[2] Even today, those surgeons who use the transabdominal and transvaginal tubal sterilization approach prefer the Pomeroy or modifications of the Pomeroy method. It is no wonder, then, that innovative laparoscopists have dealt with the problem of a safe and easy method for resection, as well as coagulation, of the fallopian tube. Also, the medicolegal security of a pathologic specimen has been a motivating factor. This requirement, of course, introduces more technical complexity to the procedure, and to some extent increases the risk of potential bleeding problems.

One of the earliest laparoscopic biopsy instruments, designed by Raoul Palmer, M.D., and known as the Palmer drill biopsy forceps, was intended primarily for ovarian biopsy. It has been adapted by many surgeons for tubal sterilization, using the two-hole puncture technique. The specimen received is usually quite generous—1 to 2 cm in length—but it may be severely coagulated, making histologic recognition impossible. If the instrument is not properly maintained and sharpened, twisting and tearing of the mesosalpinx can occur. The reader is referred to the manufacturer's brochure for the specific mechanics of this biopsy forceps.

Punch biopsy forceps have been designed that are similar to those used by the gynecologists in cervical punch biopsies. One of these, the Siegler biopsy forceps, resects a 90 cu mm segment of the tube. In the hands of an experienced operator, the specimen can frequently be kept histologically normal despite the use of electrocoagulation.

Siegler points out that the rotation of the jaws, independently of the handle position is a technical advantage in performing the punch biopsy method of sterilization. He cautions against vigorous grasping of the tube with the biopsy forceps in preparation for coagulation and biopsy. If the operator wishes, multiple biopsies are, of course, possible.[9]

Kleppinger utilizes the operating laparoscope, with either the 3 mm or the 5 mm instrument channel and a grasping forceps. Once adequate coagulation has taken place, he introduces the Frangenheim punch biopsy scissors, makes two transections, and resects a wedge of fallopian tube. Donald C. Smith uses the operating scissors to coagulate, cut and resect a wedge of uncoagulated tissue, working with an operating laparoscope. Those two physicians make the following points about this approach: They feel that the one-hole technique is easier to teach, but not all laparoscopists agree. Smith and Kleppinger do point out, and most would agree, that for those using local anesthesia, the operative laparoscope is a distinct advantage.[3,10] All authorities using the operating laparoscope stress the importance of retraction of the telescope for a panoramic view of the operative field prior to the use of electrosurgery. They specifically stress that the physician visualize enough insulation on the operating forceps to ensure protection against the hazard of arcing between forceps and laparoscope. The proper position of the forceps prior to electrosurgery is demonstrated in Kleppinger's figure (Figure 2).

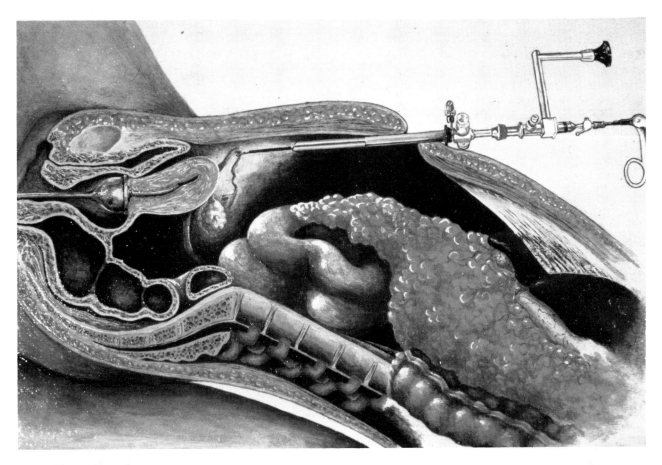

Figure 2
The proper position using the operating laparoscope
for tubal sterilization when using electrosurgery.
(Figure courtesy of Richard K. Kleppinger, M.D.)

In 1971, I introduced a method of partial tubal resection which guaranteed pathologic confirmation. This technique requires an operating laparoscope with its associated grasping forceps, and an insulated rectal polyp snare, placed through a secondary trocar. This snare is specifically designed to prevent gas leakage during the laparoscopic procedure. The instruments are placed in the abdomen under direct vision and the surgeon passes the grasping forceps through the open snare and withdraws, back through the snare, the desired amount of fallopian tube to be resected. When the snare is drawn tight around the knuckle of the tube, electrocoagulation current is applied until adequate hemostasis has occurred. Once he-mostasis has been confirmed, complete closure of the snare, using a cutting blend current, transects the base of the specimen. Retrieval of the specimen is accomplished by withdrawing the laparoscope, grasping forceps, and specimen—as a unit—through the laparoscope trocar sleeve.[12]

Since Yuzpe and others have shown that adequate coagulation is the key to a low failure rate, recoagulation of the isthmus portion of the tube, following resection, is highly desirable. Though repetitious, it is important to emphasize once again that only low-voltage, high frequency electrocoagulation with isolated ground circuitry should be used.

In summary, then, the snare technique of laparoscopic tubal resection is a two-hole technique that guarantees adequate transection and resection of the fallopian tube. In addition, it is the only method yet described that guarantees pathologic confirmation of the resected specimen. Of all the methods described, however, it is the most complex to teach and learn, and should not be attempted by the novice in laparoscopy (Chapter 15).

Bipolar Electrical Sterilization

Because of some of the grounding principles and problems of unipolar electrocoagulation units, Jacques E. Rioux launched a search for an effective bipolar electrical forceps in 1973. Since that time, Stephen L. Corson, Richard K. Kleppinger and others have helped to design bipolar forceps. The principles of bipolar surgery are discussed in Chapter 4, but the major feature is the elimination of the unipolar groundplate so that the current will run only between the grasping jaws of these forceps. When the bipolar forcep is used with an isolated ground circuitry unit, there is no possibility of alternate paths of ground-seeking. One jaw of the forceps is the active electrode and the other jaw is the ground electrode; therefore, current density is quite confined, and the spread of electrocoagulation is less than with unipolar forceps. Only low-voltage, high frequency units can be used with these forceps, thus increasing their safety.

The following suggestions have been made by Rioux, Corson, and Kleppinger. Rioux points out, as mentioned before, that a 3 cm segment of coagulation is adequate for tubal occlusion. To increase safety he has located the activating switch in the handle of his bipolar forceps, thus preventing accidental discharge of current by someone other than the operator. His forceps is unique in that the tips of the forceps are disposable. He cautions that bipolar forceps may not be sufficient to control unexpected bleeding and that unipolar capabilities should be available during all bipolar sterilization procedures.[8]

The Corson bipolar forceps does not have external insulation, which reminds us that bipolar electrical systems create their own internal insulation. This, of course, is an advantage from the standpoint of equipment maintenance. Corson agrees with Siegler that rotation of the forceps is a technical advantage to the operator. He emphasizes that grasping the tube lightly, rather than

heavily, is the method of choice in bipolar forceps surgery to allow adequate spread of current. In most cases, his instrument can be used for mechanical transection of the tube once coagulation has been completed.[1]

Though Kleppinger's bipolar forceps has been designed only for coagulation, he uses either the Frangenheim biopsy forceps or operating scissors to transect the tube. His studies have shown that bipolar coagulation requires less voltage and less current flow than unipolar techniques. The disadvantage, however, is that it takes longer to coagulate the same amount of tissue. As desiccation increases, so does tissue resistance, and self-insulation of the coagulated area will eventually occur. Occasionally, the tissue will adhere to the bipolar forceps jaw, but it can easily be released by rotating the jaws 90°. All authorities recommend that the jaws of the forceps be kept meticulously clean for proper functioning.[4]

Puerperal Sterilization

Puerperal laparoscopic sterilization was initially thought to be technically difficult and inadvisable. Steptoe, in his monograph, cautioned against the use of laparoscopy in the puerperium, although he has since endorsed the procedure.[13] Other authors supported his early opinion, frequently without the benefit of personal experience.

Keith and Houser, in 1970 and 1971, reported their experience with puerperal sterilization via laparoscopy at the Cook County Hospital in Chicago (Chapter 15). By 1975, Keith had collected approximately 5,000 successful cases of puerperal laparoscopic sterilization. He strongly recommends that the patient be adequately atropinized and that circulating blood volume be supported with Ringer's lactate solution. He also suggests using intravenous oxytocin (Pitocin) to ensure a firm, contracted uterus.

Keith seldom finds the need for deep Trendelenburg position, as the lax abdominal wall allows more than enough pneumoperitoneum to perform the procedure. He points out that because of the lax abdominal wall, it is quite easy to manipulate to either side of the fundus of the uterus with rigid instruments.

Operative Sterilization Combined With Abortion

Patients seeking abortion should have available information and methods of contraception. For some, permanent sterilization is the method of choice. Courey, Horowitz, and others have demonstrated the success of laparoscopic sterilization in patients undergoing voluntary termination of pregnancy (Chapter 15). They feel that the combination of laparoscopic sterilization and abortion should be limited to twelve weeks' gestation and less. Though laparoscopic sterilization can be performed after first trimester abortion, they prefer to defer sterilization for four to six weeks. The uterine manipulator should be blunt to avoid perforating the softened uterus. The operator should be aware that the fallopian tubes are often displaced posterolaterally away from the uterine fundus, which may occasionally require a third puncture for proper manipulation.

Their technique of sterilization does include transection, but many laparoscopists agree that the greater vascularity and varicosities increase the risk of bleeding. More and more authorities are therefore choosing the technique of coagulation alone. As mechanical occlusion devices are improved and become available, they will most likely be chosen for this group of patients.

Nonelectrical Methods

Three mechanical occlusion devices have been studied in sufficient numbers to be mentioned in this chapter. The first is the hemostatic metal clip, which has been available to surgeons for years. Unfortunately, the clip was designed for occlusion of blood vessels that are smaller than the fallopian tube; and although it seems attractive, the failure rate with this clip has been unacceptable. If the metal clip is used, two clips should be placed on each tube in such a way that the vessels supplying the portion of the tube between the clips are completely occluded, so that this tissue atrophies.

Jaroslav Hulka has designed a plastic spring clip (Chapter 15). At the time of this writing, it is still considered a research method, but present statistics look most promising. The Hulka clip consists of two plastic jaws made of Lexan, hinged by a small metal pin 2 mm from one end. Each jaw has teeth on the opposite surface, and a gold-plated, stainless steel spring holds the clip jaws in the open position. A silastic rubber filler at the far end of the clip fills all the potential dead space left when the jaws are closed. When the clip is closed, there is a 1 mm gap between the upper and lower jaws of the clip, which prevents tearing of the tube or the blood vessels. This space will become obliterated by the action of the spring 48 to 72 hours after application. A special laparoscope for one-hole application has been designed, though the Hulka clip may be used in a two-hole procedure.

InBae Yoon has designed and field tested a nonreactive silicone rubber band (Chapter 15). This silicone band has an elastic memory of 100% if stretched to no more than 6 mm. A special applicator instrument, 5 to 6 mm in diameter, can be placed either through a specially designed operating laparoscope or through a second puncture trocar sleeve. The instrument is designed to grasp a knuckle of tube and "fire" the silicone band onto the knuckle of tube, similar to the Madlener technique. If desired, the avascular knuckle of tube can be resected with biopsy forceps.

Neither the Hulka clip nor the Falope-Ring has been available long enough to determine accurate failure rates. Both authors point out the advantage of eliminating electrosurgery and its inherent risks. Though they stress that these methods should not be performed as a reversible sterilization method, experience may show that reanastomosis, if occasionally desired, will be easier and more successful.

Both authors have found this method most successful with the use of local anesthesia. They emphasize that anesthetic solution must be sprayed on the tube prior to application, and that 10% to 15% of the patients will experience postoperative cramping from the occlusive device itself.

Minilaparotomy

Every laparoscopist will occasionally have a patient in whom technical problems or equipment failure will make laparoscopy unsuccessful. Rather than canceling the surgery, the laparoscopist who finds himself in this situation should be knowledgeable about minilaparotomy sterilization.

The patient is already positioned and prepared for minilaparotomy when one does laparoscopy. The following steps can be simply performed. The uterus, with its manipulator in place, is pushed up against the abdominal wall. A 2 to 3 cm incision is made over the top of the fundus and through the fascia and peritoneum. By displacing the uterus from one side to the other side, it is possible to bring each tube into direct view. Any of the methods described in this chapter may be used in this situation. Routine abdominal closure then completes the procedure, and frequently the patient is able to go home the same day.

Complications and Failures

Complications unique to laparoscopic sterilization include electrical burns and tears of the mesosalpinx (Chapter 21). Failures following laparoscopic sterilization in a survey by the AAGL in 1975 were reported as 2.51 per 1,000 cases. Of interest was the finding that more than 50% of patients who become pregnant following tubal sterilization do not report their subsequent pregnancy to the laparoscopic surgeon. Temperance in reporting failure rates must be observed until a minimum of two years has passed from the date of surgery.[7]

Conclusion

Laparoscopic sterilization is the most popular method of female sterilization in the United States today. In the hands of the experienced laparoscopist, the three basic approaches of female sterilization (occlusion, occlusion and transection, and occlusion and resection) work well and cause minimal complications. Respect for the knowledge of electrosurgery is the key to any successful laparoscopic sterilization program. Development of nonelectrical mechanical occlusion devices shows promise for the future.

References

1. Corson SL: Personal communication

2. Garb AC: A review of tubal sterilization failures. Obstet Gynecol Surv 12:291, 1957

3. Kleppinger RK: Laparoscopic tubal coagulation and segmental resection. (unpublished data)

4. Kleppinger RK: Personal communication

5. *Manual of Standards in Obstetric-Gynecologic Practice*. 2nd ed, April, 1965

6. Official Statement of the American College of Obstetrics and Gynecology. May, 1969

7. Phillips JM, Keith D, Hulka J, Hulka B, Keith L: Gynecologic laparoscopy in 1975. J Reprod Med 16:105, 1976

8. Rioux J-E: Personal communication

9. Siegler AM: An instrument to aid sterilization by laparoscopy. Fertil Steril 23:367, 1972

10. Smith DC: Personal communication

11. Soderstrom RM, Butler JC: A critical evaluation of complications in laparoscopy. J Reprod Med 10:245, 1973

12. Soderstrom RM, Smith MR: Instrument and method—tubal sterilization, a new laparoscopic method. Obstet Gynecol 38:152, 1971

13. Steptoe PC: *Laparoscopy in Gynecology*. E&S Livingstone, Ltd, London, 1967

14. Steptoe PC: Recent advances in surgical methods of control of fertility and infertility. Br Med Bull 26:152, 1971

15. Wheeless CR, Jr.: Instrument and method—elimination of second incision in laparoscopic sterilization. Obstet Gynecol 36:208, 1970

16. Wheeless CR, Jr.: The status of outpatient tubal sterilization by laparoscopy: improved technics and review of 1000 cases. Obstet Gynecol 39:635, 1972

17. Yuzpe AA, Rioux J-E, Loffer FD, Pent D: Laparoscopic tubal sterilization by the "burn only" technique. (unpublished data)

The Spring Clip*

J. F. Hulka, M.D.

With grateful recognition of those doctors who participated in the collaborative clinical study both in the United States and overseas:

Richard Beard, M.D.
William E. Brenner, M.D.
Vernon Madrigal Castro, M.D.
James R. Dingfelder, M.D.
John I. Fishburne, M.D.
Suporn Koetsawang, M.D.
Thampu Kumarasamy, M.D.
T. H. Lean, M.D.
Hugh T. Lefler, M.D.
Brian Lieberman, M.D.
Jack P. Mercer, M.D.
K. F. Omran, M.D.
D. N. Pai, M.D.
E. P. Peterson, M.D.
Jordan M. Phillips, M.D.

The popularity of laparoscopic sterilization has increased since 1940, when this technique was first proposed.[8] Complications as a result of electrocoagulation (the first established laparoscopic method of tubal occlusion) have stimulated interest in nonelectrical techniques.

A promising alternative was the development of a clip which, when applied correctly to the fallopian tube, resulted in permanent occlusion, thus preventing passage of egg and sperm. Basic biologic principles of tubal occlusion had to be established through animal studies before this new approach could be tested ethically in humans. For this purpose the common pig was chosen because of the similarity of its tubal structure to that of humans.

A series of clip designs was tested, beginning with the Tantalum clip.[5] A comparison of these clips with a spring-loaded prototype, however, showed that there were pregnancies in those pigs with Tantalum clips because of recanalization through the gap between the jaws of the clip. Other clips that were not spring-loaded became dislodged after application because of the muscular contractions of the tubes or extensive adhesions with omentum caused by their irregular surfaces. Based upon these experiences, an effective tuboocclusive clip was developed.

Clip Design

The clip finally designed has a metal spring which acts to open and close two jaws which are made of 3 mm-wide Lexan plastic (Figure 1). Once the jaws are closed and the metal spring is advanced over them, they are held firmly closed with a constant pressure exceeding 75 g (Figure 2). A laparoscope was designed to incorporate both the optics and clip applicator in a single, 10 mm-diameter instrument. The function of the applicator is shown in Figures 3, 4, 5, 6.

* Partly supported by USAID, number csd/2979, and the Rockefeller Foundation.

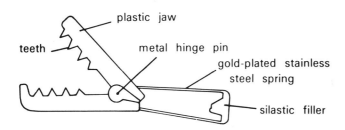

Figure 1
A diagram of the spring clip.

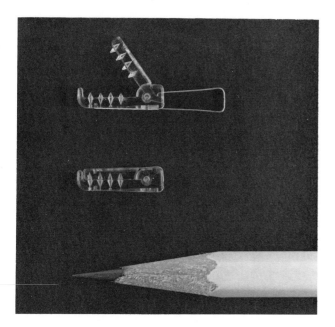

Figure 2
Closed clip with pencil in background for comparison of relative size.

Technique of Clip Application

No premedication is administered. The patient empties her bladder just before entering the operating suite. Either no sedation or 5 to 15 mg of diazepam (Valium) alone or in combination with 0.05 to 0.1 mg of fentanyl (Sublimaze) is injected intravenously. The patient is prepared and positioned as for all laparoscopic sterilization procedures. If local anesthesia is to be employed, 10 to 20 ml of 1% lidocaine (Xylocaine) are used to infiltrate the subumbilical skin, abdominal wall and peritoneum. The abdomen is inflated and the combined laparoscope applicator inserted. Manipulation of the uterus by means of the controlling tenaculum (Chapter 10) permits the operating laparoscope to approach the tubes at an appropriate angle for applying one clip under direct vision.

One clip-reloading procedure is required to place the second clip on the opposite tube. At the completion of the procedure, the uterus and tubes are inspected to confirm proper application of the clips. The laparoscopic procedure is then terminated in the usual fashion. When local anesthesia is employed, patients generally leave the operating room in a good condition varying from drowsy satisfaction to relieved cheerfulness; all are conscious throughout the procedure. The patient is observed in the recovery room for approximately one-half hour until she is able to walk unassisted, and she then goes to a clinic recovery room where she rests until she is ready to leave the hospital, generally within an hour or two following the procedure.

Human Clip Studies

A. Pain Studies: When local anesthesia is applied to the tubes, pain is experienced at the time of clip application in less than 5% of patients. Over half of the patients described the overall discomfort as equal to or less than that of the intravenous needle. Postoperatively, 8% of patients experienced a vagal reflex, characterized by hypotension and bradycardia, which was relieved promptly with atropine. When treated in this manner, patients complain of the discomfort of the start of the intravenous line itself, then of the discomfort from the insertion of a sound and tenaculum into the uterus and occasionally of discomfort from insertion of the trocar.[2]

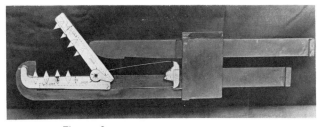

Figure 3
Diagrammatic scheme of spring clip application. Clip is in open position. The metal holder for the tube is designed to prevent the tube from rolling back away from the clip while upper jaw is being pressed down.

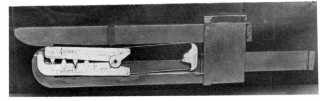

Figure 4
As the upper ram closes the jaw, a 1 mm gap remains between the upper and lower jaws of the clip. This has been designed deliberately to prevent tearing of the tube, venous or arterial blood vessels which might be in the clip. This space will become obliterated by action of the spring over the next two- or three-day period, again ensuring maximal safety in terms of prevention of hemorrhage and maximal effectiveness in terms of preventing recanalization.

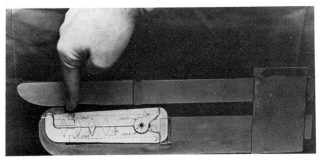

Figure 5
When the lower ram is advanced, the spring clip is caught in two notches of the upper and lower jaw, in such a way that the clip cannot be dislodged accidentally. These notches are shown by the index finger on the diagram.

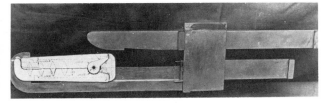

Figure 6
When the clip is applied, both the upper and lower rams are retracted, permitting the tube and applied clip to fall free into the abdominal cavity. There is minimal residual dead space to attract fluid or bacteria.

Our currently recommended premedication is 0.5 mg atropine and 0.06 to 0.1 mg fentanyl intravenously just as the abdomen is being prepared. This premedication lasts 40 minutes and virtually eliminates the discomfort and vagal reactions during surgery.

B. Respiratory Studies: With full anesthesia coverage, the clip application procedures were moved to a room outside of the operating room in the clinical research unit of the hospital. The prime purpose of this move was to document blood gas changes during laparoscopy under local anesthesia with minimal systemic medication since it became apparent that full operating room facilities were not necessary for clip application. Blood gas studies consisted of measuring PaO_2, $PaCO_2$, end-expired O_2, end-expired CO_2 and ventilatory capacity (VC, V_T, respiration rate) at base level, after the fentanyl sedation, after introduction of the Trendelenburg position, after induction of the pneumoperitoneum and at the completion of the procedure. The results of these studies indicated that the single, effective variable which changed blood gas was the sedation (fentanyl).[1] Trendelenburg and pneumoperitoneum had no effect on these changes. It was decided originally to compare nitrous oxide to carbon dioxide as a means of inducing pneumoperitoneum, but carbon dioxide was discontinued rapidly when, at this light level of medication, it became apparent that patients experienced considerable discomfort because of the absorption of CO_2 onto the surface and its transformation to carbonic acid, which apparently irritated the peritoneal surfaces. Nitrous oxide was used thereafter for induction of the pneumoperitoneum in all cases.

C. Outpatient Feasibility: After it was documented that respiratory difficulties and pain are minimal during laparoscopy under local anesthesia, a series of 100 cases was performed in the clinical research unit with full emergency equipment available but no formal anesthesia coverage. The purpose of this study was to see if laparoscopy, in skilled hands, carried with it any greater or lesser hazards than other gynecologic procedures, such as vacuum aspiration for pregnancy termination. In this series, four attempts to apply clips were discontinued because of obesity, inadequate sedation or inability to establish the pneumoperitoneum. No complications were encountered which would have justified the performance of immediate laparotomy

Table 1
Collaborative Sites

Location	Sterilizations as of March 1974	1-year follow-up
Chapel Hill, North Carolina	429	375
Los Angeles, California	31	26
Fort Worth, Texas	36	32
Ann Arbor, Michigan	15	10
London, England	106	93
San Salvador, El Salvador	137	128
Bombay, India	105	100*
Bangkok, Thailand	113	113
Singapore	107	100*
Total	1079	977

* Approximate

Table 2

Local anesthesia: lidocaine plus	Number performed
No medication	14
0.1 mg fentanyl alone	120
0.1 mg fentanyl + 5 to 10 mg diazepam	340
50 mg meperidine + 50 mg promethazine	380
Combined with abortion	166
Total	1020

in an operating room. This early series suggested that laparoscopic sterilization with clips could be done in a hospital facility other than the operating room.

International Collaborative Studies
1,000 Patients with a One-Year Follow-Up

After the first prototype applicator was tested,[4] nine "second generation" prototypes were manufactured and distributed throughout the world in 1973 (Table 1). All collaborators were required to maintain accurate admission and follow-up data on their patients on forms developed for this purpose by the International Fertility Research Program (IFRP). At the end of both the six-month[6] and one-year periods,[3] data were collected from both the central computer at IFRP and by letter, cable and phone from each individual collaborator, with the exception of the workers in Singapore and Bombay, from whom only indirect information was available.

All but five of the procedures in Chapel Hill were done under minimal local anesthesia. More sedation and local anesthesia were used in Bangkok, Bombay and El Salvador. A mixture of local and general techniques was used in Los Angeles, Fort Worth, Ann Arbor and London. Excellent general anesthesia was available and therefore used in Singapore. A summary of the medications used with local anesthesia is presented in Table 2.

Postabortal: All applications in Bombay were in combination with first-trimester abortion. At Chapel Hill 41 were done at the time of first-trimester abortion and eight were done following second-trimester abortion. In England 12 were performed after first-trimester abortion.

Patient selection: All patients requesting sterilization at Chapel Hill were offered the clip as an experimental alternative to other accepted methods with a promise of having a pregnancy interrupted in the first trimester without charge if there was a failure. No patients were turned down because of obesity or recent pregnancy; only one patient was rejected because of previous pelvic surgery (multiple abdominal scars and a functioning colostomy from diverticulosis).

Results

Operative time: Table 3 presents the ranges of operative and recovery times experienced in those centers that had developed this technique into an outpatient procedure under local anesthesia. Room turn-over time (time required from start to finish of a series of cases in one room) is a sensitive measure of both the doctor's true surgical speed and the efficiency of his or her operating team. The most efficient service was in El Salvador, where four or five patients were operated upon routinely each hour; at Chapel Hill three patients an hour are scheduled routinely for the procedure. Postoperative recovery and hospital stay are a function of long-acting medication. The average recovery time was three hours; longer-acting medication, such as Phenergan, prolonged the recovery to an average of five hours in other centers.

Complications:

a. *Because of Laparoscopy:* One laparotomy was required because of a retroperitoneal hematoma caused by the Veress needle's grazing the sacrum. The hematoma was self-limiting and the patient merely observed. No further surgery was necessary. One death occurred because of massive myocardial infarction in a patient with artificial mitral and aortic valves after a delayed abdominal wall hemorrhage forced the discontinuation of anticoagulation therapy. At autopsy, the sites of clip application were intact.

b. *Because of Prototype Equipment:* Fogging of the optics was a constant nuisance and was partly a result of the design of the prototype equipment. The defect, a metal ridge against which the optics could be forced with a resultant break in the seal, has been eliminated in the "third generation" designs.

Deviations from specifications in the manufacturing process by an early manufacturer led to failure of the applicator to free itself of the clip in several centers. As a result, laparotomy was necessitated in one case. Reapplication of a second clip was required in two cases to arrest tubal oozing. The manufacturing defects have been identified and eliminated in the "third generation" manufacturing designs.†

Table 3
Average Operative and Recovery Times Under Local Anesthesia

Surgery	15 to 18 minutes
Room turnover	15 to 30 minutes
Recovery	3 to 5 hours
Hospital stay	4 to 8 hours

Table 4
Complications

Laparotomy	
malfunction of applicator	1
Veress needle hematoma	1
Tubal tear due to applicator malfunction (corrected by second clip)	4
wound discharge	6
postoperative vagal reflex	2%–8%
postoperative cramps	4%–26%
bowel burns or injury	0

Table 5
Pregnancies

Ectopic	0	surgical or
Pregnant at surgery	3	manufacturing
Ampullary application	6	error rate; 19
Structure other than tube	5	to 23/1,000
Poor isthmic application	2	
Weak spring	3	
Unknown	4*	method failure
Correct application,	2	rate; 2 to
good spring		6/1,000

* 1 delivered, to undergo repeat laparoscopy;
  1 aborted, vasectomy chosen;
  2 no data, Singapore and Bombay.

---

† Richard Wolf Medical Instruments Corp, Rosemont, Illinois.

c. *Because of the Clip:* Pain at the time of clip application was noted early in the study. Therefore, a technique for anesthetizing the tube was devised.[2] Local anesthesia is transient, and 26% of the patients with light sedation experienced postoperative cramping similar to menstrual cramps for 24 to 48 hours as the spring crushed the viable tubal tissue between the closed jaws. With longer-acting antihistaminics, only 4% of the patients in England reported this symptom. Also noted with light sedation was a vagal reflex characterized subjectively by nausea, clamminess and faintness and objectively by bradycardia and hypotension. These symptoms responded promptly to atropine and were noted less frequently when antihistaminics were the only medication.

A summary of complications experienced is presented in Table 4. There were no bowel burns or injuries. Table 5 summarizes pregnancies and their cause in this study.

Pregnancies:

a. *Because of Surgical Error:* Three patients were pregnant at the time of clipping and subsequently delivered or were aborted. In the first six months of the study, clips were placed on the distal, or ampullary, portion of the tube. It was subsequently found that the clip would not reach across this broad portion of the tube and thus that pregnancies would result. Instructions to the collaborators therefore emphasized placing clips on the proximal, or isthmic, portion of the tube only.

New optics, partial obstruction of the visual field by the clip-applying apparatus and fogging contributed to application of the clip to structures other than the tube, including the round ligament and varicosities of the broad ligament, as well as to incomplete isthmic application. Anatomic difficulties were encountered in some obese women in whom epiploic folds of fat made anatomic identification difficult. Recent midtrimester abortion made application of the clip to the left tube impossible in two women because of the combination of obesity, enlarged uterus and tubal edema. One of these women returned for application in two months, when uterine enlargement and edema had subsided. The second became pregnant because of poor isthmic application.

b. *Because of Manufacturing Error:* The springs were designed to exert a tension greater than double the arterial pressure necessary to maintain tissue viability between the jaws of the clip. This minimal pressure was specified as 75 g at the ends of the spring. Simple manufacturing quality-control-testing devices were given to the manufacturers of the clips. Nevertheless, a number of springs which fell well below these specifications were distributed during the early months of 1974. This error was detected in August 1974, and all clips were promptly recalled by IFRP. The Soderstrom snare technique was employed to remove clips when pregnancies occurred in patients from Chapel Hill despite apparently proper clip application. Testing of springs from four of these patients in the laboratory revealed tensions well below the minimum 75 g in three. The current manufacturer of these springs has improved the tension to well above the minimum level.

c. *Correct Application, Good Springs.* It has been documented that two pregnancies have occurred with proper application of good springs. In one, a clip applied close to the uterus had not been covered with epithelium, but rather the tubal endothelium had grown around the clip and had created a passage for sperm and egg open to the peritoneum. In the second, dye insufflation and serial sections of the removed clips failed to reveal any passage for sperm and egg to unite and implant in the uterus; the explanation for this pregnancy is unknown.

d. *Ectopic Pregnancy:* To date, no ectopic pregnancy subsequent to clip application has been detected.

e. *Unknown Causes:* Two women became pregnant and have not been studied further to date: one woman is currently deciding between laparoscopy and hysterectomy by her private physician after a normal delivery, and one woman declined laparoscopy after abortion in favor of her husband's undergoing vasectomy. Two patients overseas have become pregnant, and there is no additional information available.

f. *Method Failure Rate:* Two pregnancies occurred when good clips were applied properly to the isthmic portion of the tube. Four pregnancies occurred which may have been the result of either surgical error or manufacturing error, but the actual reason is unknown. Other pregnancies occurred because of documented surgical or manufacturing error. Excluding pregnancies known to be a result of such errors, there was a method failure rate of 2 to 6 per 1,000 cases after one year of application follow-up.

g. *Reversibility:* Animal studies[7] have documented restoration of normal fertility after clip removal and end-to-end anastomosis (Figure 7). Because of the minimal tubal destruction (3 to 4 mm of tissue) by the clip, enough functioning tissue should remain to allow reversal in humans. However, to date reversal has not been requested.

Summary

This report reviews studies undertaken to develop simpler, safer and more acceptable methods of female sterilization. A clip was designed which would have a spring load, be wide enough to cause true tissue necrosis, have a firm grip on the tube in order to avoid becoming dislodged and have a smooth external surface. The result of extensive human trials of the clip and applicator is that as of March 1974 there were over 1,000 patients with clips applied by 27 physicians in 10 centers throughout the world. Most of these procedures were performed under local anesthesia in an outpatient setting and with no fixed contraindications. Complications and pregnancy rates based on a one-year follow-up are presented. Complications because of the clip appear limited to postoperative cramps for 24 to 48 hours in 26% of all patients. No ectopic pregnancies were reported. Pregnancies, corrected because they were unsuspected initially or because of misapplications as a result of the clip itself, appear to be few. Performance of this operation under local anesthesia in a hospital facility other than the operating room has been documented as feasible.

References

1. Brown DR, Fishburne JI, Hulka JF: Ventilatory and blood gas changes during laparoscopy with local anesthesia. Am J Obstet Gynecol 124:741, 1976

2. Fishburne FI, Omran KF, Hulka JF, Mercer JP, Edelman DA: Laparoscopic tubal clip sterilization under local anesthesia. Fertil Steril 25:762, 1974

3. Hulka JF: Sterilization by spring clip: a report of 1,000 cases with a one year follow-up. Workshop on Advances in Female Sterilization Techniques, Minneapolis, MN, 1975

4. Hulka JF, Fishburne JI, Mercer JP, Omran KF: Laparoscopic sterilization with a spring clip: a report of the first fifty cases. Am J Obstet Gynecol 116:715, 1973

5. Hulka JF, Omran KF: Comparative tubal occlusion: rigid and spring-loaded clips. Fertil Steril 23:663, 1972

6. Hulka JF, Omran KF, Phillips JM, et al: Sterilization by spring clip: a report of 1,000 cases with six month follow-up. Fertil Steril 26:1122, 1975

7. Hulka JF, Ulberg LC: Reversibility of clip sterilization. Fertil Steril 26:1132, 1975

8. Power FH, Barnes AC: Sterilization by means of peritoneoscopic tubal fulguration: preliminary report. Am J Obstet Gynecol 41:1038, 1941

Silicone Ring*

InBae Yoon, M.D.

The development of a silicone rubber ring and a simple laparoscopic technique for its application has resulted in a safe and effective tubal sterilization technique. This unique form of sterilization may be performed on an outpatient basis under either local or general anesthesia. Furthermore, the instrumentation and technique may be adapted to either single- or double-puncture laparoscopy, suprapubic miniincision, transvaginal colpotomy or culdoscopy.

Materials

The Applicator

The applicator consists of two concentric cylinders (Figures 1 and 2). Within the inner cylinder is a forceps for grasping and elevating a segment of the fallopian tube. The outer surface of the inner cylinder is fitted with the silicone ring, which is applied by means of a ring loader and ring guide. The outer cylinder is designed to extrude the loaded ring from the inner cylinder onto the tube, which is held within the grasp of the forceps.

The applicator must be kept clean and dry when not in use. Before use, the major parts must be separated and each part cleaned. This separation and cleaning should be done at least once a day if the applicator is in constant use. The ring applicator, especially the inside of the inner cylinder and grasping forceps, must be cleaned before each operation and tested to be sure it is in good working order. It is important to eliminate infection of the fallopian tube and postoperative adhesions on the loop of tubal segment. Whenever the applicator is malfunctioning, separate and clean each part and reassemble the applicator. This usually solves the problem of an applicator that is difficult to adjust and operate. The applicator should be handled carefully. If it is dropped, the tip must be inspected to make certain wrinkling has not occurred.

The grasping forceps of the single-incision laparoscopic applicator is angled to one side so the operator has full view of it. Therefore, the operator should be sure that the grasping forceps is within the viewing field or on the lens side. The grasping forceps of the second incision, suprapubic miniincision and transvaginal ring applicator are not angled, but the end, not the grasping forceps, of the culdoscopic ring applicator is curved.

---

* All of this published data and testing has been with the Falope-Ring^R rings and systems. The proper name for the Falope-Ring^R rings would be dimethylpolysiloxane with 5% barium sulphate. This is a special formulation which is proprietary to KLI, Inc., Ivyland, Pennsylvania.

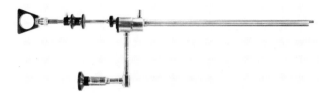

Figure 1
The Falope-Ring single incision applicator

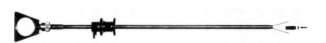

Figure 2
The Falope-Ring second incision applicator

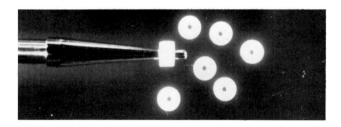

Figure 3
The Falope-Ring with loader

The Ring

The ring, composed of nonreactive silicone rubber impregnated with 5% barium sulfate (Figure 3), possesses an inner diameter of 1 mm, an outer diameter of 3.6 mm and a thickness of 2.2 mm. It has an elastic memory of 100% if stretched to not more than 6 mm. If the ring is stretched beyond 6 mm, the memory power decreases 90% to 95%; if it is stretched to more than 8 mm, rupture or microfracture of the ring occurs.

Technique

Basic laparoscopic technique is observed. The ring is made more pliable by placing it in warm saline or anesthetic jelly. It is then easily loaded onto the applicator without breaking and is inspected carefully to be certain that it is neither twisted nor torn.

If local anesthesia is employed, 2% lidocaine jelly is applied to the inner cylinder of the forceps. Alternatively, the tube may be sprayed or infiltrated with a similar substance. A latent period of 15 minutes is generally required to effect total anesthesia.

Upon entry into the pelvic cavity by an approach (by laparoscopic single puncture, laparoscopic double puncture, suprapubic miniincision, postpartum miniincision, postpartum laparoscopy, transvaginal colpotomy or transvaginal culdoscopy), a complete pelvic inspection should be done to determine whether or not there is an abnormal pathologic finding; also, the location of the fallopian tube should be determined.

The grasping forceps should always remain inside the applicator until the operator is ready to pick up the tube. Whenever the operator is not looking inside the pelvic cavity, the grasping forceps should be inside the applicator.

The ring can be dropped accidentally into the pelvic cavity because of improper manipulation of the applicator or when the operator is loading two rings onto the applicator. Instructions should be followed carefully in order to prevent premature firing of the ring into the pelvic cavity even though the operator may be able to retrieve it.

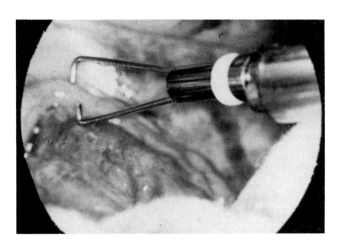

Figure 4
Identification of the fallopian tube with the grasping forceps

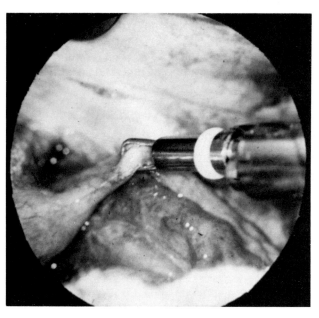

Figure 5
Lifting of the fallopian tube as it is drawn into the inner cylinder of the applicator

After confirmation of the location of the fallopian tube, the ring-loaded applicator approaches the tube at 3 cm from the uterotubal junction, and the grasping forceps is exposed from the applicator. One tip of the grasping forceps lifts the tube without touching, grasping or scratching the mesosalpinx. Thereafter, the two tips of the grasping forceps securely hold the fallopian tube, and the tube is drawn slowly into the cylinder. At the same time, the ring applicator or scope ring applicator should be moved inward in order to prevent tension on or tearing of the tube and thus pain.

The operator may elect to use a local anesthetic agent or postoperative analgesic medication for one or two days; it will usually eliminate postoperative discomfort as experienced in other tubal surgical procedures.

When the tube is drawn into the cylinder, the operating slide must be moved backward to the indicator completely in order to fire the ring onto the tube. Then the operating slide is gently pushed forward to release the loop of tube from the grasping forceps, making the loop 1 or 1.2 cm long (Figures 4–9).

If the operating slide is not drawn backward completely to the indicator, the ring may be applied on the grasping forceps with the loop of tubal segment inside the grasping forceps. If this should occur, the loop of the tube should be alternately drawn into and let out of the inner cylinder two or three times with the grasping forceps until the ring moves from the forceps to the loop of fallopian tube. This procedure usually works. A problem of this type generally does not occur when the operator has a complete understanding of the mechanism of the applicator.

If the patient is young, is a possible candidate for tuboplasty or has one child, the ring-loaded applicator should approach, if possible, at a point 2.5 to 3 cm from the fimbrial end in order for the operator to do a simple tuboplasty.

If the ring application is too close to the uterotubal junction or if the tube is not drawn slowly into the cylinder even though the ring is applied in the proper location, transection or a too small loop of segment can result.

In the event of pelvic adhesions, peritubal adhesions or acute or chronic salpingitis, ring application should be avoided, as should any other tubal surgical procedure.

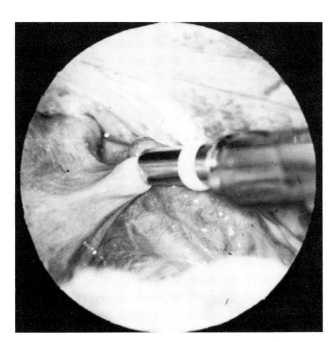

Figure 6
The fallopian tube being drawn into the inner cylinder of the applicator

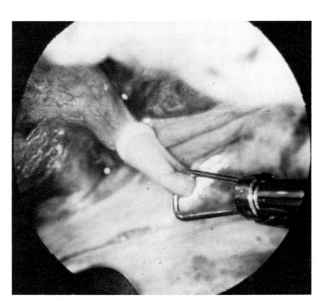

Figure 8
Release of the fallopian tube from the grasping forceps

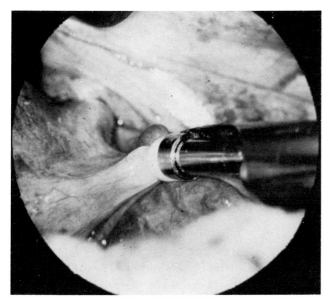

Figure 7
The application of the Falope-Ring to the fallopian tube

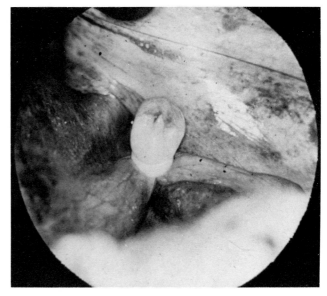

Figure 9
Falope-Ring applied to the fallopian tube

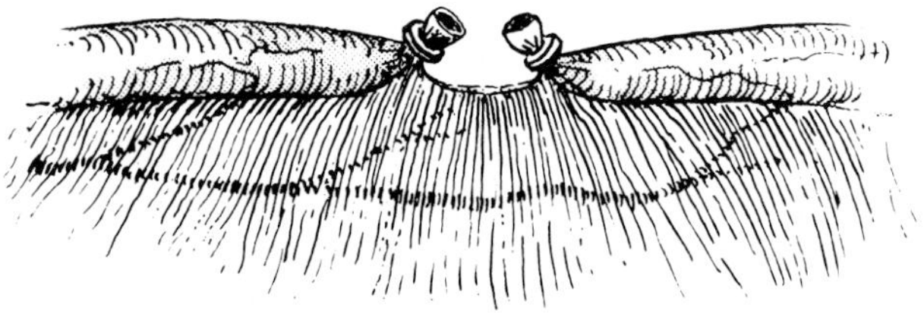

Figure 10
Bilateral proximal and distal reapplication of the ring after transection

In the event of resistance because of a thick or swollen tube, the loop of the tube should be alternately drawn into and let out of the inner cylinder two or three times with the grasping forceps in order to create an adequate loop of segment (1 or 1.2 cm).

In the event of transection or bleeding caused by grasping or scratching the mesosalpinx, the proximal and distal ends of the transected tube or bleeding point should be gently picked up with the grasping forceps and the ring applied to control bleeding (Figure 10). This procedure requires skill. Therefore, the operator must learn how to apply and remove the ring at the time of surgery in case of improper application to the round ligament, ovarian ligament, infundibulopelvic ligament or bowel. This experience can eliminate unnecessary pelvic laparotomy.

Results

From October 1973 to October 1975 the number of cases at Johns Hopkins was 902; the number done by domestic investigators, 1,741; by foreign investigators, 1,747. Therefore, the total number of recorded cases was 4,390. In the Hopkins series of 902 cases, there have been no true failures; there were, however, six cases of pregnancy: three were due to surgical error and three were luteal phase pregnancies. In the domestic series of 1,741 cases there were four cases of pregnancy; two were due to surgical error and two were luteal phase pregnancies. The foreign data shows 1,548 cases of interval sterilization and 249 cases of postabortal sterilization, bringing the total number of recorded cases to 1,747. Postpartum cases have not yet been recorded. Most cases were done with local anesthesia; mean surgical time was 11 to 13 minutes. Most surgical difficulties were incidental findings of massive pelvic adhesions prior to surgery and technical error, resulting in tubal transection. The complications recorded at Hopkins were mainly tubal transection, in 2.6% of the cases, and lower abdominal cramping, in 3.9% of the cases. Pain was probably caused by strangulation of the tube, resulting in ischemia.

There have been 13 repeat laparoscopic examinations, which showed either complete detachment, partial detachment or a fibrotic loop of segment in a period from three to 12 months after the operation. On microscopic examination, the area of ring application showed gradual fibrotic necrosis and the loop of segment showed small hemorrhagic hydrosalpinx shortly after the operation; later microscopic examinations showed fibrosis or detachment formation.

Conclusion

With the proper technique, the Falope-Ring provides safe, mechanical occlusion of the fallopian tube for sterilization. The procedure is simple to learn, easy to use and adaptable to numerous anatomical approaches.

A major advantage of this procedure is that the ring may be removed in case of application to an improper structure such as bowel, round ligament, ovarian ligament or mesosalpinx. The silicone rubber band procedure eliminates the possibility of bowel burn and reduces the amount of pneumoperitoneum, which may be associated with electrocautery, and reduces the extent of damage to the fallopian tube, which may have a positive result in cases where restoration of tubal patency is desired.

The Snare Method

Richard M. Soderstrom, M.D.

This method, first described by Soderstrom and Smith,[1] uses an operating laparoscope with its grasping forceps and a wire snare to coagulate, transect, and resect a tubal specimen adequate for pathologic confirmation. It requires a second trocar puncture. The operating time, however, is equal to that of other methods of laparoscopic sterilization.

Advantages

1. It produces adequate and uniform coagulation (using low voltage, high frequency coagulators).
2. It guarantees adequate transection.
3. It guarantees adequate resection.
4. It is the only method yet described which removes a normal (uncoagulated) specimen for pathologic confirmation.
5. It exposes the abdominal viscera to the smallest active electrode yet designed, thus reducing risk of visceral burn.

Disadvantages

1. It is a two-hole technique (debatable).
2. An operating laparoscope must be available.
3. The technique is technically more complicated to learn — it should be reserved for the skilled laparoscopist.
4. It is more difficult to teach than other methods.

Special Instruments

1. Operating laparoscope.
2. Operating laparoscope grasping forceps. It should be spring-loaded to remain *closed* when not actively manipulated; a rubber band intertwined between the finger holes suffices.
3. Insulated, self-opening laparoscope snare (Cameron-Miller; Figure 1).

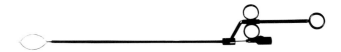

Figure 1
Self-opening laparoscopic snare (Cameron-Miller)

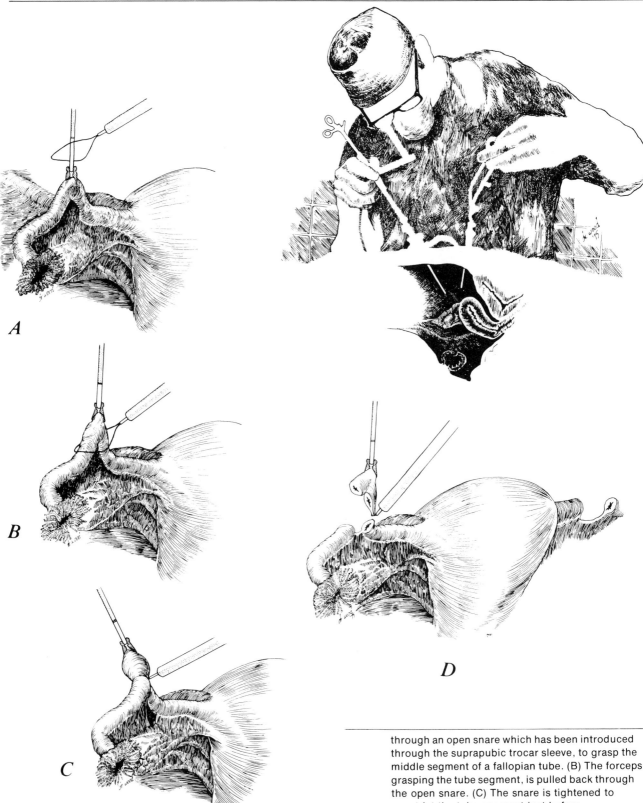

Figure 2

The Soderstrom-Smith technique of midtubal resection. (A) A grasping forceps, introduced through the operating laparoscope, is guided through an open snare which has been introduced through the suprapubic trocar sleeve, to grasp the middle segment of a fallopian tube. (B) The forceps, grasping the tube segment, is pulled back through the open snare. (C) The snare is tightened to constrict the tube segment just before electrocoagulation is applied. (D) Once the tube blanches white, low voltage, high frequency cutting current is applied and the tube segment is resected. The resected tube segment is removed with the grasping forceps and the laparoscope through the umbilical trocar sleeve. (Figure courtesy of the Bulletin of The Mason Clinic.)

Technique

After proper insufflation and introduction of the operating laparoscope, the second 6 mm fiberglass trocar sleeve with trocar is placed suprapubically in the midline under direct vision. The snare is inserted through the 6 mm trocar sleeve (Figure 2).

1. Open the snare completely and place it over the middle third of the tube.
2. Thread the tip of the grasping forceps through the open snare. Advance the tip until it touches the tube.
3. Grasp the tube. Once the tube is secure, the operator frees his hand from the grasper to steady the laparoscope. (The rubber band will maintain the grasping forceps in the closed position.)
4. Slowly withdraw the laparoscope. This ensures a wide view of the operating field and usually will pull a sufficient knuckle of tube (1 to 2 cm) through the open snare wire.
5. Once an adequate specimen has been snared, tighten the snare wire snugly. The resection site should be at least 2 cm from the uterine cornu.
6. Attach coagulator cord.
7. Use low voltage, high frequency blended coagulation (a setting of 40 watts on most models). Apply a steady current until blanching extends 5 mm into the mesosalpinx.
8. Close the snare slowly but completely while applying *continuous current*.
9. Disconnect coagulator cord.
10. Holding the laparoscope trocar sleeve trumpet *open,* remove the laparoscope and the grasping forceps from the abdomen *as a unit*. The specimen will be held securely in the jaws of the grasper because of the spring-loaded handle created with the rubber band.
11. Submit the specimen to a pathologist.
12. Inspect the resection site and repeat on the opposite side.

Complications

Complications usually occur during the learning phase and in most instances involve bleeding from the resection site. It is recommended that the technique be practiced on a few benign hysterectomy patients at the time of open laparotomy. Then practice on ten benign hysterectomy patients via laparoscopy just prior to the laparotomy incision. Common errors during the learning phase are: (1) attempting to resect too close to the uterus; (2) resecting too much specimen; (3) closing the snare wire completely before adequate coagulation of mesosalpinx has occurred; or (4) closing the snare wire without continuous current.

It is mandatory that the tube be identified definitely at the outset since resection of a segment of small bowel could result in disastrous consequences.

Summary

The Soderstrom-Smith technique of laparoscopic tubal resection is a two-hole technique which guarantees adequate transection and resection of the fallopian tube. In addition, it is the only method yet described that guarantees pathological confirmation of the resected specimen. Of all the methods described, it is the most complex to teach and learn, and should not be attempted by the novice in laparoscopy.

Reference

1. Soderstrom RM, Smith MR: Instrument and method — tubal sterilization, a new laparoscopic method. Obstet Gynecol 38:152, 1971

Sterilization Combined with Abortion

Norman G. Courey, M.D., C.M.
Arthur J. Horowitz, M.D.
Rafael G. Cunanan, Jr., M.D.

Introduction

Tubal sterilization combined with pregnancy termination is often desirable. Since the advent of laparoscopy, it can be effected with a minimum of inconvenience and morbidity, at moderate expense and with minimal hospitalization (24 hours or less). The patients suffer negligible postoperative discomfort and are able to resume daily duties rapidly.

Prior to 1969 most experiences with combined sterilization and abortion procedures were limited to the use of hysterectomy, transabdominal hysterotomy combined with traditional tubal ligation and sharp or aspiration curettage combined with abdominal or vaginal tubal ligation. Most of these procedures resulted in prolonged hospitalization and recovery times.

Steptoe[8] was the first to suggest the combination of aspiration curettage and laparoscopic sterilization. Since then many others have published their findings in similar situations.[1, 2, 3, 4, 5, 7, 9, 10]

Indications and Contraindications

Tubal sterilization is a method of permanent sterilization and consequently the indications must be considered seriously. Patients requesting sterilization at the time of abortion must be adequately counseled so they realize that the intent of the sterilization procedure is to produce permanent and irreversible termination of fertility. It is vital that sterilization *not* be presented as a requirement for pregnancy termination.

Timing

This procedure is currently feasible in association with either first- or early midtrimester abortion. Provided that no major contraindication to laparoscopy exists, it seems reasonable that morbidity from the combination of laparoscopic sterilization and abortion should not be greater than the sum total of morbidity from either procedure. With gestational length beyond 14 weeks there is an increase in morbidity, largely dependent upon the morbidity inherent in the abortion technique. For practical purposes, laparoscopic sterilization with concomitant abortion is usually limited to gestations of 12 weeks or less. In the hands of those extremely skilled in the technique of aspiration and sharp curettage as well as laparoscopy it is sometimes feasible to perform the procedure as late as 14 weeks. With pregnancies advanced beyond 14 weeks it is more prudent to defer sterilization for approximately four to six weeks after a conventional abortion.

Preoperative Preparation

The procedure may be performed on an outpatient or inpatient basis, depending upon the local customs governing hospital services and/or the patient's general medical condition. The average, healthy woman of childbearing age is certainly a candidate for an outpatient approach, but the woman with complicating medical conditions should have proper preoperative preparation.

Blood should be crossmatched, especially when the gestational length is above 12 weeks. Rh immune globulin should be given to nonsensitized Rh negative women in the rare event that tubal sterilization fails or for some reason is not completed. Another, often-neglected indication for Rh immune globulin is the possibility that subsequent to sterilization the patient may be involved in an accident for which transfusion is necessary but when type specific Rh negative blood is not available. Laminaria digitata tents may be inserted into the cervical canal six to 12 hours prior to the procedure; however, when general anesthesia is employed and gradually-tapered dilators are used, it is not absolutely essential to use a laminaria tent to achieve cervical dilatation.

Anesthesia

All patients undergoing a combined sterilization and abortion procedure should have general anesthesia since the procedure may be prolonged and uncomfortable, especially in more advanced gestations. Halothane and its derivatives and any major anesthetic gases which predispose to uterine atony should be avoided.

Pregnancy Termination

Abdominal perineal preparation is the same as that employed for laparoscopy without abortion. The patient is placed in the dorsal lithotomy position, with mild flexion of the thighs, as is usually employed in routine laparoscopic procedures. The bladder should be emptied prior to performance of the procedure. The cervix and vagina are cleansed with an appropriate antiseptic and a weighted speculum is placed in the posterior fornix. The cervix is grasped transversely with a single- or double-toothed tenaculum. The cervical canal is then dilated to the same number of millimeters as the corresponding gestational age (up to a maximum of 12 to 13 mm). The uterus is sounded to confirm uterine size and direction. Gradually-tapered dilators (Pratt, Hanks or Hawkins-Ambler) are preferable to Hegar dilators. With the tapered dilator cervical dilatation is achieved without undue force whereas the blunter Hegar dilators require more pressure, even under general anesthesia. The extra pressure increases the risks of uterine or cervical perforation as well as cervical laceration from tearing away of the tenaculum from the cervix.

Depending on the brand and type of aspiration tip used, it may be necessary to dilate the cervix slightly more than the diameter of the cannula. After dilatation is achieved the uterine cavity is evacuated at 60 to 70 cm of mercury negative pressure with a clear plastic cannula corresponding in diameter to the number of weeks' gestation. At 12 weeks' gestation it is occasionally necessary to use an ovum forceps to remove parts of the gestation which will not fit through the cannula. Beyond 12 weeks it is invariably necessary to use these forceps. Once the uterus appears to have been completely evacuated, the uterine walls should be curetted with a sharp curette.

Oxytocics are generally not necessary, even under general anesthesia, if uterine-relaxing anesthetic agents are avoided. However, if desired, one of the oxytocic agents may be added to the intravenous infusion. It will decrease blood loss to less than 200 cc even in the more advanced first-trimester and early second-trimester patients.

After completion of the abortion a manipulator must be inserted into the uterus in order to mobilize it during the laparoscopic procedure. A tubal insufflation cannula, vacuum cannula, Sargis or Hulka uterine manipulators[6] may be used.

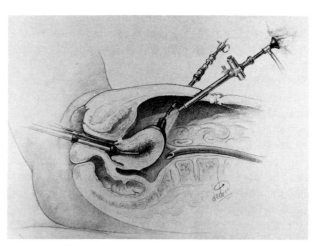

Figure 1

Laparoscopic Sterilization

The method of inserting the laparoscopic cannula and trocar is very critical since improper technique may damage the enlarged uterine fundus, especially after termination of an advanced pregnancy. Beyond nine weeks' gestation it is strongly recommended that the double-puncture laparoscopic technique be employed. A single-puncture laparoscope, though entirely appropriate for interim sterilization, is not sufficiently flexible for the positioning of instruments that is necessary when the uterus is enlarged. The immediately postabortal uterus beyond eight or nine weeks' size is usually more globular and bulky and occupies considerably more of the pelvic cavity than in the nonpregnant state. In addition, the fallopian tubes are often displaced posterolaterally away from the uterine fundus. Furthermore, the fundus is often higher than the uterine cornua, whereas in the nonpregnant state it is at approximately the same level as the tubes. As a result, it frequently becomes necessary to tease the fallopian tube up and away from the uterus with a grasping forceps (Figure 1).

The lower (second) puncture is usually made one-third the distance between the symphysis and the umbilicus or higher, depending on the height of the uterus. If this puncture is made too low, extremely awkward positioning of the operating instruments may result, which hampers the operator. In the rare event that satisfactory exposure of the fallopian tube is hindered by a bulky uterus in spite of the usual precautions, a third puncture may be made in the opposite lower quadrant. A blunt probe or manipulator is inserted and used to push the uterus aside, thus enabling the fallopian tubes to be grasped more easily. After careful visualization of the intraabdominal structures the appropriate forceps are inserted in order to grasp, manipulate, coagulate and, if desired, cut or resect the tubes. Significant varicosities in the mesosalpinx are generally not encountered until 16 weeks' gestation, despite the pregnancy. Anastomosis of the ovarian and uterine arteries occurs near the cornual angle and close to the tube at this point. There is a danger of inadvertently grasping and injuring the artery; such damage is difficult to control by coagulation, especially in the presence of an enlarged uterus.

Table 1
Complications With Combined Procedures

Authors	Number of patients	Number of complications and rate	Type of complication
Steptoe, Imram 1969[8]	101	7(6.9%)	4 mild pyrexia 1 incomplete aspiration 1 pelvic abscess 1 damage to mesosalpinx vessels
Gudgeon 1971[5]	19	2(10.5%)	1 incomplete aspiration 1 wound infection
Whitson, Ballard, Israel 1973[10]	100	8(8.0%)	5 "major" 1 subrectus hematoma 1 bowel perforation 3 failed laparoscopies 3 "minor" 1 endometritis 1 wound inflammation 1 seroma
Amin, Neuwirth 1973[1]	63	4(6.3%)	4 pyrexia
Cunanan, Courey 1974[3]	439	3(0.7%)	1 bleeding point in omentum 1 uterine perforation 1 pyrexia
Leong, Gillett, Kinch 1974[7]	65	2(3.1%)	1 pyrexia 1 incomplete abortion
Fishburne, Edelman, Hulka, Mercer 1975[4]	108	10(9.2%)	4 uterine perforation 1 cervical laceration 1 vasovagal hypotension 1 incomplete abortion and endometritis 1 salpingitis 2 wound infection

Postoperative Care

Upon leaving the recovery area the patient is allowed a diet by mouth; when she is alert and awake she may be discharged. She is cautioned not to operate any machinery or drive a motor vehicle for 24 hours. If someone does not come to take her home, she is kept overnight. All patients subjected to a combined laparoscopic sterilization and abortion procedure may be placed on prophylactic antibiotic and oxytocics. Generally a broad-spectrum antibiotic may be employed, and methylergonovine grain $1/320$ is given four times a day by mouth for eight doses. The patient is instructed to report any complications, such as bleeding, pain not relieved with aspirin, fever or persistent shoulder pain, and is seen two to three weeks after discharge to ensure that there is adequate involution and that the wounds are well healed and to reassure her that the results are satisfactory. Sutures, if nonabsorbable, are removed prior to discharge. Intercourse is permitted two weeks after the procedure to allow adequate involution.

Results

Complications accompanying the combined procedure of laparoscopic tubal ligation and aspiration curettage are no more serious or frequent than those accompanying either of the procedures alone. Reported complication rates range from 0.7% to 10.5%, with pyrexia the most common complaint (Table 1).

In contrast, complication rates for other combined procedures are much higher. Tubal ligation by laparotomy with suction termination had a morbidity rate of 17.6% in one series,[7] and a combination of Pomeroy tubal ligation and pregnancy termination by hysterotomy resulted in a 40% rate of complications in another.[3]

References

1. Amin HK, Neuwirth RS: Further experience with laparoscopic sterilization concomitant with vacuum curettage for abortion. Fertil Steril 24:592, 1973

2. Courey NG, Cunanan RG: Combined laparoscopic sterilization and pregnancy termination. J Reprod Med 10:291, 1973

3. Cunanan RG, Courey NG: Combined laparoscopic sterilization and pregnancy termination II: Further experiences with a larger series of patients. J Reprod Med 13:204, 1974

4. Fishburne JI, Edelman DA, Hulka JF, Mercer JP: Outpatient laparoscopic sterilization with therapeutic abortion versus abortion alone. Obstet Gynecol 45:665, 1975

5. Gudgeon D: Sterilization and abortion. Lancet 1:1240, 1971

6. Hulka JF: Controlling uterine forceps for laparoscopic sterilization after abortion: a new instrument. Am J Obstet Gynecol 116:884, 1973

7. Leong MKH, Gillett PG, Kinch RAH: Therapeutic abortion with concurrent sterilization: comparison of methods. Can Med Assoc J 111:1328, 1974

8. Steptoe PC: Laparoscopic sterilization during termination of pregnancy. Proc R Soc Med 62:833, 1969

9. Steptoe PC, Imram M: Combined procedure of aspiration termination and laparoscopic sterilization. Br Med J 3:751, 1969

10. Whitson LG, Ballard CA, Israel R: Laparoscopic tubal sterilization coincident with therapeutic abortion by suction curettage. Obstet Gynecol 41:677, 1973

Puerperal Sterilization

Louis Keith, M.D.
Keim T. Houser, M.D.

Puerperal Laparoscopy

Puerperal laparoscopic sterilization initially was thought to be technically difficult and inadvisable. Steptoe, in the original English monograph, cautioned against the use of laparoscopy in the puerperium though he has since endorsed the procedure. Other authors supported his early opinion, frequently without the benefit of personal experience.

At Cook County Hospital in Chicago a few puerperal laparoscopic sterilizations were done as early as 1966 and the first published series reported in 1970 and 1971.[1,2] Additions to that series and unpublished data, which includes the experience of postgraduate students trained at Cook County Hospital, place our cumulative cases at over 3,500.[3] Other reports in the literature and unpublished data added over 1,300 more cases to the international experience.[3]

It is our opinion that postpartum laparoscopic sterilization can be accomplished by the experienced laparoscopist without increasing patient morbidity and with some saving of hospital time and patient discomfort. Furthermore, this operation can also be instructive when used in teaching situations with large obstetrics services.

A summary of the Cook County Hospital technique is presented:

1. Anesthesia is begun and the patient washed, prepped and draped. She is then placed in 8° to 10° Trendelenburg position.

2. CO_2 is insufflated via a Veress needle at or near the umbilicus at a rate of 1 liter per minute. Three to four liters of CO_2 are generally needed to distend the lax abdominal wall.

3. The skin lateral to the umbilicus may be stabilized using towel clips. The site of insertion of the major trocar may be below or even slightly above the umbilicus, depending on the fundal height.

4. The trocar is inserted slowly and with care to avoid the fundus if it is high. This is facilitated by confining the major thrusting action to the wrist.

5. The auxiliary trocar is inserted in the midline, two or three inches below the major trocar or, after transillumination, in an area lateral to the rectus muscle at the level of fundus but never below that level.

6. The tube is identified, grasped, tented and coagulated and a specimen removed bilaterally, if desired.

7. Skin closure is accomplished via clips or sutures; subcuticular sutures may be used.

These points are of particular interest in postpartum laparoscopy:

1. The patient should be atropinized adequately. If there is a question about it, or if 90 minutes have elapsed prior to induction of anesthesia, an additional intravenous dose should be administered.

2. Five hundred to 750 cc Ringer's lactate or appropriate intravenous solution is given prior to induction of anesthesia. It rapidly expands the circulating blood volume and helps prevent hypotension.

3. Pitocin added to the intravenous fluids at the beginning of anesthesia helps to ensure a firm, contracted uterus.

4. Avoid deep Trendelenburg position: it embarrasses respiration and is usually not necessary because of the height of the fundus and lax abdominal wall.

5. An indwelling catheter used during surgery will help keep the uterus in the pelvis.

6. The lax abdominal wall can be manipulated to either side of the fundus with the rigid trocars so that the telescope and cautery forceps are directly above the tube and the fundus does not obscure sight lines.

Clinical experience with a large number of cases has demonstrated that puerperal laparoscopic sterilization can be accomplished successfully with morbidity no greater than that of interval sterilization.

References

1. Keith L, Houser K, Webster A, Lash AF: Postpartum laparoscopy for sterilization. J Int Fed Obstet Gynecol 8:145, 1970

2. Keith L, Houser K, Webster A, Lash A: Puerperal tubal sterilization using laparoscopic technique: a preliminary report. J Reprod Med 6:133, 1971

3. Keith L, Simonelli J, Webster A: Laparoscopic sterilization in the puerperium: worldwide experience. Presented before the Second European Congress of Endoscopy, Konstanz, Germany, April 18, 1975

Editorial Comments

The wide variety of laparoscopic sterilization techniques has been reviewed thoroughly in this section.

The ideal method of sterilization should be 100% effective and carry with it very little morbidity or mortality, if any. This ideal method has yet to be found. As stressed, the dangers of electrosurgical injury are obviated by the use of nonelectrosurgical occlusive techniques, including clips and rings or bands. However, the efficacy of these newer techniques and their effect upon postoperative adhesion formation has yet to be evaluated in the long term.

Electrosurgical destruction of tissue beyond what is apparent at the time of surgery does occur. Thus, the future ability to reestablish patency and subsequent function in such tubes is questionable. With the increasing numbers of women requesting restoration of fertility, the ring and clip techniques seem to offer a better prognosis since there is less tissue destruction with them. Very little information is available on individual experiences with tubal reanastamosis after electrosurgical or mechanical occlusion. Behrman has achieved some pregnancies by resection and reanastamosis or reimplantation after electrocoagulation.[1]

Electrosurgical occlusion is still the most popular technique. Bipolar instruments have decreased the dangers of electrical burns, but long-term follow-up studies of such procedures are not yet available, either.

The techniques which have withstood the test of time include those of coagulation only, coagulation and cutting, and coagulation and resection. The results of some published data are presented in Table 1. It appears that in many cases the only failures encountered followed the combined procedures of sterilization and first-trimester abortion. As Soderstrom stressed at the beginning of this chapter, increased vascularity and tubal edema increase the possibility of failure due to inadequate or incomplete electrocoagulation.

From the long-term follow-up of the large series of cases presented in Table 1 it appears that the "burn only" technique is adequate, providing that 2 to 3 cm of the tube are electrocoagulated sufficiently. In addition, as shown by Phillips and co-workers,[7] the incidence of hemorrhage due to mesosalpingeal and tubal tears is lower with the "burn only" technique.

With great anticipation I await the long-term follow-up study on the nonelectrical occlusive techniques of Yoon and Hulka.

One of the major concerns associated with all forms of tubal sterilization is the apparent subsequent increase in dysfunctional uterine bleeding. If this is the case, then the degree of mesosalpingeal injury which occurs with the various techniques may be a factor; it may be due to damage to the anastamotic arcade of vessels which lies within this structure. The validity of this assumption may be clarified at least in part by current investigations. Many variables in such a study, however, must first be excluded before any valid conclusions can be extracted.

A.A.Y.

References

1. Behrman SJ: Personal communication

2. Cunanan RG, Courey NG: Combined laparoscopic sterilization and pregnancy termination. In *Gynecological Laparoscopy: Principles and Techniques* (JM Phillips, L Keith, Eds.) Stratton Intercontinental Medical Book Corp, New York, 1974, p 233

3. Edgerton WD: Experience with laparoscopy in a nonteaching hospital. Am J Obstet Gynecol 116:184, 1973

4. Fishburne JI, Edelman DA, Hulka J, Mercer JP: Outpatient laparoscopic sterilization with therapeutic abortion versus sterilization alone. Obstet Gynecol 45:665, 1975

5. Liston WA, Downie J, Bradford W, Kerr MG: Female sterilization by tubal electrocoagulation under laparoscopic control. Lancet 1:382, 1970

6. Peterson EP, Behrman SJ: Laparoscopic tubal sterilization. Am J Obstet Gynecol 110: 24, 1971

7. Phillips JM, Keith D, Hulka J, Hulka B, Keith L: Gynecologic laparoscopy in 1975. J Reprod Med 16:105, 1976

8. Soderstrom RM: Personal communication

9. Thompson BH, Wheeless CR: Failures of laparoscopy sterilization. Obstet Gynecol 45:659, 1975

10. Yuzpe AA, Rioux J-E, Loffer FD, Pent D: Laparoscopic tubal sterilization by the "burn only" technique. Obstet Gynecol (In press)

Table 1
Follow-up of Laparoscopic Sterilizations

Technique	Length of follow-up (in months) Minimum	Maximum	Total number of cases	Surgical failures	Pregnancies Intrauterine	Ectopic	Failures with combined procedures
Thompson[9] Wheeless							
Coagulate and resect large segment	36	66	1000	3	2	1	
Single burn and resect small segment	24	36	1000	12	12	0	
Burn, resect and recoagulate proximal stump	12	27	2200	6	4	2	
Soderstrom[8]							
Burn and resect	24	*	1000	4	4	0	4
Cunanan Courey[2]							
Burn and resect	*	*	439	1	1	0	1
Liston[5]							
Burn and resect	*	*	760	1	0	1	?
Edgerton[3]							
Burn and transect	*	*	959	0	0	0	
Peterson Behrman[6]							
Burn and transect	6 80 cases	12 80 cases	186	1	1	0	
Fishburne[4]							
Burn and transect	*	*	76	0			0
Yuzpe et al[10]							
Burn only	6	66	2857	1	0	1	1

* Unspecified

Section
7

Diagnosis
and
Management
of
Infertility

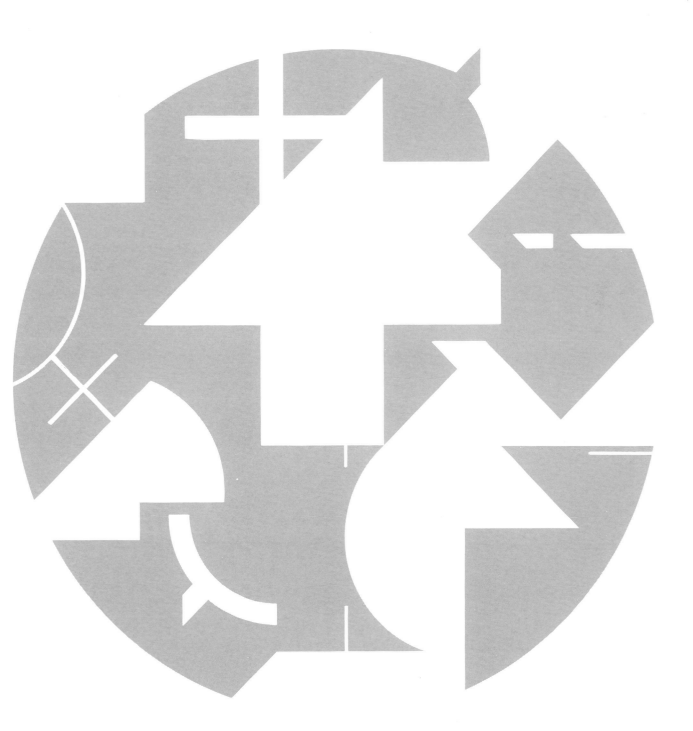

Editorial Introduction

Some years ago I had the privilege of reviewing Dr. Cohen's monograph on laparoscopy for *Obstetrics and Gynecology*. At that time I referred to him as a doyen of laparoscopy; I can't think of a more appropriate term now. In the following chapter he has given us a philosophic overview of laparoscopy and its role in infertility based on a wealth of personal experience.

John Esposito's section deals more with specifics and therefore lends itself to discussion. I frequently perform laparoscopy if pregnancy has not occurred after three apparent clomiphine-induced ovulatory cycles. The reason for this is that some of these patients have had prior wedge resection of the ovaries and 15% may be expected to be infertile as a consequence of perifimbrial adhesions. Also, enlarged ovaries help to create confusion about the proper spread of opaque medium following hysterosalpingography. On the other hand, while Albano's guidelines are useful, I see no reason for early laparoscopy in a patient seeking donor insemination provided the gynecologic history is negative.

We have relegated the Rubin's apparatus to a dusty shelf in our office; for us it creates more obfuscation rather than insight into true tubal function.

The infertility authors mention the discordance rate between salpingography and laparoscopy. Remember that cornual spasm can be encountered under general anesthesia and in the presence of skeletal-muscle-relaxing agents as well as in the x-ray department. One reason for false negative results with either procedure is insertion of the cannula too far in the uterus, thus causing the tip to penetrate the endometrium. Use of a balloon catheter may cause apparent cornual obstruction if the balloon is inflated beyond 2 cc. The hysterogram, for all its inaccuracy, gives information about the uterine cavity and tubal lumen not obtainable by laparoscopy. It is not, however, the final answer and we should feel free to reassess the situation with an endoscopic approach.

In his book *Hysterosalpingography* Siegler[1] has the following table, based on 1,000 consecutive salpingograms for infertility, of which 60% indicated bilateral patency:

Sites of Tubal Obstruction

Location	Unilateral	Bilateral	Total
Cornua	15.2%	5.3%	20.5%
Midpoint	4.9	0.8	5.7
Ampulla	7.6	5.0	12.6

Since the clinical incidence of cornual obstruction doesn't begin to approach these figures, this diagnosis should be made with great care and certainly not without confirmatory findings at laparoscopy.

I prefer to time diagnostic laparoscopy/tubal lavage to coincide with the eighth postovulatory day in order to obtain an endometrial biopsy. I doubt that lush secretory endometrium or polyps could completely occlude the cornual area. It is important to finish the tubal flushing procedure prior to endometrial biopsy in order to avoid regurgitation of endometrial fragments into the peritoneal cavity. Indigo carmine is preferable since it seems less irritating than methylene blue and passes through tissue planes more slowly.

If one tube seems to pass dye promptly and the other not at all, it is helpful to temporarily occlude the "good tube" with a blunt probe or atraumatic forceps placed at the isthmus. Often dye will be seen to flow from the other side suggesting normal but dissimilar patency.

I was very intrigued by John Esposito's description of the cul-de-sac postcoital test. This is a truer physiologic endpoint than cervical sampling and might be helpful in cases of "cervical factor infertility" where no other cause is found. Serial tests with office culdocentesis could be employed to assess treatment results.

Personally, I find that laparoscopy is indicated and helpful in patients who have been infertile for at least one year and whose initial workup demonstrates three months of apparently ovulatory temperature charts in the presence of normal semen analysis, normal postcoital exams and normal hysterosalpingography. Approximately 35% of these "negative" patients have unappreciated, asymptomatic endometriosis. Another 30% have minimal tubal disease such as tubal phimosis or peritubal adhesions, missed by x-ray but of physiologic importance. Phimosis may be treated by hydrotubation, laparoscopic surgery or laparotomy, if needed. The salutary effect of hysterosalpingography or laparoscopic lavage on fertility probably occurs in those patients who need a simple, mechanical cleansing of the gelatinous, inspissated mucus which has collected at the fimbrae.

Roland and his group have had great experience in this area and the data contained in his Table 1 support the philosophy of resorting to laparoscopy early in the fertility workup. Within three months a diagnosis can be made and proper treatment begun. I echo his plea for complete reporting of laparoscopic findings. Standard charts, such as those used by Roland or Cohen, are helpful. Pictures, if skillfully taken, are better. We have had to reinvestigate patients laparoscopically who were referred for further study because of poor reporting and because tubal lavage had not been performed at the first procedure. The statement that "the tubes appeared grossly normal" is insufficient for accurate evaluation.

Gomel's chapter considers laparoscopy as a therapeutic tool in addition to a diagnostic aid. I am not yet certain if fulguration of multiple endometriotic implants is preferable to sharp excision. Many of us are enthusiastic about ovarian biopsy during laparoscopy for diagnosis. It is becoming apparent that at least some of these patients begin to ovulate after this procedure, which might more correctly be called "mini-wedge resection." Actual salpingostomy and extensive salpingolysis performed via laparoscopy demand great skill and much patience. As evidenced by pregnancy rates and pictures, Gomel has achieved a high degree of success with this technique.

S.L.C.

Reference

1. Siegler AM: *Hysterosalpingography.* Medcom Press, New York, 1974, p 136

Chapter 16

Laparoscopy and Infertility

Melvin R. Cohen, M.D.

Laparoscopy is usually necessary for the diagnosis of obscure pelvic disease in every infertile woman 30 years of age or older and for any patient, regardless of age, who has been infertile for three or more years. Laparoscopy is unnecessary when overt pathology, such as large leiomyomata, exists or when the man is judged infertile.

Laparoscopy should not be performed prior to an adequate diagnostic survey. The majority of the tests outlined in Figure 1 are performed in the office. The following points should be covered in the initial interview of the couple:

1. Age, occupation and education
2. Length of marriage and prior marriages of either partner
3. Duration (years) of infertility; whether or not birth control was used and the exact method of contraception
4. With secondary infertility in this marriage or with prior fertile marriages, it is important to know the number and outcome of each pregnancy and whether complications occurred
5. Menstrual history; leukorrhea
6. Coital history including frequency and difficulties, such as dyspareunia
7. Prior diagnostic studies, with reports in depth
8. General history (medical, surgical and nutritional) of each partner in childhood, adolescence and adulthood.

There must be a general examination of each partner, including genital examination of the husband and pelvic examination with a Papanicolaou smear of the wife. General laboratory tests are performed on both partners.

The actual survey of the infertile couple usually begins with semen analysis unless the couple present themselves near ovulation time. At ovulation time it is more rational to observe the effect of spermatozoa *in vitro* in the woman. Although theoretically it only takes one normal, motile spermatozoon to achieve conception, a highly fertile man will have millions of actively motile spermatozoa in his ejaculate.

1. Initial interview
   Medical and marital history of couple
   Physical and pelvic examination of the wife

2. Laboratory tests of husband and wife
   Urinalysis
   Complete blood count and erythrocyte sedimentation rate
   Blood type and Rh factor
   Blood profile including thyroid function
   Rubella H. I. immunity in the wife

3. Bacteriologic examinations and Papanicolaou smear

4. Semen analyses — minimum of two examinations
   Split analysis if the semen count is low
   With this technique, the first drop or two of ejaculate is collected in one container and the remainder in a second container. Usually it is possible to concentrate spermatozoa from five to ten times with the most concentrated sample in split number 1.

5. Ovulation timing during two cycles to determine:
   a. whether the secretions of the wife are receptive to her husband's spermatozoa
   b. the degree of ascent or penetration of spermatozoa
   c. the exact time of ovulation
   d. whether the lining membrane of the uterus is capable of receiving a fertilized egg

6. Special endocrine assay, when indicated for disturbances of ovulation and spermatogenesis

7. Tubal patency tests and x-ray studies of the female organs

8. Urologic examination of the husband

9. Immunologic tests, when indicated

10. Laparoscopy, when indicated

11. Consultation

Figure 1
Outline of the fertility survey

Optimal Time for Laparoscopy

The optimal time for performing laparoscopy in the infertile woman is after ovulation has occurred. Immediately prior to ovulation a Graafian follicle may be seen. After ovulation a corpus hemorrhagicum with a typical stigma is seen. With failure of ovulation, on the other hand, laparoscopy may be performed at any time during a period of amenorrhea. Although numerous tests of ovulation have been suggested, e.g., the Farris rat test, glucose reaction and vaginal smear cytology, at the Fertility Institute we rely chiefly on the basal body temperature chart and cervical mucorrhea.

The woman is instructed to take her basal body temperature, rectally if possible, each morning before rising, beginning shortly after a menstrual period is over and continuing daily until menstruation ensues. She is instructed to report to the office daily from the ninth to the 15th day of a typical 28-day cycle. A patient with an irregular cycle may have to be seen more frequently over a longer period.

A vaginal speculum is inserted without lubrication and the following routine is performed: the tip of a glass or metal cannula is inserted into the endocervix and, by means of gentle suction, a quantity of endocervical mucus is obtained for examination. It is blown out on a glass slide and the amount is estimated from 0 to 4+ (profuse). A glass cover slip is placed on this glob of mucus, and the spinnbarkeit or stretch phenomenon is measured in centimeters. The cover slip is replaced and the slide examined for the presence of white blood cells and spermatozoa. The cover slip is again removed, the mucus is allowed to dry and the fernleaf reaction, or crystallization of the cervical mucus, is noted.

We believe that ovulation occurs at the low point in the temperature cycle, on the day before this low point, or on the rise from low to high. Prior to ovulation the cervical mucus becomes profuse and thin and shows a stretch phenomenon from 10 to 20 cm in length. Normally at this time large numbers of spermatozoa are recovered postcoitally. Figure 2 indicates the time of optimal fertility.

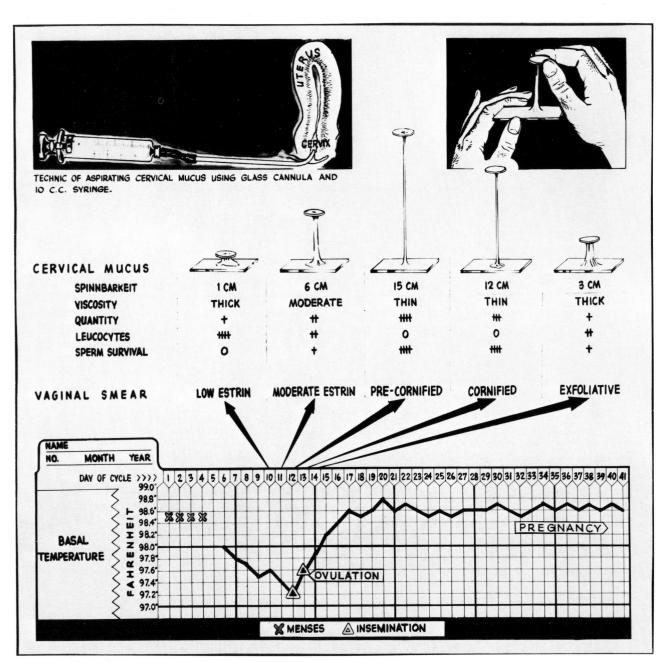

Figure 2
Time of optimal fertility. Basal body temperature
graph indicating presumptive ovulation at low point
(day 12) of cycle. The vaginal smear cytology and
cervical mucus findings on days 10 through 14 are
shown.

Laparoscopy is usually scheduled immediately after the mucorrheic phase of the cycle. In a patient with a typical 28-day cycle, laparoscopy could be performed from day 14 through day 21 of the cycle. Inasmuch as the patient is hospitalized for this endoscopic procedure, it is feasible to obtain an endometrial biopsy, a 24-hour urine for pregnanediol and 17-ketosteroids, and thyroid function tests as routine procedures in the infertile patient. During a period of amenorrhea there is no definite time for performing this technique. However, occasionally the amenorrheic patient will suddenly demonstrate a spurt of mucus with an elevation of the basal body temperature, and in such patients we have been able to obtain visual (endoscopic) evidence of ovulation.

Ovulation Failure

Ovulation failure per se may not require laparoscopy. Overt ovarian failure, such as premature menopause, may be diagnosed by a history of secondary amenorrhea, hot flashes and evidence of a hypoestrogenic state with elevation of follicle-stimulating hormone. Laparoscopy is usually unnecessary for the diagnosis of gonadal dysgenesis unless the typical stigmata of this disorder, as described first by Turner (1938), are absent. Laparoscopy in these patients reveals streak ovaries with a hypoplastic uterus and elongated fallopian tubes. Biopsy of the streak ovaries reveals ovarian stroma devoid of follicles but with hilar cells and rete structures.

Laparoscopy may be helpful in diagnosing hypothalamic and postpill amenorrhea or that due to the polycycstic ovarian syndrome.

In the polycystic ovarian syndrome, laparoscopy is indicated for a feasibility study prior to contemplated surgical wedge resection. Laparoscopy immediately after Pergonal treatment may be hazardous: the hyperstimulated ovary has a very fragile capsule, and trauma from the laparoscope or a second puncture instrument could produce rupture and hemorrhage.

Uterine Pathology

Uterine tumors usually present no diagnostic problems. Occasionally laparoscopy may be helpful as a feasibility study prior to myomectomy. Uterine malformations are usually diagnosed by means of hysterosalpingograms. However, it is sometimes difficult to differentiate the septate from the double uterus. Certainly, laparoscopy would be helpful as a feasibility study immediately prior to a metroplastic procedure.

Endometriosis

Prior to August 1966, culdoscopy was the only endoscopic procedure performed at Michael Reese Hospital. With culdoscopy, patients who might have had very advanced endometriosis were deleted because of technical problems, viz, fixed retroversion or cul-de-sac masses. Since August 1966, laparoscopy has been the endoscopic procedure of choice. During this period, ending December 1974, 1,380 patients from the Fertility Institute were examined laparoscopically.[1] Three hundred and twenty of them, or 23%, had mild, moderate or severe endometriosis. Of this group there were 240 who had symptomless endometriosis.

Therefore, if one relied upon the diagnosis of endometriosis as suggested by a history of dysmenorrhea, dyspareunia or menometrorrhagia plus pelvic findings of adnexal mass or cul-de-sac nodularity, one would miss an enormous number of patients with early, mild endometriosis. Textbooks usually state that active endometriosis is found most commonly between the ages of 30 and 40 years, rarely in teenagers and almost never in postmenopausal patients. We have found a large number of patients in their early and late 20s with minimal, moderate or even severe endometriosis. Certainly it is not uncommon for a teenager to have a chocolate cyst. The evidence of endometriosis among infertile patients may be as high as 30%, and this incidence increases with the age of the patient.

Pelvic Inflammatory Disease

In the past, the diagnosis of tubal obstruction has been made either with the original Rubin gas patency test or by hysterosalpingogram. Such procedures are frequently inconclusive, and laparoscopy may be required for clarification of whether tubal disease exists either as a true hydrosalpinx, tubal phimosis, patency into a pocket or adhesions, or of whether there are peritubal adhesions or endometrial implants that could interfere with ovum transport. Certainly as a feasibility study just prior to contemplated tubal plastic procedures, laparoscopy is required.

The Miniinfertility Survey via Laparoscopy

At times, the infertility specialist is pressured to perform an infertility survey for an out-of-town couple. Inasmuch as time is a factor, it is possible at least to evaluate tubal and ovarian factors via laparoscopy.

Surgical Laparoscopy

We recently reported a series of 1,093 laparoscopies in infertile patients from the Fertility Institute.[2] From this group 163 had surgical procedures which included lysis of adhesions, liberation of adherent ovaries, biopsy of ovaries for the diagnosis of amenorrhea and endometriosis, biopsies of other areas of suspected endometriosis, cautery of endometrial implants, retrieval of tubal splints and dilatation of fimbria.

Endometriosis was our most frequent finding in this group of patients. At laparoscopy the gross appearance of the pelvic organs is usually sufficient for diagnosis. Biopsy is rarely needed. Brownish hemorrhagic or purplish to black areas are typically found (1) at the vesicle uterine fold, (2) in the cul-de-sac or uterosacral ligaments, and (3) involving the ovaries. Implants may be found on the surface of the ovary, but endometriosis should be suspected when an ovary is found adherent to the cul-de-sac or posterior leaf of the broad ligament.

My most gratifying results have been in patients with moderate endometriosis involving one or both ovaries; in them it is possible to liberate these ovaries from their attachments to the posterior leaf of the broad ligament or cul-de-sac. Usually during this procedure there is minimal bleeding, and it can be controlled by simple cautery.

Medical treatment is indicated after surgical laparoscopy for endometriosis. Many patients have had diagnostic laparoscopy followed by suppressive therapy for endometriosis and a repeat laparoscopy with laparoscopic surgery of residual implants or adhesions. Several of our patients had as many as three laparoscopies for the diagnosis and management of this frustrating illness.

Documentation

There is an old Chinese proverb to the effect that one picture is worth 10,000 words. Figure 3 should be completed, with a drawing, preferably in color, immediately at the conclusion of every laparoscopic examination. Documentation must be as accurate as possible; should operative laparoscopy be performed, a before-and-after drawing is advisable. Further, the gynecologic laparoscopist should be able to take still photographs in color as a routine procedure.

Summary

Gynecologic laparoscopy has become an accepted procedure for the diagnosis of obscure pelvic disease. It is indicated (1) in every infertile patient 30 years of age or older, (2) in any patient, regardless of age, infertile for three years or more, (3) for suspected endometriosis suggested by acquired dysmenorrhea, dyspareunia, plus suspicious pelvic findings, (4) for suspected residual pelvic inflammatory disease, (5) for the diagnosis of ovulation failure, (6) for preoperative feasibility studies prior to contemplated tuboplastic procedures or ovarian resection, (7) for the evaluation of medical therapy for endometriosis or ovulation failure, and (8) postoperatively to evaluate the results of prior surgery. At this time, revision of the operative site with lysis of recurrent adhesions and cautery of endometrial implants may be made under laparoscopic control.

References

1. Cohen MR: Recent advances in the diagnosis of endometriosis—Endoscopy. Excerpta Medica, 1976

2. Cohen MR: Surgical laparoscopy in infertility. J Reprod Med 15:51, 1975

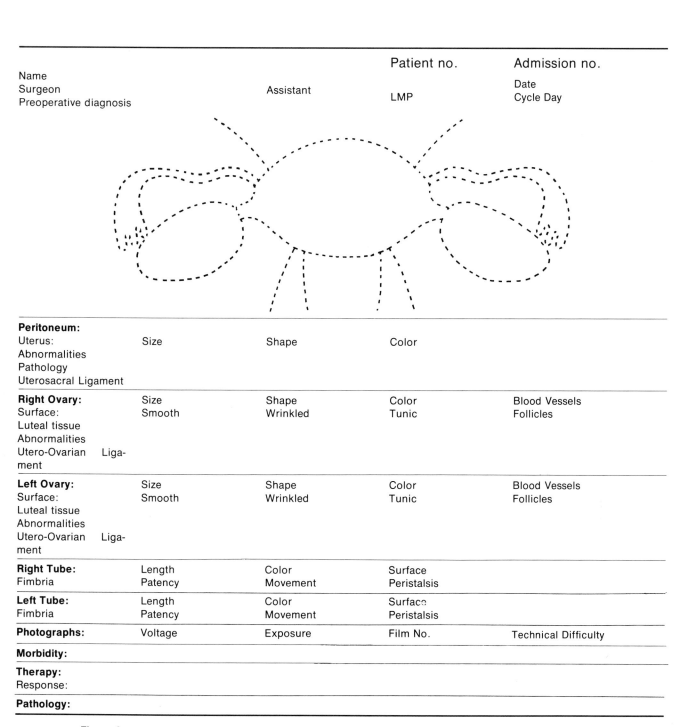

Peritoneum:

Uterus:	Size	Shape	Color	
Abnormalities				
Pathology				
Uterosacral Ligament				

Right Ovary:	Size	Shape	Color	Blood Vessels
Surface:	Smooth	Wrinkled	Tunic	Follicles
Luteal tissue				
Abnormalities				
Utero-Ovarian Ligament				

Left Ovary:	Size	Shape	Color	Blood Vessels
Surface:	Smooth	Wrinkled	Tunic	Follicles
Luteal tissue				
Abnormalities				
Utero-Ovarian Ligament				

Right Tube:	Length	Color	Surface	
Fimbria	Patency	Movement	Peristalsis	

Left Tube:	Length	Color	Surface	
Fimbria	Patency	Movement	Peristalsis	

Photographs:	Voltage	Exposure	Film No.	Technical Difficulty

Morbidity:

Therapy:
Response:

Pathology:

Figure 3
Peritoneoscopy (laparoscopy) report form

Chapter 17

Diagnosis of Infertility

Maxwell Roland, M.D.
David Leisten, M.D.

Introduction

This chapter outlines the use of laparoscopy in an infertility survey. Since the techniques of laparoscopy are described elsewhere in this volume, only a few special considerations will be mentioned here.

1. A laparoscope of 5 mm diameter allows adequate visualization of the pelvic organs and minimizes potential trauma to the abdominal wall.

2. To elevate the distal portion of the oviduct one may use either the grasping forceps, a solid palpator or an atraumatic suction cannula through a secondary incision.

3. Beginners often insert the laparoscope to its maximum, the result of which is a magnified view of a very small segment of the pelvic structures. The operator thus fails to achieve a panoramic view, which facilitates identification of all structures, especially when anatomy is distorted. To avoid these difficulties the laparoscope should be inserted about half way—i.e., with the lens just beyond the rim of the cannula. At this point the view of the pelvis is panoramic. The cervix can then be moved with the cannula, permitting exact identification of the corpus.

4. In the presence of multiple pelvic adhesions, especially those involving the omentum, the expert can often pass the laparoscope through without causing bleeding, thus attaining a view of most of the pelvic contents.

5. While one is testing tubal patency by injecting dilute indigo carmine solution through partially obstructed tubes, the increased pressure on the plunger occasionally breaks the suction between vacuum cannula and cervix, allowing dye to escape into the vagina. When dye is in the tubes, an assistant should elevate the corpus with the cannula. This movement allows the laparoscopist to see the fimbria. Occasionally the dye is seen through the anterior aspect of the lower uterine segment, indicating that the tip of the cannula has penetrated this structure. To allay concern the bladder may be recatheterized: clear urine is reassuring. Ordinarily, lower-segment punctures heal without complication and do not interfere with subsequent pregnancy.

6.   Although many clinicians do not routinely administer prophylactic antibiotics after laparoscopy, infection in the infertile patient can be catastrophic. Whenever the possibility of pelvic infection is considered, cul-de-sac fluid can be cultured. Then an antibiotic can be selected on the basis of sensitivity studies. Usually, however, tetracycline, 250 mg four times daily for seven days, is sufficient to diminish the risk of postoperative inflammation from manipulation. Unless lysis of adhesions has been performed, do not use steroids in combination with the antibiotics. Frankly, we are not convinced that corticoids really prevent reformation of adhesions. However, we use the mild combination of antibiotics and antihistamines after tuboplasty (more on an empirical basis). In our opinion, more controlled studies are needed before this question is resolved.

The Plan of the Infertility Investigation

It is convenient to organize the investigation of the infertile woman under the following headings:

Gamete Formation
Transportation of Ova and Spermatozoa
Reception and Deposition of Spermatozoa

The Nidatory and Postconceptional Factors: The conduct of these steps in the infertility investigation has been described by many clinicians. In the following comments, errors of interpretation and omissions are emphasized, especially as they pertain to studies at laparoscopy.

Gamete Formation: Occasionally neither the 21- nor 23-day endometrial morphologic features nor the results of radioimmunoassay of serum progesterone along with basal body temperature clearly indicate the status of the patient's ovulatory function. In such circumstances the direct ovarian visualization with laparoscopy may resolve the issue. A clear, fully formed corpus luteum, as seen on day 21 to 23 of a 28-day cycle, is rarely misdiagnosed by a trained observer. The laparoscopist must bear in mind, however, that intrafollicular luteinization can lead to a biphasic temperature record, secretory endometrium and, occasionally, moderate levels of progesterone in the serum. Accordingly, when the appearance of a swollen follicle is ambiguous, biopsy resolves doubt. With regard to the so-called Steinoid (microcystic) ovary, the macroscopic appearance is readily detected at laparoscopy. Since accurate diagnosis is based on histologic examination, biopsy is also desirable (the technique is described elsewhere in this text). Obviously important, but often neglected, is a thorough ovarian examination in the face of unilateral tubal abnormality. The hasty examiner may be content to diagnose normal gamete formation and transportation on the basis of signs of follicular activity in the contralateral ovary although it is the ipsilateral ovary that now will tell the story. It is necessary to obtain data on its status as well in order to assess *relevant* gamete formation. Biopsy is desirable if the visual appearances do not indicate follicular activity.

Gamete Transportation: The usual indicators of tubal status, such as tubal insufflation, hydrotubation combined with carbon dioxide insufflation, and hysterosalpingography, are all of limited diagnostic value in assessing this factor in infertility. In the case of tubal insufflation, spasm may play a great factor if the test is negative. Hysterosalpingography may be misleading at times. Laparoscopy therefore has become the most reliable means of not only determining tubal patency but also of observing any other abnormalities as well.

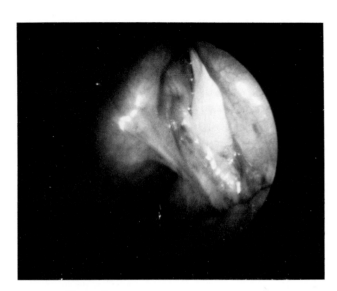

Figure 1
Peritubal adhesions and kinks

The importance of transitory saccule formation in the oviduct during instillation of dilute indigo carmine solution is not well recognized. In our experience this finding often suggests the presence of fimbrial adhesions or phimosis of the distal portion of the ampulla. Many gynecologists do not recognize fimbrial phimosis as an entity, or they doubt its pathophysiological importance. We believe, however, that phimosis can seriously compromise ovum pickup. This opinion is shared by other workers, including Gomel, Decker and Clyman.

The treatment for tubal phimosis, in our opinion, is, first, dilatation with indigo carmine solution at laparoscopy followed by preovulatory hydrotubation, with normal saline, antibiotic and corticosteroids. It is our opinion that the effective dilatation can be accomplished during laparoscopy while the patient is under general anesthesia. Postlaparoscopic hydrotubation follow-up is a means of retaining the dilated effect. It is performed in the preovulatory state, once or twice per month. In this text, Gomel describes laparoscopic dilatation of phimotic tubes utilizing ancillary instruments. The following conditions are similarly-neglected considerations in the causes of infertility related to gamete transportation:

1. Peritubal adhesions, with or without kinks (Figure 1), may delay transport of the fertilized ovum past the time when implantation is possible. Some clinicians, such as Frangenheim, prefer to lyse these adhesions via laparoscopy. However, we recommend laparotomy for lysis of some types of adhesions if pregnancy is not established after six months of hydrotubation.

2. When the oviduct is occluded at the fimbria and a hydrosalpinx is present, one may see indigo carmine behind the serosa of the distal portion of the tube. In such cases, relatively intact fimbriae are often behind the serosa. If this is so, salpingectomy should not be considered. Instead, the operator should perform tuboplasty or salpingolysis and incise the serosa carefully. In many instances numerous fimbrial structures will be encountered.

Reception and Deposition of Spermatozoa

This process involves the male's ability to deposit the ejaculate in the vagina: here the physician has to look for hypospadias, impotence, premature ejaculation and other factors that interfere with semen deposition near the external cervical os. Most frequently, defects in this area can be detected by history, physical examination and office procedures. Occasionally, hysteroscopy may help with the diagnosis of gamete reception.

Nidation: When the endometrial date does not correspond with the day of the cycle on which tissue was obtained, visualization of the corpus luteum may help to confirm its inadequacy, thus strengthening the rationale for postovulatory administration of progesterone.

Accurate Recording of Visual Observations in Infertile Patients

The subject of laparoscopy in infertility would be inadequately presented if the criteria for reporting observations were not mentioned. Inadequate reporting is common and may account for a high degree of repeat endoscopic examinations. The accompanying chart and line drawing (Figures 2 and 3) indicate our conception of an adequate report of findings at laparoscopy for the infertile patient. We often receive abstracts or reports from gynecologists who performed laparoscopy on an infertile patient in which the description of the findings is so meager that the second physician can scarcely draw any inferences from it. For example, one report simply states, "The tubes were found patent." No mention is made of the exact condition

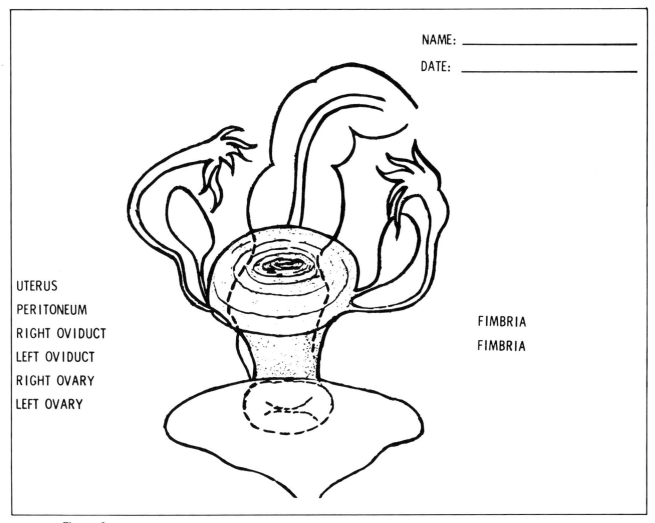

NAME: _____

DATE: _____

UTERUS

PERITONEUM

RIGHT OVIDUCT

LEFT OVIDUCT

RIGHT OVARY

LEFT OVARY

FIMBRIA

FIMBRIA

Figure 2
Line drawing of pelvic organs for laparoscopic description.

Findings at Laparoscopy for Infertility Investigation

Date...................... Clinical signs of absence of tubal infection,
                              including TB, verified: ....

Day of Cycle.................

                    (Tine test date : ....)

                    (Endometrial culture & biopsy: ....)

I. Gamete Formation

    Ovaries: Both present? .... Size: Right...........Left........

      Normally positioned or displaced (specify) : ....

    Appearance: Normal reproductive...............If no, explain ....
                       (Yes, No)

                        ....Follicular activity: Right.......Left.........

    Corpus luteum present: (Left.......... (Right ....
                       (Maturity....... (Maturity............................

    Condition of capsule: Sclerotic.............Stein-Leventhal....................
                       (right, left)   (right, left)

      Surface lobulated: .... Steinoid..........................
                       (right, left)   (right, left)

    Endometrial Implants.................... Cysts.........................
                       (right, left)   (in cm, right, left)

    Adhesions between ovary and ....
                  (specify structures involved)

    Other: ....
            (Dermoid, Turner's syndrome, etc.)

    Biopsy taken? ....
            (right, left)

II. Oviducts (Transportation of Gametes)

    Both present: .... Gross appearance: Normal as to: length.....
                                                  (R, L)
                                        location...............
                                                  (R, L)

    Fimbriae: Grossly normal: .... Adhesions...................
                           (right, left)   (If "yes", specify structures
       Not visible..........   ....
                                        ....
                                        Kinks.....................
    Ampullae normal as to size....................   (right, left)
                         (right, left)

      Hydrosalpinx:.........................
             (Acute, subacute, chronic;
              right, left)

      Midportion: distortion.................   Kinks.....................
                    (right, left)   (right, left)

        Isthmica dosa......................   Other: ....
                    (right, left)

    Cornua: appearance: ....   Myoma...................
                       (right, left)   (right, left)

II A. Tubal perfusion

      Solution: ....
            (Indigo carmine, Methylene blue)

      Occlusion....................Complete............ Site...............
          (right, left)   (right, left)

        Partial............   Site: ....
        (right, left)

       Sacculation: ....   Location: ....
        (right, left)

       Duration: ....
        (> , < 30 sec; > 30 sec = phimosis)

       Phimosis ....
        (right, left)

Type of occlusion (layers involved) : ....
                             (right, left)

Adhesion visualization after dye instillation: changed? ....
                                      (Yes, No)

     If so, how : ....

Grasping forceps used for visualization of distal oviduct:

     ....
              (right, left)

             Observations after side puncture:

             ....
                (right, left)

II B. Cul-de-sac aspirated postcoitally: ....
                               (Yes, No)

     If yes Aspirate clear or bloody....................

       Motile sperm present : ....

       Endometrial implants: ....

         Sacrouterine: .... Other: ....

      Adhesions: ....
                (specify structures involved)

III. Other Anatomic Observations

    Uterus: Location................... Size : ....

    Gross abnormalities: Fibroids......................
                         (give type)

      Endometrial implants...........................
               (location and size)

      Adhesions: ....
               (specify structures involved)

      Identify any other abnormalities detected ....

IV. Hysteroscopy: .... Defects seen: ....
              (Yes, No)   (polyp, submucous fibroid,
                                       synechiae, uterine anomalies,
                                       "suspicion" lesions)

    biopsy done: .... If "yes", why: ....
             (Yes, No)

    D & C : .... Amount of curettings...................
             (Yes, No)   (scant, moderate, hyperplastic)

Figure 3
Suggested chart for reporting findings at
laparoscopy for infertility investigation.

of each oviduct with regard to distorted anatomy, adhesions, phimosis, kinks and so on. The exact appearance of the ovaries frequently is not described. That blue dye comes through the fimbrial portion of the oviduct does not necessarily mean that there is normal physiologic function. For instance, the observation of the formation of one or several sacculations proximal to the ampulla that do not disappear within 30 seconds is an excellent indication that there is not complete patency, but this observation is rarely mentioned.

Special Hints and Observations

The therapeutic value of tubal perfusion under direct vision must be emphasized. In cases of partial tubal occlusion at the fimbria the surgeon can apply a higher pressure to the piston of the syringe containing the blue dye than is feasible in the office. In numerous instances we have observed the saccules vanish and the dye flow through with ease. About 50% of a series of 208 patients having partial tubal occlusion, which was observed at laparoscopy, maintained tubal patency after "high pressure" tubal perfusion under direct visual control. This was demonstrated via hydrotubation followed by tubal insufflation postoperatively. One hundred and eighteen of this group subsequently conceived without further tubal surgery. For this reason we disagree with those who are of the opinion that if partial or complete occlusion is detected at laparoscopy, one should proceed, at the same sitting, to perform tuboplasty. For the patient who does not conceive within six months after laparoscopy, tuboplasty may be considered.

After our encouraging results with the use of the spiral stents, this has become our routine procedure. For fimbrioplasty the senior author has designed a special cone-shaped spiral teflon tubing, stiffened at its distal portion by thin, highly malleable copper wire approximately 10 cm in length, which provides just enough rigidity to retain the spiral form. After fimbrioplasty the proximal end of the cone-shaped spiral is placed within the lumen of the ampulla and held there by three 4–0 chromic sutures. The distal ends are brought out of the abdominal cavity through a flank puncture, tied and left immediately beneath the subcutaneous fat. A Pfannenstiel incision covers the tubing with subcuticular suture. The prosthesis is left in place for eight weeks and removed under local anesthesia in the office.

Briefly, our short-term infertility survey includes:

1.   Complete history and physical examination of the couple.
2.   Semen analysis and semen penetration performed at the beginning of the survey.
3.   Endometrial biopsy taken on day 21 to 23 of the cycle; serum drawn on the same day for serum progesterone by radioimmunoassay and compared with the basal body temperature record.
4.   Hydrotubation followed by preovulatory tubal insufflation.
5.   Laparoscopy, tubal perfusion with indigo carmine solution and dilatation and curettage.
6.   Biopsy of ovaries whenever indicated.
7.   Lysis of adhesions when indicated.

The patient is then followed in the office with a course of action predicated on findings obtained during the workup. Our experience with the use of the short-term approach in these 328 infertility patients has persuaded us to continue with this regimen.

Table 1
Pelvic Pathology Found in 328 Infertile
Patients During Laparoscopy

Total Abnormalities	
Uterus:	95
Fibroids:	
Less than 1 cm	11
More than 2 cm requiring myomectomy	42
Intramural fibroids	31
Submucous fibroids	11
Congenital Anomalies:	13
Bicorate uterus	8
Septate uterus	3
Septate vagina	2
Ovaries:	272
Pathologic	136
Stein-Leventhal	6
Steinoid type	82
Follicular cysts	24
Simple-physiologic	16
Pathologic-requiring surgery= partial or complete	8
Endometriosis:	106
Implants on ovaries	22
Chocolate cysts	16
Implants in cul-de-sac	68
Adhesions:	163
Between:	
Ovary and tubes	31
Ovary and cul-de-sac	28
Tube and lateral wall	23
Omentum and cul-de-sac	39
Omentum and corpus	42
Tubes:	
Hydrosalpinx	38
Partial tubal occlusion at fimbria	115
Complete tubal occlusion	78
at fimbria	62
at cornua	11
at midportion	5
Adhesions:	257
Peritubal	115
Between:	
Cul-de-sac and tube	42
Ovaries and tube	67
Lateral wall and tube	33

Chapter 18

Infertility Management

John M. Esposito, M.D.

I. The Routine Workup.

There is no doubt about the usefulness of laparoscopy in the workup of the infertile couple. The editor of the *Obstetrical and Gynecological Survey,* commenting on an article by Peterson and Behrman,[14] stated that "no patient with unexplained infertility may be considered to be completely studied until the pelvic organs are visualized." In spite of such categorical approval, some basic questions still must be answered. They include: (a) Should laparoscopy be a routine part of the infertility workup? (b) Should laparoscopy be done only when the workup is completed and negative, and, if so, should it be done immediately, or should six to eight months be allowed to pass? (c) Should a set of guidelines be instituted to determine who should have laparoscopy?

Roland,[15] in his short-term infertility study, has used laparoscopy as a focal point of the workup. In such circumstances, the patient's initial visit is usually scheduled for the 14th to 16th day of the cycle. A semen analysis will have been performed previously; a fern test, spinnbarkheit and semen penetration are performed at this visit. Three months of basal body temperature records are reviewed. If there is a history of amenorrhea, a 24-hour urine analysis for 17-ketosteroids, 17-hydroxycorticosteroids and pregnanetriol and serum follicle-stimulating hormone (FSH) level are performed. On the sixth postovulatory day, judged by temperature, laparoscopy is performed and direct evaluation of tubal patency and internal genitalia obtained.

Another authority, Frangenheim,[8] believes that the Rubin test and hysterosalpingogram are of no use for infertility and that laparoscopy should be done in all cases. He believes that only in this way can adequate information be obtained on the condition of the internal genitalia. Others, including Siegler,[16] Swolin[19] and Maathuis,[10] feel that hysterosalpingography is worthwhile. They believe that laparoscopy should be done when indicated or when the initial workup is negative. The question in the minds of many is, what are the indications, and when should it be done?

It is my opinion that in the majority of cases of primary and secondary infertility, a negative infertility workup should be followed by an additional six to eight months of attempting pregnancy prior to laparoscopy. At the same time, however, Albano's[1] guidelines are useful for determining if laparoscopy should be a part of the initial workup:

1. If pregnancy has not taken place after one year of therapy.
2. If cycles are irregular, or the basal body temperature is monophasic.
3. If the patient is older than 28 and/or has been involuntarily infertile for more than three years.
4. If there is history of previous laparotomy.
5. If hysterosalpingography has been done with an oily contrast medium.
6. If there has been a history of pelvic inflammatory disease.
7. If there is a history of appendicitis.
8. Repeatedly abnormal Rubin's test.
9. Suspected endometriosis.
10. If the patient is a candidate for insemination.

If any of these factors is present, then laparoscopy should be done immediately as an integral part of the initial workup.

What information can be obtained from laparoscopy?

A) Tubal Patency

1. Should a Rubin test be performed first?

There is some feeling that a Rubin test may, in fact, be therapeutic.[12] As far as reliability of results is concerned, Sobrero[17] reported an 8.4% false negative rate and more than 31% normal, but misleading, results.

2. Should a hysterogram be done?

Maathuis[10] reviewed a series of hysterograms: there was only a 46% agreement between laparoscopy and hysterosalpingography, with 17% false patency with the latter. Coltart[6] reviewed hysterosalpingograms showing nonpatency. He found that when the blockage was isthmic, the hysterogram and the laparoscopy agreed in 72% of the cases. When it was fimbrial, there was only 21% agreement. Swolin[19] noted agreement in 78% of the cases.

These four studies combined yield 68% agreement. I believe, however, that hysterosalpingography should be performed for two reasons: (a) because of its possible therapeutic effect, and (b) because of information which one obtains about the configuration of the uterine cavity and endosalpinx. If pregnancy does not occur in six to eight months in the absence of other etiologic factors, laparoscopy should be performed and further therapy based upon the findings.

Timing: when should laparoscopy be performed?

The decision on timing is often difficult and should be based on the history and clinical findings in the individual patient and the information which the physician wishes to obtain.

Should it be preovulatory? If done at this time, information cannot be obtained on the ovulatory status of the patient. However, this is the standard time which has been recommended for doing tubal patency tests.

Should it be postovulatory? Only at this time can further information on the ovulatory status of the patient be obtained. Laparoscopy done at this time must recognize that endometrial "valve" action may interfere with any tubal patency test and that apparent cornual blockage found at this time should be confirmed by hysterosalpingogram in the preovulatory phase of the cycle. If one suspects endometriosis, however, the best time to perform laparoscopy is in the menstrual phase of the cycle.

Technique for chromotubation: Many methods have been recommended for injecting dye through the cervix into the uterine cavity and eventually through the tubes. These methods include:

1. Rubin cannula or a variation of it
2. Suction cannula (Semm, etc.)
3. Pediatric Foley catheter
4. Combined hysteroscopy and laparoscopy with insufflation of the dye through the hysteroscope
5. Laparoscopy and hysterosalpingography using fluoroscopic control, as recommended by Brooks[2]

In our opinion, a pediatric Foley catheter is less traumatic and obtains a satisfactory seal except under high pressures when the bag is extruded through the cervical os. This serves as a safety valve and makes it impossible to inject the dye at pressures which could cause damage to the fallopian tubes.

Solution: Methylene blue 1% or indigo carmine (1:5) is used most commonly. Cognat[4] has recommended a combination of one of these dyes with cortisone and/or penicillin. The solution should be injected under manometric control with maximum pressure of 200 mm per Hg. Others have recommended that carbon dioxide insufflation and chromotubation be performed simultaneously.

Pneumoperitoneum: nitrous oxide versus carbon dioxide

Nitrous oxide is the better choice for pneumoperitoneum if diagnostic procedures alone are to be performed; carbon dioxide is irritating to the peritoneal surface, and the resulting hyperemia and occasional tubal spasm can often be confusing. However, if one anticipates electrosurgical intervention, such as electrocoagulation of areas of endometriosis, then carbon dioxide is preferred.

Anesthesia: It is important that the examination be performed systematically, and for this reason the procedure may take longer than tubal sterilization. Therefore, it is best performed under general anesthetic with intubation. Immediate documentation is important so that future references to the operative findings are accurate. It may be done by sketches, photography and special postoperative forms.

Tubal findings: Palmer has classified hydrosalpinx as small, medium or large.[11] The *small* variety presents with the fimbria preserved; however, with insufflation, decreased perfusion is noted, and the dye distends the tubal lumen (phimosis). The *medium* variety usually has multiple constrictions; frequently, adhesions fix these constrictions to the peritoneal surface. The *large* are multilobulated and usually larger than 2 cm in diameter. Palmer[11] considers only the small variety operable, and when the tubes are enlarged more

than 2 cm, tuboplasty is contraindicated. Siegler,[16] however, is of the opinion that tuboplasty is also possible in the medium and large groups if there is leakage of dye from the terminal clubbed portion.

Isthmic block: In this condition there is no tubal filling, and blanching of the isthmus is often noted along with back flow of dye through the cervical os and uterine distension as pressure is exerted in the syringe. If isthmic filling is observed and there is no spillage of dye into grossly normal tubes, it indicates inadequate instillation and not tubal blockage. In cases of isthmic block, surgery should be performed only if the ampullary segment and fimbriated end of the tube are free and healthy in appearance; this occurs in about one-third of the cases (Thoyer-Rozat).[20]

Other findings: Peterson and Behrman,[14] reporting on 204 cases with unexplained infertility, found endometriosis in 33%, pelvic adhesions in 16% and tubal disease which had not been appreciated on hysterosalpingography in 5%. Pawson[13] found major pelvic pathology in 36.1% (i.e., endometriosis, tubal pathology, small myomata, ovarian dermoid cysts) and minor pathology in 11.1% of infertile patients. Frangenheim[8] feels that laparoscopy can give information on the status of the uterus (i.e., presence of isthmic myomas and congenital malformation) which may explain infertility.

B) Postcoital Test
Technique: Best done on day of ovulation. The patient has coitus 12 to 18 hours prior to laparoscopy. Fluid is taken from the cul-de-sac and from each tubal ostium. In order to accomplish the latter, it may be necessary to irrigate the tubes through the uterine cavity with saline. A small polyethylene catheter is used to collect the aspirate. In each aspirate there should be approximately 200 mobile sperm. The sperm migrate to the tubes within a few minutes to three hours after coitus and normally remain motile for approximately two to three days. Although there is still much work to be done in order to standardize this technique, it shows promise and gives information on the ability of sperm to migrate to and through the fallopian tube.

C) Ovarian Evaluation

This can be a visual evaluation. Adhesions are noted, and the effect on ovum pickup is assessed. Adhesions from endometriosis may fix the ovary to the broad ligament. Often, lysis of adhesions can be done at this time.

Biopsy for more accurate histologic and diagnostic karyotyping can be performed with a needle or with modified Palmer or Siegler forceps. (Details of this procedure are discussed in Chapter 14.) Biopsy provides useful information about primary amenorrhea, vaginal agenesis and certain chromosomal anomalies. Turner's syndrome, Savage syndrome and true ovarian dysgenesis may be differentiated by this technique. Patients with secondary amenorrhea, as well as those who are anovulatory, also are candidates for ovarian biopsy.

Sykes[18] has suggested that a germinal cell count per millimeter be performed and that this count be used to determine the prognosis for ovulation. Zographos[21] has discussed the problems of interpretation of these specimens. More work must be done in this area before a definite statement on this matter can be made.

II. Pretuboplasty Evaluation

Laparoscopy prior to tuboplasty or reanastomosis permits better selection of cases. The question arises whether surgery should be concomitant with laparoscopy or done at a later date. If delayed, how long should the interval be between the two procedures? In our clinic, corrective surgery is performed at the same sitting, thus sparing the patient a second anesthetic. Those who are of the opinion that it should be done as a separate procedure state that at least six weeks should elapse before one attempts the tuboplasty.

III. Procedures under Laparoscopic Vision

Diagnostic and therapeutic fertility-promoting procedures include:

1. Lysis of adhesions
2. Ovarian biopsy—mini wedge resection
3. Salpingostomy—see Chapter 19 for technique
4. Hydrotubation
5. Electrocoagulation of endometrial implants
6. Removal of tubal stents or hoods
7. Uterine suspension
8. Aspiration of peritoneal fluid
9. Collection of ova

IV. Evaluation of Tubal Surgery

If the patient is not pregnant within one year of reconstructive surgery, it is important that a reevaluation be made. A discussion of the prognosis for pregnancy, based on objective findings, may then take place.

Summary

There definitely is a place for laparoscopy in the workup of the infertile patient. It is our opinion that laparoscopy should not be a routine part of every workup but that guidelines should be followed in order to determine who should undergo the procedure. Laparoscopy is helpful in determining tubal patency and the condition of the internal genitalia and surrounding milieu. It is also an ideal method for performing certain operative procedures which may aid the infertile patient.

All patients having tubal surgery should have pretuboplasty evaluation by laparoscopy; better selection will increase the pregnancy rate following these operative procedures. Laparoscopy may also give important information about sperm viability and ability to migrate to and through the fallopian tubes. No negative infertility workup is complete without laparoscopic examination, but the patient should be given an additional six to eight months to achieve pregnancy prior to diagnostic laparoscopy.

References

1. Albano V, Cittadini E: *La Celioscopia in Gynecologia.* G. Denaro, Palermo, 1972, p 277

2. Brooks P, Berci G, Adler D: The simultaneous and combined use of laparoscopy and hysterosalpingography using image amplification. J Reprod Med 10:285, 1973

3. Cittadini E, Rossi T: *Celioscopy and Ancillary Techniques.* Piccin Medical Books, Padua, 1974

4. Cognat M.: *Coelioscopie Gynecologique.* Simep Editions, Villeurbanne, 1973, p 59

5. Cohen MR: *Laparoscopy, Culdoscopy and Gynecology: Technique and Atlas.* W. B. Saunders Co, Philadelphia, 1970, p 87

6. Coltart TM: Laparoscopy in the diagnosis of tubal patency. J Obstet Gynaecol Br Commonw 77:69, 1970

7. Editorial. Obstet Gynecol Surv 26:257, 1971

8. Frangenheim H: *Laparoscopy and Culdoscopy in Gynecology.* Butterworth, London, 1972, p 49

9. Keirse MJNC, Vandervellen R: A comparison of hysterosalpingography and laparoscopy in the investigation of infertility. Obstet Gynecol 41:685, 1973

10. Maathuis JB, Horbach JGM, Gall EV: A comparison of the results of hysterosalpingography and laparoscopy in the diagnosis of fallopian tube dysfunction. Fertil Steril 23:428, 1972

11. Palmer R: Abdominal coelioscopy in the diagnosis and treatment of sterility. International Congress of Gynecology, Dublin, 1974

12. Parsons L, Sommers SC: *Gynecology.* Saunders Co, Philadelphia, 1962

13. Pawson ME: The diagnostic and therapeutic role of laparoscopy in infertility. Med Gynaecol 8:6, 1975

14. Peterson EP, Behrman SJ: Laparoscopy of the infertile patient. Obstet Gynecol 36:363, 1970

15. Roland M, Leisten D, Kane R: Fertility study by means of laparoscopy. J Reprod Med 10:233, 1973

16. Siegler AM: Laparoscopy as a prelude to tuboplasty. In *Gynecological Laparoscopy: Principles and Techniques.* (JM Phillips, L Keith, Eds.) Stratton Intercontinental Medical Book Corp, New York, 1974, p 253

17. Sobrero AJ, Silberman CJ, Post A et al: Tubal insufflation and hysterosalpingography, a comparative study in 500 infertile couples. Obstet Gynecol 18:91, 1961

18. Sykes DW, Ginsburg J: The use of laparoscopic ovarian biopsy to assess gonadal function. Am J Obstet Gynecol 112:408, 1972

19. Swolin K, Rosencrantz M: Laparoscopy vs hysterosalpingography in sterility investigations: a comparative study. Fertil Steril 23:270, 1972

20. Thoyer-Rozat J: Celioscopy and Sterility. Abbottempo 1:24, 1963

21. Zographos G, Zakarian S, Bergier G, Varette-Dauvergne Y: Problems in the interpretation of ovarian biopsies in functional gynecologic disorders and sterility of ovarian origin. J Reprod Med 10:295, 1973

Chapter 19

Fertility Surgery

Victor Gomel, M.D.

Laparoscopy is an integral part of most infertility investigations. Although the value of laparoscopy as a diagnostic technique is well established, its role as an operative mode has not attained the same degree of recognition.[2]

In 300 consecutive infertility cases subjected to hysterosalpingography and subsequent laparoscopy, discrepancies between the two procedures were present in over 40% of the cases. Almost three-quarters of these discrepancies were related to adhesions, the remainder being related to discrepancies in tubal patency. In the latter group, the most common radiologic error was associated with tubes that appeared relatively normal and patent on hysterosalpingography, while in fact at laparoscopy they were found to have only a pinhead-sized opening at their distal end (tubal phimosis).[3] Other authors have reported a similar discrepancy rate between the two procedures.[5, 8]

Laparoscopy permits complete visualization of the internal genitalia and thus allows direct assessment of the fallopian tubes and surrounding structures. Otherwise undetectable pelvic adhesions may be diagnosed and their nature and distribution ascertained. Their apparent relationship to the clinical problem thus may be evaluated more accurately.

In the management of infertility problems related to tubal or ovarian factors one or more laparoscopic procedures may be of value:
1. Electrocoagulation of pelvic endometriosis and aspiration of endometriotic cysts
2. Multiple ovarian biopsy—may be both diagnostic and/or therapeutic
3. Salpingolysis and ovariolysis
4. Dilatation of phimotic tubal ostium
5. Salpingostomy

Laparoscopy is essential prior to embarking upon open laparotomy for promoting fertility. In the series of 300 cases previously described, open laparotomy was avoided in 68 (22.7%). In 12 of these cases the pelvis was found to be essentially normal despite contrary findings on hysterosalpingogram. In 21 prognosis for improvement with laparotomy was deemed exceedingly poor and was thus avoided. Among these 21 were six cases of unsuspected genital and intraperitoneal tuberculosis. In the remaining 35 one or more surgical procedures were performed via the laparoscope.

Techniques

General anesthesia with endotracheal intubation is employed. The bladder must be empty and is catheterized routinely. Adequate Trendelenburg position and pneumoperitoneum are essential. An intrauterine cannula is essential both to manipulate the uterus as well as to introduce the dye solution when testing for tubal patency. The cannula is secured by attaching it to a tenaculum placed on the cervix or by a vacuum when a suction type cannula is employed. For chromopertubation either methylene blue or indigo carmine, diluted in normal saline, may be used.

In performing fertility-promoting procedures the multiple puncture technique is preferable. By separating the visual and mechanical axes better visualization and greater facility in manipulation of the operative instruments is possible.

The basic steps in performing the routine laparoscopic procedure are described in the section dealing with basic techniques. The left and right McBurney points are preferable for insertion of the ancillary instruments. Depending upon pelvic findings, however, an alternate site of entry in the lower abdomen may be necessary.

Pelvic Endometriosis

When infertility is associated with endometriosis, varying degrees of involvement may be encountered.

1. Endometriotic seedings, appearing as raised purple spots ("powder burns"), may be encountered on the surface of the ovary, the uterosacral ligaments, etc. The ovaries may be adherent to the posterior surface of the uterus or pelvic sidewall or in the cul-de-sac. When released with the aid of a probe or grasping forceps, escape of small amounts of chocolate-colored material may be observed. These endometriotic seedings may be coagulated using an insulated conical electrode or the closed tip of a biopsy forceps introduced through an appropriate sheath.

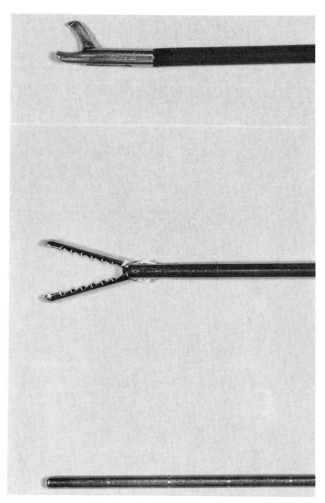

Figure 1
Instruments: scissors, alligator forceps and probe.

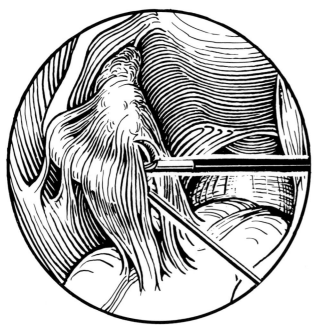

Figure 2
Adhesions stretched before division with scissors.
From: Gomel V: Laparoscopic tubal surgery in
infertility. Obstet Gynecol 46:47, 1975

2. Adnexal masses may be present. They
are usually related to endometriotic cysts of the
ovaries. These masses are generally adherent to
adjacent structures. The cysts may be aspirated, by
means of a 3 mm suction cannula or a large caliber
needle.[1] After evacuation of the cysts more satisfactory visualization and assessment of the ovaries
and tubes become possible. A free tubal fimbriated
end is usually present, whereas a large portion of
the ovary and the fallopian tube are involved in
brownish adhesions. Many of them may be divided,
as will be described subsequently. Progestational
therapy may then be initiated for an appropriate
period of time.

With these combined measures Palmer[6]
has been able to report a pregnancy rate of 20%. If
pregnancy does not result in the subsequent year,
one may resort to laparotomy and further conservative surgery.

Ovarian Wedge Resections

This term refers to a large single biopsy or
multiple ovarian biopsies which are intended to
simulate the effects obtained at open laparotomy.
The actual technique is described in Chapter 14, a
section of which is devoted to the topic of ovarian
biopsy.

Palmer[7] has reported 30 cases of Stein-
Leventhal syndrome studied between 1960 and
1967. Biphasic menstrual cycles were observed in
60% of the cases, and pregnancy occurred in 20%
following unilateral ovarian biopsy.

Salpingolysis and Ovariolysis

In the presence of patent tubes, pelvic
adhesions may still be extensive, totally isolating
the fimbriated end of the tube and/or the ovary and
thus impeding ovum pick-up. In such cases hysterosalpingography may demonstrate patent tubes
with loculation of the dye and eventual spill into the
peritoneal cavity.

A 3 mm grasping forceps or probe is inserted through a left lower quadrant puncture.
Through the right lower quadrant a second trocar
and sleeve of appropriate size to accommodate a 3
mm or 5 mm insulated scissors is introduced. The
adhesions are stretched with the grasping forceps
or the probe and divided with the scissors (Figures
1 and 2). Thin, veil-like adhesions, when divided,
retract and almost disappear. Minute bleeding
points may require coagulation. Thicker, more vascular adhesions usually require coagulation prior
to division. Frequently, numerous layers of adhesions are present. They should be divided individually (Figures 3, 4 and 5). If bleeding occurs and
blood has accumulated in the pouch of Douglas, it
may be removed by means of a suction cannula
introduced through one of the trocars. This procedure also permits lavage of the pelvis with normal
saline, to be performed at the completion of the
procedure.

Following the salpingolysis and/or the
ovariolysis, hydropertubation is carried out using
hydrocortisone acetate solution. This step, which
is carried out by instilling the material through the
uterine cannula, is meant to prevent reformation of
these adhesions. This procedure should be repeated one week later.

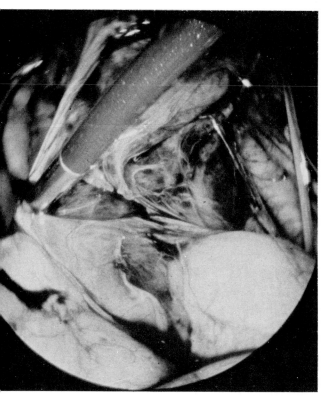

Figure 3
Coagulation of thick adhesions.

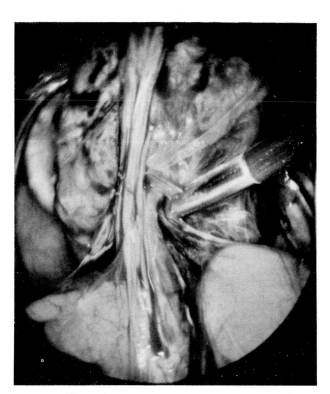

Figure 4
Thick multiple adhesions.

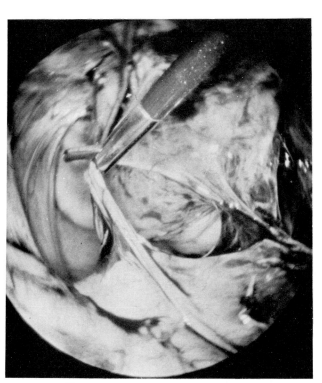

Figure 5
Division of individual adhesion.

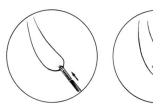
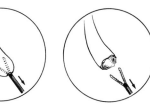

Figure 6
Alligator forceps introduced, opened and removed.
From: Gomel V: Laparoscopic tubal surgery in
infertility. Obstet Gynecol 46:47, 1975

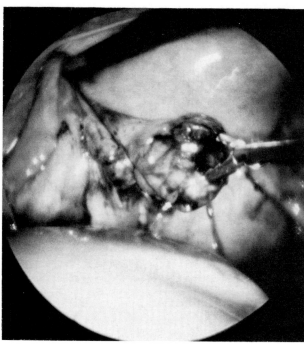

Figure 7
Removal of forceps.

Dilatation of Phimotic Tubal Ostium

In some cases, a somewhat distended
tube is encountered, the distal end of which has a
pinhead-sized opening. Minimal passage of dye occurs during chromopertubation. This condition
may be the only single finding, but more often it is
associated with peritubal and periovarian adhesions.

If adhesions are present, they may be divided as previously described. The phimotic tube is
immobilized by manipulating the uterus with the
uterine cannula and with the aid of the grasping
forceps which generally is inserted through the left
lower quadrant.

To dilate the phimotic ostium a 3 mm
grasping forceps with alligator jaws is employed
(Figure 1). It is usually inserted through a right
lower quadrant puncture. The alligator forceps is
introduced into the tube in the "closed" position
through the existing small opening. The jaws are
then opened within the tube and drawn out in the
"open" position (Figure 6). This maneuver is repeated several times. With gentle manipulation of
the tube, bleeding is seldom encountered (Figure
7).

This procedure is followed by hydropertubation with hydrocortisone acetate solution at the
time of the surgery and repeated one week later.

Personal Experience

Thirty-seven patients treated by salpingolysis and ovariolysis were followed for a minimum
of one year. Seventeen also had unilateral or bilateral dilatation of fimbrial phimosis performed.

All 37 patients had an adequate preoperative period in which to achieve pregnancy (18 to
144 months). Also, for a case to be included in this
series ovum pick-up had to be deemed impossible.[4]

One case in this series has been lost to
follow-up. One patient was separated from her husband within two months and thus pregnancy was
not desired. Of the remaining 35, 20 subsequently
conceived *in utero*. This result represents a ratio of
57.1% (Table 1). In all there were 26 intrauterine
pregnancies (three of which terminated in spontaneous abortions) and two ectopic gestations.

Six of the 13 women who have not conceived to date have been found to have other factors related to their infertility problem.

When no other cause for infertility was present, those who became pregnant did so within the first year after the procedure, with the majority of them having conceived within the first six months.

Peritubal and periovarian adhesions without true occlusion of the fallopian tube are the principle cause of infertility in about 15% of patients.[6] Salpingolysis, ovariolysis and dilatation of phimosis of the fimbriated end of the tube by laparoscopy was used as the primary approach. Fifty-seven percent of the patients have had a live birth or are presently pregnant. This rate may improve with longer exposure and by overcoming the other factors of infertility which affect some.

Salpingostomy

Salpingostomy via laparoscopy has been performed on seven patients. All but one patient represented failure of previous tubal surgery, with a postoperative pregnancy trial period varying between 18 and 96 months. The findings were either bilateral hydrosalpinx, or unilateral hydrosalpinx with absence or cornual occlusion of the opposite tube.

The tube is distended with dye solution injected via the uterine cannula and immobilized as described previously. Using the 3 mm or 5 mm scissors the tube is first entered at its distal end by puncturing it in its thinnest point. This is followed by extending the incision in an inverted (Y) fashion, using the scissors (Figure 8). Bleeding occurs at many points. The bleeding points are visualized by irrigating the area with normal saline and are coagulated individually with either insulated scissors or a fine electrode. The whole line of incision is not coagulated prior to cutting for fear of producing extensive tissue destruction. This procedure is followed by hydropertubation using hydrocortisone acetate solution and is repeated one week later.

Three intrauterine pregnancies have been achieved so far. This procedure is not proposed as a primary method of managing a hydrosalpinx. Furthermore, the numbers are as yet too small to formulate any conclusion.

Table 1

Salpingolysis and Dilatation of Tubal Phimosis: 37 Cases

Lost to follow-up	1
Not pregnant	13
Separation (contraception)	1
Ectopic gestation	2
Patients with intrauterine pregnancies	20 (57.1%)

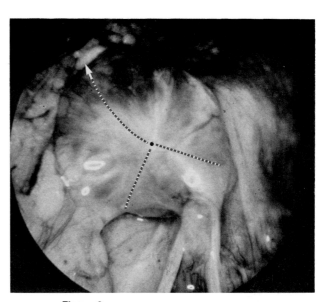

Figure 8
Inverted "Y" incision.

Conclusion

Aside from its diagnostic value, laparoscopy has become an important adjunct to the surgical treatment of female sterility.

In several instances laparotomy may be replaced by a laparoscopic procedure, which offers the following distinct advantages:

1. Avoidance of laparotomy with its associated complications and other drawbacks,
2. Minimal discomfort,
3. Brief hospital stay,
4. Reduced patient and hospital cost,
5. Good results — due, at least in part, to minimal tissue trauma.[4]

References

1. Cognat M: *Coelioscopie Gynécologique*. Simep Editions, Villeurbanne, 1973, p 37

2. Gomel V: Laparoscopy. Can Med Assoc J 111:167, 1974

3. Gomel V: Unpublished data

4. Gomel V: Laparoscopic tubal surgery in infertility. Obstet Gynecol 46:47, 1975

5. Maathuis JB, Horbach JG, Van Hall EV: A comparison of the results of hysterosalpingography and laparoscopy in the diagnosis of fallopian tube dysfunction. Fertil Steril 23:428, 1972

6. Palmer R: Laparoscopy in the diagnosis and treatment of endometriosis and pelvic adhesions. Symposium Laparoscopie in de Gynaecologie. Ned Tijdschr Verloskd Gynaecol 70:295, 1970

7. Palmer R, De Brux J: Résultats histologiques, biochimiques et thérapeutiques obtenus chez des femmes dont les ovaires avaint été diagnostiqués Stein-Leventhal à la coelioscopie. Bull Fed Soc Gynecol Obstet Lang Fr 19:405, 1967

8. Swolin K, Rosencrantz M: Laparoscopy vs hysterosalpingography in sterility investigations. Fertil Steril 23:270, 1972

Section 8   Complications

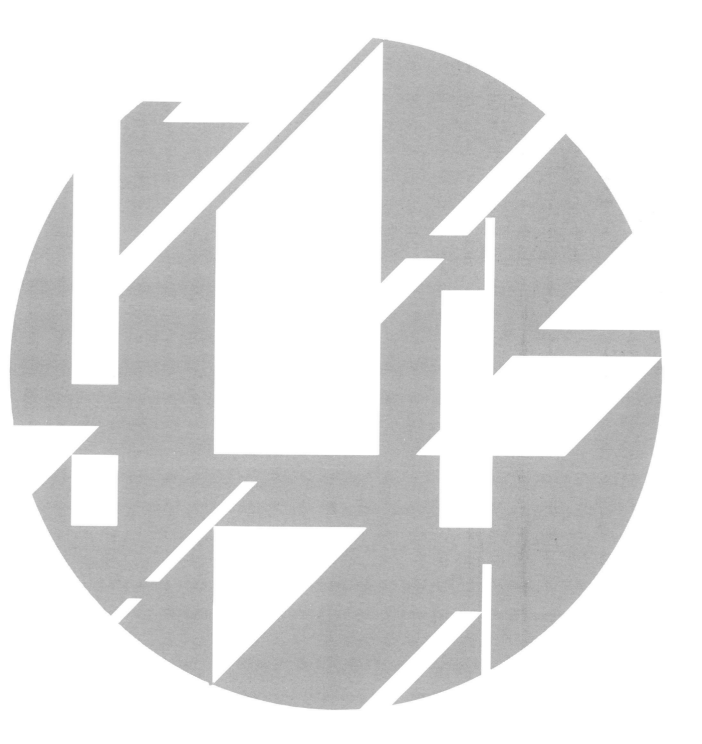

Chapter 20

Complications

Carl J. Levinson, M.D.

Introduction

Laparoscopy is a procedure involving highly technical equipment: it makes the operator prone to errors and the patient susceptible to complications. Laparoscopy was used initially for diagnostic purposes; however, it soon became obvious that many operations could be performed more easily under laparoscopic control. The most commonly performed laparoscopic operation is sterilization of the female by some form of cauterization and/or cutting of the fallopian tubes. The combination of operative instruments with the use of electrosurgery contributes to the patient risk.

The more frequently any operation is performed, the more likely it is that complications will occur. This is particularly true when the instruments are new, sophisticated and rapidly changing, when the technique is not accepted or universally well established and when the quality of teaching is variable. This chapter has two purposes: (1) to indicate the general categories in which complications tend to occur, and (2) to provide the reader with a step-by-step review, illustrating those points at which errors might be made (along with suggestions as to how they might be avoided or managed).[5]

Contraindications

Some complications are the result of "errors" committed in the course of the surgery. In retrospect, many of them could have been avoided by adherence to basic principles (Chapters 4 and 10). Laparoscopy is contraindicated in the excessively obese patient not only because of the thickness of the abdominal wall but also because of the frequent presence of redundant omentum and bowel in the pelvic cavity. Even if pneumoperitoneum is well established, the situation remains fraught with potential problems, particularly if electrosurgery is used. Previous abdominal surgery generally is not a contraindication to laparoscopy, but the presence of massive adhesions (following even one prior surgical procedure) can provide problems for the novice. On the other hand, failure to establish an *adequate* pneumoperitoneum may result in even greater hazard to the patient since the physician often feels compelled to proceed with the operation. In these circumstances visualization is poor, working space is inadequate, "everything seems to be wrong" and the operator encounters numerous and considerable difficulties.

A lack of experience by itself may be the single "contraindication" of the greatest magnitude. Statistics (Chapter 23) indicate that all manner of complications are much more common in the hands of the inexperienced, possibly more so in laparoscopy than in most operative procedures. Whereas the difficulty of obesity, relatively poor pneumoperitoneum and prior surgery may prove to be of no consequence to the laparoscopist with skill and experience, they may prove to be insurmountable obstacles in the hands of the relative novice.

Equipment

Adequate illumination is an absolute necessity for the performance of laparoscopy. This is particularly true if operative procedures are to be performed, though numerous authorities have personally reported participating in laparoscopic operations as observers or teachers where the principal operators have been satisfied with truly *inadequate* illumination. If, at any time during laparoscopy, no light is available, then one of the following must be reviewed (Figure 1):

1.   The electrical outlet is not providing AC current.
2.   The electrical cord for the light source is not properly inserted into the wall socket.
3.   There is a break in the electrical cord.
4.   There is a defect in the light source box.
5.   The light cable is not properly secured to the light source.
6.   The light cord is not properly secured to the laparoscope.
7.   The bulb is defective.

Under these circumstances the correction is obvious. (One admonition: extra light bulbs should always be readily available.)

On the other hand, should the illumination be present but inadequate, there are fewer possibilities (Figure 2):

1.   Generally the light bulb is defective and must be replaced.
2.   The light cable has been twisted and bent, with resultant damage to the glass fibers which transmit the light.
3.   The ends of the cable may be damaged.

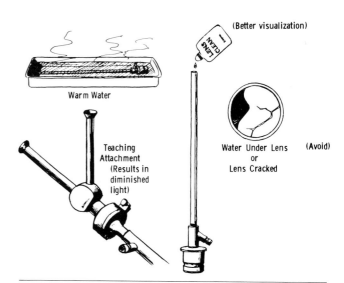

Figure 1
Visualization
Problems interfering with proper visualization.

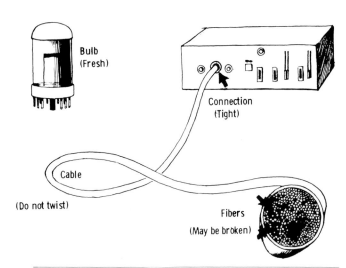

Figure 2
Light Source
Problems associated with diminished or absent light.

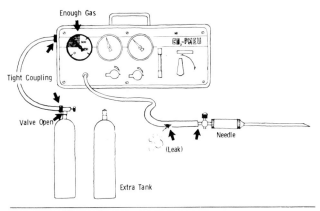

Figure 3
Insufflator Supply
Evaluation of adequacy and possible leaks of gas.

It is our experience that with a single light source, a single cable and a single laparoscope, the light may diminish in a gradual fashion so that neither the operator nor the hospital personnel are aware of it. For this as well as many other reasons, it is suggested that two pieces of equipment be available in each category so that the intensity of illumination can be compared periodically to determine whether deficiencies exist.

Insufflation

Insufflation is simple and performed expeditiously. However, problems can develop when it is improperly or inadequately performed. All equipment should be tested and checked in sequence prior to use: the storage or reservoir tank, the insufflator, the tubing and the Veress needle. If no gas flows from the needle tip, the following must be checked (Figure 3):

1.   There must be residual gas in the reservoir tank (the appropriate meter on the insufflator should be checked).
2.   The gas tank valve must be open (it is amazing how often this is overlooked).
3.   An extra tank of gas should always be available.

The tip of the Veress needle should be inspected to be certain that the apertures of the inner and outer portions are superimposed, thereby ensuring a free flow (Figure 4).

Inadequate insufflation results in restricted visibility. It may occur early in the procedure or develop during its course. In the former case, it may be due to a leak: the insufflator should be checked by a qualified mechanic or, preferably, by the operator. If there is *no* gas in the insufflator, the coupling device between the storage tank and the insufflator should be checked; in addition, the appropriate valves should be observed to determine if they are open.

The nurses should understand the mechanics of insufflation as well. The apertures should be checked for cleanliness; plastic tubing and any areas of coupling should be checked for leaks (preferably under water). Occasionally a small fragment of fascia will be inspissated into the lumen of the Veress needle during the process of abdominal wall puncture, thereby obstructing free flow of gas. Exceptionally slow insufflation will also result if the handle on the insufflator is turned to "automatic" during the initial filling.

The dials on the insufflator apparatus (Figure 2) are among the best safety devices in laparoscopic equipment. The dial to the observer's left indicates the presence or absence of gas within the system. The center dial records the amount of gas within the insufflator itself, generally ranging from 0 to 5 or 0 to 10. In reality, the unit is filled when the reading is at 0; the subsequent dial readings indicate the amount of gas released from the insufflator to the tubing into the patient. The right dial may be the most significant of all. Before use on a patient the terminal pressure should be recorded with a free flow of gas through the apparatus, the tubing and the Veress needle directly into the operating room atmosphere. This gives the inherent resistance of the system and generally results in a reading between 6 to 10 mm. When the insufflation needle is inserted into the peritoneal cavity with the patient fully relaxed under anesthesia, the reading is approximately 6 to 10 mm higher. An increase of more than 10 mm should make the operator suspicious that the end of the needle is located somewhere other than the peritoneal cavity. (Note: if the patient is not fully relaxed under anesthesia or is under local anesthesia, the intraperitoneal pressure is higher and may falsely indicate incorrect placement of the needle.)

The Electrosurgical Unit

There is no substitute for understanding, fully and in depth, the mechanism whereby electrical current is distributed to the patient for the purposes of electrosurgery (Chapter 4). If, at any time, the apparatus being used has been the source of a shock to either the patient or the operator, that apparatus should not be used again until it has been examined and the deficiency found and corrected. The machine must be checked for "shorts," and there must be proper grounding of the patient. Problems will also occur if the operative instruments are insulated improperly. Trocar sleeves should be made of a nonconductive substance such as fiberglass. The instrument carrying the electrical current should be insulated throughout, except at the operating tip. If a single-puncture operating laparoscope is used, then the tip of the electrical instrument should project some small distance from the metallic end of the lens before cautery is attempted.

Failure of the electrosurgical equipment to function properly generally results from a mechanical failure within the apparatus itself. This apparatus should be inspected and repaired by someone familiar with it. Not infrequently, a loose connection to the ground plate or the cautery instrument either at the power source or at the instrument itself is the problem. If a proper dial setting for the power source has not been established, the machine may be set at too low a value. All other factors must be examined prior to increasing the setting because no amount of adjustment will compensate for loose connections. More important, the current may prove excessive if the settings are adjusted at a high level and *then* the loose connections are corrected. Application of current should be brief so as not to overheat the tip of the forceps, which then may touch other tissue. The improper or inadvertent application of current is generally a human error. The operator must know, at all times, where the foot pedal is located; preferably it should be put in the same place each time and located on a solid base. The pedal should be conveniently located but protected so that it cannot be bumped, kicked or stepped on by accident. *Never* plug the cautery cord onto the electrosurgical instrument until the tissue to be cauterized has been grasped and it is certain that there is no bowel in the vicinity. In the case of a sterilization procedure, this may mean removing and replacing the cord several times.

Anesthesia

At this point it seems proper to invoke the caveat of "contraindications," particularly with regard to those patients with extreme obesity and/or cardiorespiratory disease. Under these circumstances it may be difficult or impossible to provide proper and truly safe anesthesia (Chapter 9).

Local anesthesia[1,2] is quite satisfactory in a large percentage of cases if the patient meets certain criteria: relatively thin, psychologically stable, fully aware of the planned procedure and willing. Should general anesthesia be chosen, then all the problems of this technique exist. The anesthesiologist must be familiar with the technique of laparoscopy, including controlled ventilation, the need to avoid hypoxia, the desirability of electrocardiogram (ECG) monitoring, the preference for intubation and the frequent need for gastric suction.

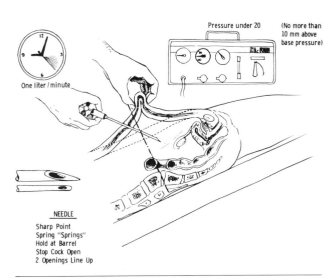

Figure 4
Pneumoperitoneum
Evaluation of adequacy of flow and intraperitoneal
pressure

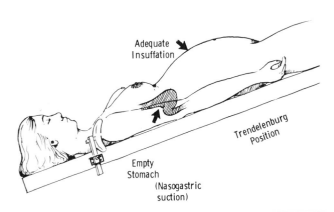

Figure 5
Positioning
Proper position and details necessary to avoid a
bowel perforation

The following anesthetic problems[4, 6] are the most directly related to laparoscopy. When the P_{CO_2} is increased, the pH decreases, and the P_{O_2} is also decreased. This is frequently a result of inadequate ventilation and the absorption of CO_2 and may result in tachycardia and arrhythmias. Additional factors contributing to these changes are increasing intraabdominal pressure, Trendelenburg position and diaphragmatic immobilization. Mild hypercarbia can be treated with adequate premedication (especially atropine) and assisted ventilation with intubation, using a minimum of 50% oxygen. The tendency to develop irregular cardiac rhythms can be observed with the ECG and monitored. Reflex vagal reactions (most often from abdominal distention) may be eliminated or diminished by the use of intravenous atropine immediately prior to insufflation.

Positioning of the Patient
Laparoscopy is often difficult because of the failure to adhere to certain basic rules of positioning (Figure 5). The legs may be (a) positioned in stirrups, or (b) placed flat upon the table once the cervical cannula has been affixed (in the latter circumstances it is necessary that the table have a cutout portion through which the vaginal instruments may protrude below the patient). The buttocks must come to the edge of the table so that the cannula can be manipulated properly. Knee straps and shoulder braces will maintain the patient properly on the table if steep Trendelenburg position is utilized. The patient's arms should be at the side rather than on an armboard, particularly if the legs are in stirrups, since this position tends to restrict lateral movement of the operator at the side of the table. The patient should be catheterized since a full bladder obscures vision within the pelvis and presents an additional hazard during the electrosurgery. The Trendelenburg position will assist by allowing the bowel to slip from the pelvis into the upper abdomen. Unless the angle is adequate, bowel pushed out of the pelvis will slide back, adding a continuous hazard to the procedure.

Establishment of Pneumoperitoneum

Prior to attempting insufflation all equipment should be checked thoroughly. If pneumoperitoneum cannot be established easily, a recheck is necessary. The needle should be withdrawn and the aperture checked for patency and then the needle reinserted at a somewhat sharper than 45° angle. In cases of previous surgery, marked obesity or failure with several attempts in the region of the umbilicus, it is of great value to insert the needle into the upper left quadrant, one fingerbreadth below the costal margin in the nipple line. The needle should be inserted at an angle of 45° across the patient's abdomen and away from the spleen; as a safety measure, gastric suction will ensure an empty stomach. The gas should flow into the abdomen at a slow rate, no greater than one liter per minute. Should a gas embolism[4] take place, a "mill wheel" murmur will be heard over the precordium. The patient should be turned into a left lateral position, and the gas may be removed by means of a catheter inserted via the subclavian route.

An incorrectly placed needle may result in insufflation of the abdominal wall, the retroperitoneal space, the mesentery, the omentum or the bowel. To prevent erroneous placement of gas, proper technique must be utilized (see Chapter 10). A few points should be stressed: the Veress needle must be open and have a sharp point and the spring mechanism must work. The needle itself must be held at the barrel during insertion so that there is no obstruction of the spring mechanism. Prior to insertion of the needle the abdominal wall is raised upward by hand or instrument. The needle is thrust through the abdominal wall with a rapid (but not spastic) thrust, hopefully avoiding "tenting" of the peritoneum. There are two basic indicators of the success of this movement: (a) the *feel* of the thrust, which can only be obtained with experience, and (b) monitoring of the intraabdominal pressure. The pressure should be no more than 10 mm (mm Hg) above the figure obtained when testing the system. The needle should be manipulated or rotated in such a manner as to keep the pressure at its lowest possible level. This requires that the operator observe the gauge at all times. Percussion of the lower abdomen is valueless since it will sound tympanitic whether the insufflation is occurring above or below the peritoneum. Percussion should be performed in the right upper quadrant to determine whether liver dullness disappears.

If there is uncertainty about whether the gas is located within the peritoneal cavity, it is best to start over, reinserting the needle at a somewhat sharper angle. Some operators prefer to aspirate the needle with a syringe, flush with saline and reaspirate; we have found this test to be of limited value. Once again, we recommend the use of the left upper quadrant for placement of the needle and reinsufflation.

If leaking gas results in depression of the anterior abdominal wall, thereby limiting visualization, more gas should be inserted periodically. This is made easier by transferring the lever on the insufflator to the *automatic* sign.

Occasionally the needle may be placed in a blood vessel, i.e. the inferior vena cava, the iliac vein, the parietal and omental vessels. Because of this possibility we insert the Veress needle prior to the attachment of the gas tubing. The hub of the needle is observed for 10 seconds in order to note the presence of blood. In addition, if the needle is located in a vessel, the pressure reading should be elevated considerably.

Emphysema may not be entirely avoidable. This may be subcutaneous or mediastinal and may result in pneumothorax. Severe complications can be avoided: do not over-inflate, monitor the intraperitoneal pressure carefully and avoid vigorous compression of the abdomen.

Insertion of the Laparoscope

Clarity of visualization is crucial for the proper performance of laparoscopy. The optical system (Figure 1) must be perfectly clear, clean and dry. A drop of water on either the eye piece or the lens results in a cloudy image (a drop of "lens cleaner" can be applied to both the eye piece and the lens). Gas sterilization is preferable, for the use of autoclaves or excessively hot washing water may result in deterioration of the lens seal, thus allowing water to seep beneath it. Cracks in the lens may result from careless handling and apparently minor knocks or drops. Diminished visibility occurs during use of the teaching attachment; under these circumstances it is helpful to have a 1,000 watt lamp (Figure 2).

Failure to maintain the trocar and sleeve in good condition results in a number of problems which occasionally lead to complications (Figure 6). If the valves of the sleeve stick, gas will be lost on removal of the trocar; the valves must be cleaned and lubricated frequently. If the rubber gasket has been used, worn or cut, there will be a continuous leak of gas around the laparoscope, resulting in diminished visibility. If the trocar has been worn to a dull point, entry will be difficult and will require excessive thrust pressure. The point should be pyramid-shaped and sharp. A sharp thrust through the abdominal wall is often preferable in order to prevent tenting of the peritoneum. After entry into the peritoneal cavity it is preferable to hold the trocar and sleeve steady, pull back the trocar 2 cm and then push the sleeve 2 cm further in, thereby eliminating any necessity for manipulation with the pointed trocar. By holding the elbow of the thrusting hand close to the bony thorax, thrust action is confined to the hand and wrist. The opposite hand should be used to steady and restrain the thrusting motion in order to prevent the thrust from going too deep, which may result in over-penetration into the retroperitoneal space.

Bleeding

Bleeding may occur from a variety of places. Bleeding at the skin incision is usually of no consequence; insertion of the trocar and sleeve usually provides enough compression to stop the skin from bleeding. Occasionally bleeding occurs from vessels within the rectus abdominus muscle. The most significant bleeding in this area comes from the epigastric vessels; unfortunately, not much can be done to avoid this problem.

Compression usually stops skin bleeding. Should a subcutaneous or subfascial hematoma develop and be recognized, it should be incised and evacuated. After the bleeder is clamped and tied, drainage can be instituted, if necessary, and the incision resutured. If a subcutaneous hematoma is found postoperatively, compression is generally sufficient although healing of the incision undoubtedly will be delayed. More serious complications result if a perforation takes place into vessels within the mesentery, adhesions or the retroperitoneal space. Under these circumstances laparotomy is indicated if there is continuous bleeding.

Second Puncture

The thrust technique with trocar and sleeve is approximately the same for the second puncture (Figure 7) as for the first. The incision is usually at the upper border of the hairline. Puncture of the bladder can be avoided by catheterization and by maintaining the puncture site at or above the hairline. Placing the laparoscope light under the abdominal wall will indicate a site free of blood vessels (but this is not always true). The thrust into the abdomen should be done under direct visualization. There is a marked tendency for the peritoneum to tent — hence the need for a sharp trocar and the sharp thrust. When there is a good deal of tenting, much manipulation is often necessary to overcome it. Obviously this should be done towards an area free of bowel and major vessels. A useful technique is as follows: aim the second trocar towards the sleeve of the laparoscope; withdraw the laparoscope 2 to 3 cm into the sleeve; push the point of the second trocar into the sleeve. The use of steep Trendelenburg position will move much of the pelvic bowel out of the field.

Electrosurgery

Whether using the single- or double-puncture technique, the problems and complications of electrosurgery are essentially the same.[5] Some authors state that the double-puncture technique offers better visualization since the lens is larger and there is no visual defect (blind spot) in any segment of the view. Others feel that the single-puncture instrument offers no specific handicaps. However, when doing electrosurgery it is much easier to move bowel away from the operative site by means of a second, freely movable instrument rather than having to move the entire unit (light, lens and operative instrument) and the bowel all at the same time. The section on electrosurgery should be read carefully (Chapter 4). There is no substitute for complete understanding of the procedure. Several repetitive comments are in order: the equipment should be checked carefully for short circuits, a fiberglass sleeve should be used instead of a metal one and insulation of all equipment must be checked for defects.

Errors may occur in visualization or judgment and will result in failure to perform the procedure properly. This, in turn, will lead to complications. The anatomy must be checked carefully (Figure 8). Even minor derangements may prove confusing. The round ligament is forward, anterior and leads to the anterolateral pelvic wall. The tube is looser, posterior and can be traced to its fimbriated end. The infundibulopelvic ligament is lateral to the tube and extends caudad. The ovarian ligament is below the proximal end of the tube. Any part of this normal anatomy may be impaired by disease processes, particularly adhesions. Cauterizing the round ligaments is relatively harmless, but attempting to cut them may result in brisk bleeding. If the tube is cauterized inadequately and then cut, bleeding may result from the mesosalpinx. The tube should be cauterized 1 cm in each direction away from the grasping forceps, including downward into the mesosalpinx. If too much of the tube is grasped initially, then the larger vessels within the mesosalpinx may be included and torn. Furthermore, these vessels must be cauterized adequately or they will bleed during the process of

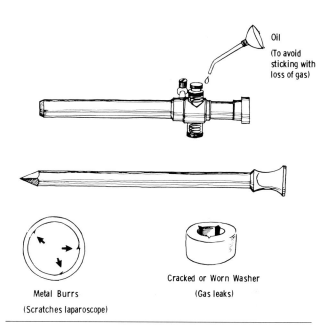

Figure 6
Trocar
Problems and proper maintenance.

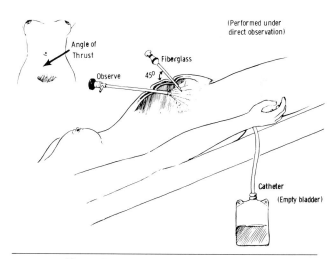

Figure 7
Second Puncture
Observation of details to avoid complications.

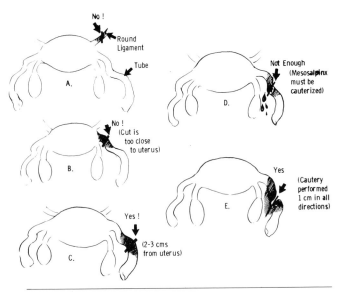

Figure 8
Sterilization
Attention to details of anatomy, particularly in regard to bleeding.

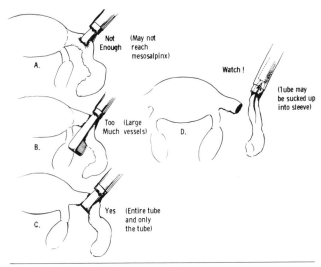

Figure 9
Electrosurgery
Proper location of cauterizing instrument.

cutting. Similarly, if the tube is cauterized too close to the uterus and then cut, the larger vessels located there will bleed (Figure 9). If the biopsy tong is utilized, cautery may be simple, but cutting the tube may be difficult if the sleeve edge is dull. This can be overcome by *mild* traction away from the uterus. Once the tube is cut, there is no purpose in continued twisting of the outer sleeve of the biopsy tong since it may result in the tube being pulled up into the sleeve, possibly even beyond the area of cautery, and thereby resulting in bleeding.

Bleeding during electrosurgical sterilization (Figure 9) may occur (a) immediately upon grasping the mesosalpinx if the grasp is too deep, or (b) during the process of cutting following cauterization. Should it occur, the area must be re-grasped and recauterized with no further attempt at cutting. (Reports indicate that multiple cauterized areas give approximately the same sterilization results as do cauterization *and* cutting.) The tubes should not be cut too close to the cornua since this is an area of confluence of ovarian and uterine vessels; the tube should be grasped 2 to 4 cm from the cornual end.

Burns

Burns may occur any time electrosurgical equipment is utilized. The severity of the complication depends on the location of the burn. Abdominal wall burns of the patient or skin burns to the operator are frightening but rarely of major consequence. Newer cautery equipment often has automatic shutoff devices. The use of bipolar equipment may reduce many of these problems since the electrical current only passes between the surfaces of the two tongs of the forceps. It does not traverse the entire body as it does in unipolar systems. Since bipolar cautery is relatively new,[7] larger series of patients need to be evaluated before the true incidence of thermal injury from this method can be determined.

Bowel burns occur by direct application of current to bowel, by touching the bowel with a hot tip or through sparking of the current across an actual or potential space. (There is some question about the occurrence of the latter.) For the most part, burns to the bowel are serious and can result in perforation with subsequent peritonitis (Chapter 21). To eliminate this devastating complication all of the fine details of laparoscopy must be observed. As much as possible, the bowel in the true pelvis should be removed prior to the use of electrosurgery (Figure 10). Good anteflexion of the uterus by means of a cervical cannula results in better visualization of the tubes in a location further removed from the bowel. There is no substitute (again!) for a good panoramic view *at the moment* of electrosurgery. Similarly, good anesthesia is necessary at this moment to provide proper relaxation and to prevent "bucking." Whatever equipment is used, the tube should be tented, i.e., pulled upward and forward away from the bowel, prior to turning on the current. This is facilitated by an adequate pneumoperitoneum, which provides sufficient working space. The cautery cord should be attached only when the equipment is used; the equipment should be calibrated so that the proper current is applied. Cauterization should be performed only under direct vision. Burns can be eliminated entirely by the use of nonelectrical techniques of tubal sterilization such as the clip or the ring.[3,8]

Nonelectrical Techniques for Sterilization

The nonelectrical techniques for sterilization are discussed elsewhere (Chapter 15). This author has had experience only with the ring. In order for this technique to be successful, it is necessary for the tubes to be free. It is preferable to manipulate the tube at a distance of at least 2 cm from the cornual end in order to provide sufficient flexibility; otherwise, cutting and bleeding may result. The tube may be cut in half if it is too thick or adherent; therefore, these circumstances may prove to be contraindications for performing this procedure.

Conclusion

Complications can be avoided by adherence to the basic principles of technique in association with a full understanding of electrosurgery. There is no substitute for experience. Students in laparoscopy should be supervised closely. When learning, the operator must do more diagnostic work prior to attempting operative procedures.

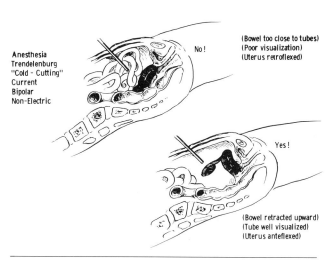

Anesthesia
Trendelenburg
"Cold - Cutting"
Current
Bipolar
Non-Electric

(Bowel too close to tubes)
(Poor visualization)
(Uterus retroflexed)
No!

Yes!

(Bowel retracted upward)
(Tube well visualized)
(Uterus anteflexed)

Figure 10
Avoid Bowel Burn
Attention to details necessary to avoid burns to the bowel.

References

1. Alexander GD, Goldrath M, Brown EM, Smiler BG: Outpatient laparoscopic sterilization under local anesthesia. Am J Obstet Gynecol 116:1065, 1972

2. Corson SL, Patrick H, Hamilton T: Electrical considerations of laparoscopic sterilization. J Reprod Med 11:159, 1973

3. Hulka JF, Fishbourne JI, Mercer JP: Laparoscopic sterilization with a spring clip. Am J Obstet Gynecol 116:715, 1973

4. Keith L, Silver A, Becker M: Anesthesia for laparoscopy. J Reprod Med 12:227, 1974

5. Levinson CJ: Laparoscopy is easy—except for the complications. In *Gynecological Laparoscopy: Principles and Techniques.* (JM Phillips, L Keith, Eds.) Stratton Intercontinental Medical Book Corp, New York, 1974, p 153

6. Peterson EP: Anesthesia for laparoscopy. Fertil Steril 22:695, 1971

7. Rioux J-E, Cloutier D: True bipolar electrosurgery for tubal sterilization by laparoscopy. In *Gynecological Laparoscopy: Principles and Techniques* (JM Phillips, L Keith, Eds.) Stratton Intercontinental Medical Book Corp, New York, 1974, p 315

8. Yoon IB, King TM: A preliminary and intermediate report on a new laparoscopic tubal ring procedure. J Reprod Med 15:54, 1975

Editorial Comments

This chapter lists, in clear and succinct details, some of the major complications associated with laparoscopy. As any experienced surgeon clearly knows, complications are not always avoidable. They happen under the best of circumstances, to well trained individuals and at the most unexpected times. Such, in my opinion, is the nature of surgery.

If the reader is not already aware of the declining rates of complications for laparoscopic operations in the United States, he or she is referred to Chapter 36. There have been substantial declines in the rates of most of the major hazards associated with this procedure. The reported death rate was zero for laparoscopic operations performed for sterilization by members of the American Association of Gynecologic Laparoscopists in 1974 and 1975. These accomplishments are due in part to improved teaching, increased experience of individual operators and continuing efforts of leading practitioners to analyze their daily performance with an eye to reducing complications.

Every effort must be made to reduce complications to a minimum. This chapter addresses itself to each area where complications have been known to occur and provides the reader with methods of prevention and management.

L.K.

Chapter 21

Thermal Gastrointestinal Injuries

Clifford R. Wheeless, M.D.

The most serious complication of laparoscopic sterilization operations has been inadvertent thermal burns to the gastrointestinal tract and abdominal wall. Other thermal injuries have been reported, but they have been less serious. It is difficult to ascertain exactly how thermal burns occur. Numerous theories have been offered, but no one has produced a scientifically controlled study that explains these injuries (Figure 1). Thermal injuries to the colon have been reported, but out of any series they are generally rare.

The most common site of thermal injury to the gastrointestinal tract has been the antimesenteric border of the terminal ileum (Figure 2). In the majority of cases no complication or difficulty was noted at the time of laparoscopy[2]. The usual pattern has been that the patient was discharged from the hospital with few, if any, significant findings. On the third or fourth postoperative day she complained of bilateral, cramping, lower abdominal pain, low-grade fever, slight nausea without vomiting and either obstipation or a slight, watery diarrhea. The clinical picture is similar to that of acute appendicitis prior to rupture.

When these patients were observed, their disease seemed similar to ruptured appendicitis: the white blood cell count rose dramatically to 20,000, the temperature became elevated to 102 F to 103 F and board-like rigidity of the abdomen ensued, as did nausea, vomiting and obstipation. This clinical picture may require several days to develop in its entirety.

Current theories on the causes of thermal injuries range from contact of the terminal ileum with the grasping jaws of the forceps to the aberrant behavior of high-intensity electrical current (Figure 1). In my opinion the one theory for which there is no conclusive scientific evidence but which appears the most likely cause of the injury is the inadvertent withdrawal of the operating forceps or tong to a point where it makes contact with the

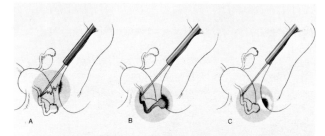

Figure 1 ——
Various theories of how thermal burns to the gastrointestinal tract occur from laparoscopy.

intraabdominal portion of the operating laparoscope or the intraabdominal portion of the second-incision trocar sheath. At this point the entire operative laparoscope or the intraabdominal portion of the second trocar sheath acts as an electrocoagulator. The heat disseminated from this contact may thermally damage the intestine lying in contact with the sheath of the operating laparoscope or the sheath of the second-incision trocar (Figure 1). Other possibilities, such as defects in the insulation and the so-called spark gap theory, also have been proposed as the causes of these injuries.

The failure to recognize spreading peritonitis and to intervene surgically has resulted in the deaths of several patients. However, it is not necessary to operate on every patient suspected of gastrointestinal injury. Many of these patients can be followed conservatively, with evaluation every four to six hours, and thus can avoid pelvic laparotomy without excessive risk. The key point is the detection of spreading peritonitis. When it occurs, surgical intervention is required immediately.

From the first reported cases of gastrointestinal injuries in the late 1960s to the present, numerous modifications of the equipment and technique have been made, all with the hope that the gastrointestinal injuries would be eliminated. Although the incidence of such injuries has been reduced, they continue to occur in sophisticated urban university centers as well as in small rural county hospitals. This is a baffling problem. It is unlikely that any one modification in equipment or technique would eliminate thermal injuries. Non-electrical techniques, of course, eliminate the problem.

In 1968 we performed a pilot series of laparoscopic sterilizations on 100 patients. After this series we began performing laparoscopic sterilizations on an outpatient basis on a broad scale. Our outpatient female sterilization program was begun in 1969, and since that time 5,350 such procedures have been performed; data on gastrointestinal injury has been accumulated on all these patients. Among these patients, 12 injuries to the gastrointestinal tract have been noted, an incidence of 0.22%. The classic two-incision technique was used on 1,230 patients (with three gastrointestinal injuries, an incidence of 0.22%). The one-incision technique was used on 4,120 patients (with eight injuries, an incidence of 0.19%). Thus, statistically, there appears to be little difference between the single- and double-puncture techniques.

In the 3,532 patients who underwent laparoscopic sterilization under *local* anesthesia, two gastrointestinal injuries occurred (an incidence of 0.05%). In the 1,818 patients who had laparoscopic sterilization under *general* anesthesia, nine injuries occurred (an incidence of 0.49%). This difference is significant. The site of injury was the ileum in 11 instances and the sigmoid colon in one instance.

Of the 12 cases of gastrointestinal injuries, six were recognized at the time of surgery. (One of these six had immediate laparotomy because of an obvious trocar injury to the bowel. It was over-sewn, without sequelae.) The remaining five patients in this group of injuries *recognized* at the time of surgery were treated by observation only. This regimen consisted of nothing by mouth with intravenous feeding, systemic antibiotics, antibiotic bowel preparation (in two cases) and an abdominal examination by the surgeon or the gynecologic house staff every six hours. If spreading peritonitis had been observed in these patients, laparotomy would have been performed. None of these house patients had spreading peritonitis; therefore, none of them underwent surgical therapy. (Since that series, 35 additional cases have been noted in consultation from other clinics. Gastrointestinal burn occurred at the time of laparoscopy; all 35 patients were observed with the idea of performing laparotomy only for spreading peritonitis. Of this group, only one required laparotomy and bowel resection.)

The remaining six cases of gastrointestinal injuries that were not recognized at the time of laparoscopy represent the worst experience we have had with laparoscopic sterilization. These patients presented on the third or fourth postoperative day with pain, minimal pelvic peritonitis and slight nausea: a picture very much like acute appendicitis. On the fourth to sixth day they developed fever, severe pain, nausea, vomiting and obstipation: signs and symptoms like those of ruptured appendicitis. All six of these patients underwent laparotomy. All of them had injuries to the terminal ileum, and all had resection of the terminal ileum with ileoileostomy. (Two patients developed postoperative pelvic abscess on the sixth and eighth postoperative days, respectively. One patient had pelvic thrombophlebitis associated with septic pulmonary emboli.) The average hospital stay for these patients was 15 days, with a range of 10 to 31 days.

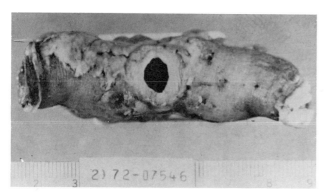

Figure 2
Burn site and perforation of terminal ileum.

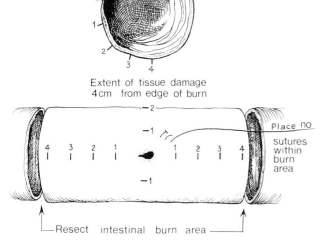

Extent of tissue damage
4 cm from edge of burn

Figure 3
Emphasis on the importance of bowel resection
because damage to the bowel wall extends 4 to 5 cm
from burn site, thereby compromising the quality of
the anastomosis in that area.

We evaluated the pathologic process occurring in the terminal ileum by making serial sections from the point of maximum thermal burn upward for approximately 10 cm (Figures 2 and 3). For the first 2 to 3 cm, gross electrocoagulation in the necrosis of the bowel mucosa as well as the muscular layers was observed (Figure 4). In addition, significant coagulation necrosis and inflammatory reaction could be seen for as far as 5 cm from the margin of the thermal injury (Figure 5). The pathologic findings described above led to several conclusions for therapeutic management of these patients (Figure 6).

First, because of the extent of thermal injury distal to the site of perforation, all such patients should have bowel resection without an attempt to oversew the thermal burn. This would avoid placing the anastomosis sutures through compromised intestinal tissue (Figure 6-1). Second, all necrotic tissue should be removed from the abdomen (Figure 6-2). It is not sufficient to do a clean bowel resection and then leave fallopian tubes in a pelvis that has been bathed in stool for as much as 12 to 14 hours. The removal of such tissue should be complete even if a hysterectomy has to be performed, for the failure to remove the necrotic tissue promotes the formation of pelvic abscess. Third, the peritoneal cavity should be lavaged of all foreign material with normal saline. It is important to remove particles of food and intestinal contents that have leaked into the peritoneal cavity through the bowel perforation (Figure 6-3). Fourth, the pelvis should be drained through the vagina, cul-de-sac or the flanks (Figure 6-4). Fifth, aggressive antibiotic therapy should be instituted. Coverage for gram-negative and gram-positive organisms can be achieved with 30 million units of penicillin and two grams of chloromycetin given intravenously each day. Cultures should be taken from the peritoneal cavity with emphasis given to the detection of anaerobic bacteria such as bacteroides. If they are found, appropriate therapy should be instituted.

Those patients treated with these five considerations in mind had the least complicated postoperative courses. The one patient in whom the necrotic fallopian tubes were left in the pelvis and in whom no saline lavage was performed had a very stormy postoperative course, with recurrent pelvic abscesses, ascites and a pleural effusion.

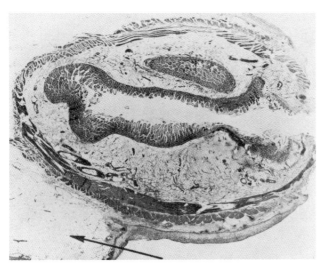

Figure 4
Bowel perforation site showing extensive
coagulation necrosis of mucosa, submucosa and
serosa.

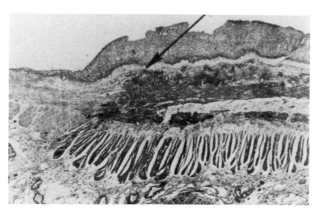

Figure 5
Five centimeters from the burn site showing
coagulation necrosis in the submucosa.

All of the injuries except for one occurred
in the terminal ileum. Knowing that most gynecological thermal injuries of the gastrointestinal tract
occur in the terminal ileum offers the surgeon an
opportunity to start the abdominal exploration at
the cecum and work backward from the ileocecal
junction. In the majority of cases, the lesion can be
found approximately 2 to 4 feet from the terminal
ileum. This also offers the advantage of a lower
midline incision rather than a paramedial incision,
which may be unattractive and may add to the
patient's anxiety about this complication.

While the incidence of electrocoagulation
gastrointestinal injury has decreased, there remains a small but consistent incidence of such
injury, at a rate of approximately one case per 1,000
laparoscopic sterilizations. In spite of a declining
incidence, with improved training of surgeons and
improved techniques, the problem has not been
eliminated. The solution to the problem of thermal
injury probably lies in the use of one of the nonelectrical techniques for sterilization, such as the
"clip" or the "ring." This would leave only the
trocar perforation injuries as potential causes of
gastrointestinal damage. There is no known technique of abdominal entry that is completely free of
gastrointestinal injuries. Poulson[1] has reported a
series of tubal sterilization procedures utilizing laparotomy and vaginal culpotomy in which the overall
incidence of gastrointestinal injury is 0.45%, approximately double that from sterilization by laparoscopy.

Gastrointestinal injury represents the
highest morbidity and mortality occurring with laparoscopic sterilization. Every attempt should be
made to reduce the incidence of such injuries. This
objective can be achieved by sound surgical practice, particularly in regard to contraindications,
comprehensive knowledge of the equipment, meticulous care in all details of the procedure and
close attention to postoperative symptoms.

References

1. Poulson AM: Analysis of female sterilization techniques.
   Obstet Gynecol 42:131, 1973

2. Thompson BH, Wheeless CR: Gastrointestinal complications
   of laparoscopy sterilization. Obstet Gynecol 41:669, 1973

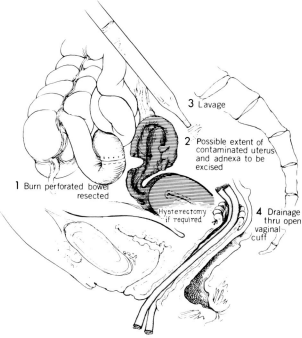

Figure 6
The four essential techniques for management of a gastrointestinal burn perforation secondary to laparoscopic electrocoagulation.

Editorial Comments

Dr. Wheeless has presented the situation fairly and squarely. Gastrointestinal burns are probably the most untoward and dangerous complications of laparoscopic sterilization, the most common procedure performed via the laparoscope. The issue is straightforward: the operator must understand the principles of electrosurgery. Prevention is far better than therapy. Early recognition of injury is of paramount importance, along with surgical intervention when indicated. The magnitude of complications from thermal injury makes a nonelectrical technique for sterilization desirable.

C.J.L.

Thermal gastrointestinal injuries are among the most dreaded complications that can occur following laparoscopy. The injury can never be considered minor, and it requires swift and decisive management. Whatever the cause of thermal gastrointestinal injuries, they represent a potential disaster for the patient and the physician.

Dr. Wheeless' experience with these injuries is probably equal to or greater than that of anyone else in the world, for in his position at a great teaching institution he became the person who reviewed complications. In addition, he has received consultations on the management of such problems from all over the country. I can add no first-hand information that would improve upon the suggestions already presented to the reader.

While it is comforting to know that the survey of laparoscopy performed by the American Association of Gynecologic Laparoscopists in 1975 showed that 2.3% of the sterilizations performed in the preceding year had utilized nonelectric methods, it is unrealistic to think that electricity will no longer be used in the abdomen a few years from now. Even if metallic clips and silastic bands are used to a greater extent than at present, physicians who perform operative surgery on the tubes and ovaries will continue to need electricity. And so it appears that the problem of burns will be with us for a long time.

L.K.

Chapter 22

Trocar and Needle Injuries

A. Jefferson Penfield, M.D.

Introduction

A rare and serious accident associated with laparoscopy is laceration of a major blood vessel such as the aorta or common iliac artery. Hemorrhage may follow needle or trocar puncture of a large artery or vein. Serious bleeding may also follow shearing forces on the mesentery, excessive traction on the infundibulopelvic ligament and ovarian artery, division of the fallopian tube without adequate prior fulguration or traction on the mesosalpinx during sterilization procedures.

The incidence of major vascular injury in laparoscopy is unknown. Neither Cohen, Frangenheim nor Steptoe discuss large vessel injuries in their textbooks, although they do comment on the possibility of bleeding from the abdominal wall or omentum.[1,2,5] Many physicians have heard of an occasional case of aortic or iliac artery laceration and of the lawsuit likely to accompany it. However, no accurate estimate of the incidence of such injuries can be made because most of these cases are not reported.

This chapter will discuss major vascular injuries caused by the needle and the trocar and some of the hemorrhagic catastrophes which have resulted. Particular attention will be given to faulty equipment and technique and to preventive measures.

Materials and Methods

In August, 1975, a questionnaire was sent to 25 of the most knowledgeable and experienced laparoscopists in the USA, Canada, Great Britain and Holland asking for details on any cases of major vessel injuries which had come to their attention (Table 1). Nineteen replies were received. Twelve of the respondents described 19 cases in varying detail. At the same time the seven remaining respondents, who had personally performed or attended at least 30,000 laparoscopies, stated that they had never experienced a major vessel injury, nor did they know of one in their medical communities.

Results

Table 2 lists the 19 injuries. The aorta was punctured in eight instances and the common iliac artery in seven. There was one injury to each of the following: the right common iliac vein, the superior mesenteric artery (a traction or shearing injury), a jejunal artery and an abdominal wall bleeder.

Table 1

Blood Vessel Injury Form

Please do not include name of patient or surgeon

Patient Information

Age	Race	Gravida	Para	Weight
Abdominal Wall:	Thin	Normal	Moderately obese	Very obese
Specify previous abdominal surgery:				
Intraabdominal adhesions:	Suspected	Confirmed	None	
Location of abdominal surgical scars:				
Previous peritonitis:				
	"P.I.D."	Wound disruption		
Other pertinent abnormalities:				

Surgeon

Experienced:	Yes	No	
Number of previous laparoscopies:	Supervised	Unsupervised	

Procedure

	Single incision	Double incision		Sterilization
			Diagnostic	
Anesthesia:	General	Local		
Pneumoperitoneum:	Adequate	Inadequate	None	

Instrument

Needle:	Veress	Touhy	Other	
	Major trocar	Secondary trocar	Unknown	
If trocar implicated:	Diameter	Pyramidal	Conical	
	Dull	Sharp		
Had trocar been sharpened since purchase?		Yes	No	How?
Insertion:	Easy	Much force needed	Number of attempts	
Angle of insertion:	Oblique	Perpendicular	Lateral, off center	

Narrative account of incident: Please specify how and when injury was detected, evidence of shock, vessel injured, time elapsed between incident and laparotomy, how repaired, number of transfusions, outcome.

What precautions or changes in technique have been introduced to prevent a recurrence?

Mail completed form to:
Carl Levinson, M.D.
Chairman, AAGL Complications Committee
Department of Obstetrics and Gynecology
Baylor College
Texas Medical Center
Houston, Texas 77025

Please do not sign this form. Thank you.

A. Jefferson Penfield, M.D., F.A.C.O.G.

Table 2 Major Vessel Injuries from Needle or Trocar	
Aorta	8
Common iliac artery	7
Common iliac vein	1
Superior mesenteric artery	1
Jejunal artery	1
Abdominal wall bleeder	1
Total	19

Table 3 Instrument Causing Vessel Injury	
Subumbilical trocar	6
Veress needle	6
Lower abdominal trocar	3
Unspecified (needle or trocar)	4
Total	19

Table 3 specifies the instrument causing the damage. The Veress needle was implicated as frequently as the major trocar.

Discovery of the injury was made under varying circumstances. In one patient, blood under pressure appeared in the gas tubing immediately after the Veress needle valve was opened. In three patients, injury was not suspected until the anesthesiologist noted a drop in blood pressure during the operation. In one patient there were no signs of intraabdominal bleeding until four hours after the operation. A laparotomy was done, and a laceration of the superior mesenteric artery was repaired. In 16 of the 19 cases the surgeon was inexperienced. He was either a junior resident or a gynecologist doing one of his first cases.

Only occasionally did the respondent analyze the factors contributing to the accident. In five cases of aortic injury, however, it was noted that the surgeon had utilized a perpendicular approach either with the Veress needle or with the subumbilical trocar. In one case of common iliac puncture it was specified that the Veress needle had been inserted in a slightly lateral or off-center direction.

In 16 of the 19 cases a laparotomy was performed promptly, and the vessel was repaired by a vascular surgeon. These patients survived, without major sequelae. On the other hand, three of the patients sustaining trocar puncture of the aorta or common iliac artery succumbed.

Discussion

Table 4 lists important factors in the causation of large vessel injuries by needle or trocar:

1. Inexperienced or unskilled surgeon.
2. Failure to sharpen the trocar. (Wheeless has cautioned that a dull trocar has frequently been an important factor in bowel and vessel injuries.[6] Even with a continuous rotational movement during insertion of a dull trocar the force required to penetrate the abdominal wall reduces the surgeon's positional awareness and sensitivity. The pyramidal trocar may be sharpened on a fine stone or emory paper.)
3. Failure to place patient in Trendelenburg position.
4. Failure to elevate or stabilize the abdominal wall.

Table 4
Factors Responsible for Large Vessel Injuries

1. Inexperienced or unskilled surgeon.

2. Failure to sharpen the trocar.

3. Failure to place patient in Trendelenburg position.

4. Failure to elevate or stabilize the abdominal wall.

5. Perpendicular insertion of needle or subumbilical trocar without adequate elevation of the umbilicus.

6. Lateral insertion of the needle or trocar.

7. Inadequate pneumoperitoneum.

8. Failure to rotate the trocar during insertion.

9. Forceful "arm-and-shoulder" thrust.

10. Failure to note anatomical landmarks.

5. Perpendicular insertion of needle or subumbilical trocar without adequate elevation of the umbilicus. (The perpendicular approach is safe only if the technique described by Drs. Loffer and Pent is followed meticulously.[3] For this technique the patient must be under general anesthesia with sufficient abdominal wall relaxation so that the umbilicus may be elevated several inches. Both needle and trocar must be introduced with proper precautions to avoid a sudden thrust upon entry into the peritoneal cavity.)

6. Lateral (off-center) insertion of needle or trocar.

7. Inadequate pneumoperitoneum.

8. Failure to rotate the trocar during insertion, with resultant inability to control its descent, thus causing an undesirable depression of the abdominal wall and an uncontrolled thrust into the peritoneal cavity.

9. Forceful "arm-and-shoulder" thrust instead of controlled wrist action during insertion of the trocar.

10. Failure to note anatomical landmarks (Figures 1 and 2).

The surgeon must have a knowledge of anatomy. The position and angles of intended insertion of both the needle and the trocar must be checked. The aortic bifurcation occurs at the level of the fourth lumbar vertebra. The level of this vertebra corresponds consistently with the summits of the iliac crests, which can be palpated even in the obese woman. The position of the umbilicus, however, is highly variable, although it may also be at the level of the aortic bifurcation. When the insufflating needle and subumbilical trocar are inserted, these instruments should, if possible, be pointed towards the center of the pelvic cavity. In the obese patient, however, penetration of the abdominal wall may require an angle of insertion as little as 10° from the perpendicular. In such a case, even if the surgeon allows the tip of the instrument to proceed as far as the vertebral column, it is not likely to puncture the aorta. Injury to either common iliac artery or vein obviously cannot occur unless the surgeon introduces the needle or the trocar in a lateral or off-center direction.

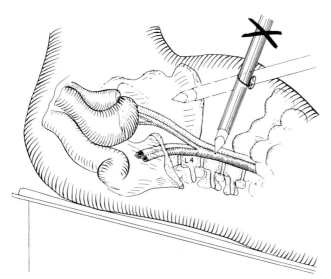

Figure 1

The patient is in Trendelenburg position. The incorrect perpendicular insertion as depicted would result in aortic puncture. Note the aortic bifurcation at *L4* which is precisely at the level of the summit of the iliac crest. The interrupted trocar line shows the correct angle of insertion.

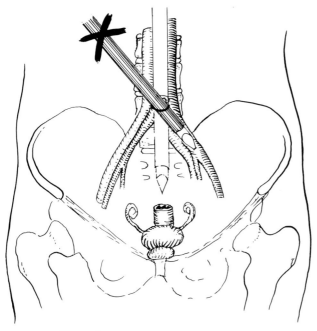

Figure 2

Puncture of the common iliac artery will occur only if there is significant deviation of the trocar from the midline.

Additional protection of intraabdominal vessels from trocar injury is provided by the initial establishment of a satisfactory pneumoperitoneum as well as by the placement of the patient in a moderate Trendelenburg position. The intraperitoneal gas elevates the abdominal wall from the aortic and iliac vessels while the "head-down" position allows the omentum and intestines to fall out of the pelvic and lower abdominal cavities. Thus, neither the large vessels, the omental vessels nor the mesenteric vessels should be in the path of the entering trocar.

The needle puncture of the jejunal artery referred to previously was, as one might expect, associated with a puncture of the jejunum itself. Either the surgeon did not elevate or stabilize the abdominal wall properly or the needle was inserted to a considerable depth in a perpendicular fashion in order to puncture the omentum, jejunum and jejunal artery in turn.

Conclusion

These 19 cases can be regarded as a random sampling of the total number of major vessel injuries which have occurred. Although no statistical conclusions can be made, certain observations have been presented and may be summarized as follows: the laparoscopist must review the anatomy and sharpen the trocar. The patient should be in a moderate Trendelenburg position, and an adequate pneumoperitoneum should be established. The proper angles for insertion of the needle and trocar should be selected, and the surgeon must be in full control of their descent and entry into the peritoneal cavity.

From the evidence presented in this chapter, major vessel injuries in laparoscopy seem to be preventable: they are associated with defects in equipment or technique. In order to safeguard the patient, the laparoscopist must avoid or eliminate these defects.

References

1. Cohen M: *Laparoscopy, Culdoscopy and Gynecography.* WB Saunders, Philadelphia, 1970, p 42

2. Frangenheim, H: *Laparoscopy and Culdoscopy in Gynecology.* Georg Thieme, Stuttgart; Butterworth and Co, London, 1972, p 42

3. Loffer F, Pent D: An alternate technique in penetrating the abdomen for laparoscopy. In *Gynecological Laparoscopy: Principles and Techniques* (JM Phillips, L Keith, Eds.). Stratton Intercontinental Medical Book Corp, New York, 1974, p 107

4. Palmer R: Security in laparoscopy. In *Gynecological Laparoscopy: Principles and Techniques.* (JM Phillips, L Keith, Eds.). Stratton Intercontinental Medical Book Corporation, New York, 1974, p 17

5. Steptoe P: *Laparoscopy in Gynaecology.* Williams & Wilkins, Baltimore, 1967, p 30

6. Wheeless C: personal communication.

Editorial Comments

Trocar and needle injuries are among the most potentially serious complications of laparoscopy. The organs most susceptible to injury from the trocar or needle are the hollow visci, such as the stomach and bowel, and the major blood vessels. A review of the literature shows that the stomach, small intestine and colon have been perforated by the Veress needle and the major trocar. Similarly, the aorta, vena cava, epigastric vessels and hypogastric vessels have been injured. To my knowledge, this chapter reviews the subject in much greater depth than has been done previously.

L.K.

Chapter 23

Statistics

Franklin D. Loffer, M.D.
David Pent, M.D.

There is a multitude of dangers lying in wait for the unsuspecting laparoscopist. In spite of them, the vast majority of laparoscopic patients tolerate the procedure well and have no problems. They are often able to return to their usual activities within 24 hours.

The careful laparoscopist, aware of potential problems, is more likely to avoid them than one who has no concept of the dangers of the procedure. For that reason it is valuable to examine: (1) those problems specifically associated with laparoscopy, (2) their time of occurrence, and (3) their incidence of occurrence. Only those problems and complications peculiar to, or whose frequency is increased by, laparoscopy will be discussed. Statistics on laparoscopic complications can be obtained by either reviewing the literature[1] or by surveying gynecologists interested in the procedure.[2, 3] Both methods have been used and give surprisingly similar results. In reviewing the statistics it must be remembered that no list is ever complete; as instrumentation and techniques change, old complications may become less frequent and new ones appear.

Pneumoperitoneum Complications

Complications during the creation of the pneumoperitoneum have been reported to occur with an incidence of 7.4 per 1,000 cases.[2] Some of these problems are life-threatening and occasionally fatal. Gas embolism (four cases) with fatality (one case) has been described in the literature.[1] Gas embolism may be more common than has been reported since 1.7% of surveyed physicians state they had experienced this event.[2] The outcome in each of these cases was not given, but it is noteworthy that all were under general anesthesia. Small amounts of CO_2 are not significant. Some neurologic diagnostic studies use 100 cc intravascularly without difficulty. In larger amounts, however, CO_2 (in spite of its greater solubility in blood) will act like N_2O or air when accumulated in the heart: it interferes with the maintenance of circulation. Intravasation, secondary to excessive gas pressures, has been suggested as a cause of gas embolism; however, misplacement of the Veress needle is a more likely reason.

Cardiac arrests (10 cases) have been reported in the literature, with three deaths.[1] Thus, it is surprising that as many as 47 physicians (representing 4.8% of surveyed respondents) reported this problem.[3] The etiology of these cardiac arrests may have been gas embolization; more probably they were the result of marked pulse and blood pressure changes. Significant cardiac arrhythmias were observed by 38.6% of all responding physicians; this complication occurs more commonly with general anesthesia than with local.

Factors contributing to cardiac instability are increased P_{CO_2}, decreased arterial pH and a decreased P_{O_2}. Although these changes may occur from CO_2 absorption through the peritoneal surface, inadvertent hypoventilation by the anesthesiologist is probably an important factor: there are fewer cases reported when local anesthesia is used. Cardiac instability has also been attributed to vagal reflexes from abdominal distension, the postpartum state and cardiac compression. The role of premedications, intubation and mechanical ventilation is still debatable. N_2O has been advocated as a means of avoiding this problem, but adequate ventilation and maintenance of an intraabdominal pressure of less than 20 mm Hg are the major safety factors.

Another potentially serious (but infrequently reported) complication is pneumothorax. It has been reported four times during gynecologic laparoscopy.[1] The presence of diaphragmatic hernia does not seem to play a significant role in the etiology of this problem, nor does excessive pulmonary ventilation since some cases have occurred with local anesthesia. Excessive pressures during creation of the pneumoperitoneum may be an important factor.

The most common complications of the pneumoperitoneum are related to insufflation of the preperitoneal space and/or omentum; it leads to "failed" laparoscopy because of the inability to create an adequate pneumoperitoneum and accounts for more failed laparoscopies than any other single factor. Only experience and the understanding of good laparoscopic technique can enable the laparoscopist to avoid this problem. "Failed" laparoscopy occurs five times more frequently with the laparoscopist who has performed fewer than 100 cases.[2]

Hemorrhage Complications

The next most common complication is some form of hemorrhage requiring further therapy. It has been recorded as occurring in 6.4 per 1,000 patients.[2] The literature reports bleeding from the mesosalpinx in the majority of patients during transection of the fallopian tube for sterilization. Strangely, among all the laparoscopists surveyed[2] the incidence was higher in diagnostic laparoscopy—4.1 per 1,000 cases. Although the majority of these patients can be managed by recoagulation, some have required a laparotomy for control of bleeding. It appears that the risks of bleeding decrease as laparoscopists become more experienced.

Other potential sources of bleeding are the abdominal wall, generally at the site of the ancillary trocar; the ovary at the time of biopsy; and the peritoneum when biopsies are performed on implants. Laceration of large pelvic vessels, even the aorta, has been reported and must be considered a result of an error in technique (Chapter 12).

Electrical Complications

Electrical injuries are a significant risk with laparoscopy because of the necessity of using complicated electrical equipment. Electrical complications have been reported to occur in only 2.2 per 1,000 patients[3]; they are potentially a more serious problem than either pneumoperitoneal or hemorrhagic complications. The majority of these problems involve burn to the small bowel, inadvertently damaged at the time of sterilization. However, it is reported that 5% of all electrical bowel injuries have occurred during diagnostic laparoscopic procedures and approximately one-fourth during teaching sessions. Thermal injuries are reported to be a complication for 7.2% of physicians surveyed.[3] Large bowel as well as small bowel can be damaged. All but seven of the 44 cases of electrical bowel injury reported in the literature[1] required laparotomy. Significant burns in the anterior abdominal wall have occurred, but the advent of insulated trocars should reduce this problem.

The seriousness of electrical injuries is due to the fact that most are not recognized when they occur. The patient with a bowel injury may be discharged and sent home only to become progressively more ill. The resultant peritonitis and its sequelae have been the cause of several deaths (Chapter 20).

Penetration Complications

Both the Veress needle and the telescope trocar must be introduced blindly into the abdomen; therefore, the risk of penetrating injuries exists continually. The incidence of penetrating injury is reported as 2.7 per 1,000 patients.[3] These injuries primarily happen to the bowel: stomach (nine cases), small bowel (five cases) and colon (six cases). The most recent survey of the American Association of Gynecologic Laparoscopists demonstrates a bowel injury rate of only 1 per 1,000 patients. The bladder has been injured at least four times.

Pregnancies

Pregnancy must be considered a complication of laparoscopic sterilization procedures. The survey indicates an incidence of 1.8 per 1,000 patients.[2] Luteal phase pregnancies are not an error of the procedure but rather of timing: they are justifiably excluded from this figure. If those pregnancies secondary to misidentification of anatomical structures are excluded, the "true" method failure rate is only 1.1 per 1,000 cases. The survey of laparoscopists[3] reports a pregnancy incidence of 0.91 per 1,000 patients but does not indicate whether these are only "method" figures.

Miscellaneous Complications

Infections in laparoscopy are surprisingly few considering the number of instruments and frequent use of photographic equipment. Pelvic inflammatory disease and pelvic abscesses have been reported in 26 patients and significant skin infections in 15 patients. It has been suggested that the removal of IUDs at the time of laparoscopic sterilization may increase the potential of pelvic infection.[1]

Other complications include incisional hernias (which have involved omentum in six patients and bowel in two), which have only been reported with the 10 mm telescopes with the larger trocar and sleeve. Postoperative adhesions in the uncomplicated case are reported rarely.

References

1. Loffer F, Pent D: Indications, contraindications and complications of laparoscopy. Obstet Gynecol Surv 30:407, 1975

2. Phillips J, Keith D, Keith L, Hulka J, Hulka B: Survey of gynecological laparoscopy for 1974. J Reprod Med 15:45, 1975

3. Phillips J, Keith D, Hulka J, Hulka B, Keith L: Gynecologic laparoscopy in 1975. J Reprod Med 16:104, 1976

Editorial Comments

Statistical reports on the performance of medical activities are somewhat like bitter-sweet chocolate: the overall effect is good, no doubt; all too often, however, there is a lingering aftertaste. In this instance the "aftertaste" is the nagging question that frequently arises about what is taking place in the areas not surveyed. In other words, do the statistics tell the reader what they are supposed to? Do they represent what is really going on in the world, or are they spurious?

My personal bias dealt with, let us now address ourselves to this chapter. What does it tell us? It shows us trends, documents changes and quantifies some of the problems, at least partially. As such, it is worthwhile reading for anyone interested in our specialty. The method selected by the authors—that is, a retrospective analysis of the published literature—is well known to most readers. To be sure, some question the value of such a review, stating that this sort of information is already in the literature; granted, but it is the interpretation, only possible when a dozen or fifteen articles are lying in front of you, that makes these activities so fascinating. The other method of survey, obtaining data directly, has been performed by the American Association of Gynecologic Laparoscopists on numerous occasions. (The reader is referred to Chapter 36 for further details.)

The authors comments are pertinent and should be particularly constructive for residents and young people in practice. Often these individuals are eager to write a paper but don't know where to begin. Here, from the pen of a very experienced physician, is the way many others have begun an interesting adventure in medicine—a review of the literature—which can become the basis of a review paper from which all colleagues can benefit.

L.K.

Loffer and Pent have done a superb job of collating the statistics on the performance of laparoscopy and laparoscopic sterilizations. They point out certain salient features:

The less experienced the laparoscopist, the more frequent the complications.

During pneumoperitoneum it is vital that there be adequate ventilation and that the intraabdominal pressure be kept as low as possible. These factors seem much more important than whether carbon dioxide or nitrous oxide is used.

The failure to establish a pneumoperitoneum or the establishment of an inadequate pneumoperitoneum leads to numerous complications, some overt, some subtle, as a result of poor visualization.

Complications resulting from electrical burns and perforating injuries are the most serious ones encountered.

There is no substitute for complete attention to detail in order to prevent the complications of laparoscopy. Each procedure is a unique experience and requires the utmost concentration and effort.

C.J.L.

Section 9

Systems for Instruction

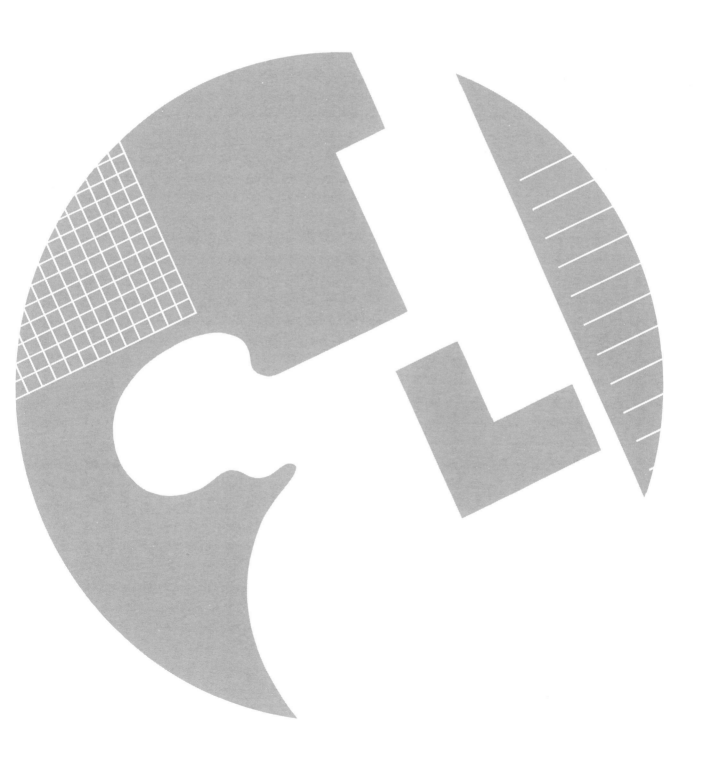

Chapter 24

Self-Instruction

Franklin D. Loffer, M.D.
David Pent, M.D.

It is impossible for any learning program, whether based on a textbook, a didactic course, audiovisual material, a preceptorship or any combination of them, to make a surgeon adequate and confident in a given area. Even a residency program cannot do so. The final ingredient must always include some element of self-instruction. The concept of self-instruction should not be foreign to surgeons. It is a never-ending process which first helps him or her to refine his or her new knowledge and then allows him or her to improve it throughout his or her entire professional life. Its basis lies not only in journals, books and lectures but, possibly most importantly, in an honest and critical assessment of his or her results as compared to others'.

It has been suggested that a long training program is required to prepare a gynecologist adequately to do laparoscopy.[12] Our opinion, and certainly the opinion of others, is that this is not always necessary for a physician learning a new technique *within* his or her specialty. This position is supported by the fact that most major authors on laparoscopy are essentially self-taught.[8] The ability of these "experts" to teach themselves did not come about simply because of their academic positions but rather by a slow and careful program of self-teaching based on whatever information had preceded them. This same type of "program" is readily available to any practicing gynecologist interested in endoscopy.

These comments should not be construed as negating the value of a training program. Such programs expedite the attainment of proficiency, and physicians would be foolhardy not to take advantage of the preexisting information offered by them. While ultimately all graduates of accredited residency programs in obstetrics and gynecology will receive endoscopic training, most practicing gynecologists are not yet so trained. This section will deal primarily with the self-instruction which follows training in one of the many formal but short courses which are available.[1] The principles can also be applied to residency endoscopic training programs.

Self-instruction can be divided into three distinct phases. They are: (1) preparation for training, (2) training, (3) posttraining. During each of these periods the student will be able to improve him- or herself in different ways.

Preparation for Training

At least some background knowledge is advantageous prior to any formal training program. Three major monographs on laparoscopy offer a point of departure. Their value lies primarily in their historical perspective and their description of early and basic techniques,[11] their description of the progression and refinement of these techniques[3] and, last, their inclusive description of the most modern laparoscopic techniques, findings and complications.[5] In addition, self-training manuals[2] and review articles[7] are available which allow one to gain an overview of laparoscopy in its entirety. More detailed information on the value of "before-and-after" training can be found in texts on laparoscopy[9] and review articles on areas of special concern.[4, 6]

A second valuable preparation for the training period is to acquire some endoscopic experience with another surgeon who is proficient in the technique. This allows written material to be placed in perspective and provides the students with some firsthand knowledge of the capabilities and limitations of gynecological endoscopic techniques. This suggestion for "previous experience" is *not* meant to imply that it is beneficial for a student to do a few cases on his or her own after only reading and prior to having formal training.

The Training Period

The training program of a short postgraduate course in gynecologic endoscopy, unlike that of a residency program, will be compact. Several points must be appreciated. First and foremost is that only the most basic material can be presented in a short training period. For this reason, **nothing** discussed should be considered trivial. Each and every point has considerable value in the mind of the teacher even though it may not be readily apparent to the student. Second, since the material being presented is abbreviated, the student must not assume that all he or she has heard in one area is the sum total of available knowledge. The student must remember that numerous articles are accumulating in the world literature pertaining to every aspect of the subject which has been discussed. Third, even if the training program includes at least some personal surgical contact on the part of the student (as we feel it should), the student must remember that he or she is not yet on his or her own. The mere presence of a teacher who has the ultimate responsibility to the patient makes the trainee's decision-making easier. This last point is especially important. Watching an expert do endoscopy or doing endoscopy directly under the guidance of an expert may appear disarmingly simple. Once on his or her own, the new endoscopist may find that he or she does not know how this seemingly simple procedure was really accomplished and for what reasons. If this point is not appreciated, the student may ignore subtle points of technique and later begin to do endoscopic procedures immediately on his or her own without the benefits of appropriate postcourse self-training.

Self-training Following the Training Period

It is most beneficial for a student of endoscopy to return to his or her community and have someone proficient in the procedure scrub with him or her on the first few cases. Not only will this preceptor provide a ready backup source of information, but he or she can also provide a critique of the new endoscopist's recently acquired skill. Of less value to the student is scrubbing on the preceptor's cases. The surgeon not operating on his or her own case finds him or herself in an entirely different position than when the ultimate responsibility is his or hers.

If endoscopy is not already being performed at the hospital where the new student practices, he or she should initially organize, with the help of the operating room staff, a crew to help on all cases. An essential part of any gynecologic endoscopic procedure is the team which supports the surgeon. They, too, must learn new techniques with him or her.

An important point in developing endoscopic ability is the proper selection of patients. For laparoscopy the ideal patient to start with is one who would require a laparotomy if laparoscopy were not available, even though preoperatively it is recognized that the chance of finding an abnormality requiring a laparotomy might be minimal. Such patients include infertility patients, those with pain or a mass of unknown etiology or those with a possible ectopic pregnancy. If this type of patient is chosen initially, no harm is done if, for some technical reason, laparoscopy cannot be accomplished or if the operator's inexperience makes evaluation of the findings questionable and a laparotomy must be done. In addition, should an untoward event occur, such as a perforation of a viscus, bleeding, etc., only the repair of the damage and not laparotomy *per se* would be added to the patient's care.

The ideal patient should have no significant medical or surgical problems and should be thin, with an unscarred abdomen. She should have none of the known contraindications to laparoscopy or any of the relative contraindications.[7] Relative contraindications add to the difficulty of procedures and should not be imposed upon the learning laparoscopist. Failure to recognize this point may be the basis for the greater number of complications found in diagnostic laparoscopy, as recently reported.[10]

If the suggestion about the type of patient is followed, none will have a planned laparoscopic surgical or operative procedure. We feel strongly about this since the addition of a surgical technique such as a tubal sterilization while one is learning to do basic laparoscopy adds much more than may be appreciated by the beginner. It is our opinion that it takes at least 20 to 30 simple diagnostic cases before the novice laparoscopic surgeon has gained enough experience to be sufficiently comfortable and proficient to add a new dimension to the operation. During these initial cases there inevitably will be problems with instruments, maintenance of the pneumoperitoneum, interpretation of findings and running out of operating room time, to mention just a few. Once these preliminary cases have been done and the laparoscopist feels comfortable with creation of the pneumoperitoneum, introduction of the trocar and telescope, manipulation of intraabdominal contents with the suction cannula and ancillary probes and interpretation of findings, then he or she can turn his or her attention to intraabdominal surgery via the laparoscope.

When the laparoscopist begins to add surgical laparoscopic procedures to his or her repertoire, it is of value to tell the patient that, under some circumstances, the planned laparoscopic surgical procedure might not be possible and it might be necessary to accomplish what is desired in the conventional manner. This allows the surgeon to have the latitude of not doing a potentially dangerous laparoscopic surgical technique unless he or she is comfortable, and it forewarns the patient that a laparotomy might be necessary.

The surgeon should recognize that the latter comments are a combination of an excuse and informed consent. He or she should *not* come to rely on this type of statement in subsequent cases any more than, as an example, he or she relies upon informing patients that he or she might have to do an abdominal hysterectomy rather than a vaginal one. Should a laparoscopist never attain significant self-confidence to drop these forewarnings in all of his or her cases, he or she should consider limiting his or her laparoscopy simply to diagnostic work or referring all cases to someone who has a special interest in endoscopy and does many cases.

Finally, the endoscopist must continue to be critical of his or her own results as compared to others'. This is especially easy using the published surveys available.[10] The field of obstetrics and gynecology now contains so many areas that subspecialization will continue to grow, as it has in internal medicine. It is appropriate that an obstetrician-gynecologist who does not do sufficient work in an area refer the patient for care to a more experienced individual.

Conclusion

The role of self-instruction in laparoscopy and other gynecologic endoscopic techniques is not dissimilar to that in other areas of medicine. The physician should take advantage of the written and didactic training programs which are available to him or her. They should be supplemented throughout his or her entire professional career by continual reevaluations of his or her own techniques and accomplishments in order to maintain proficiency.

References

1. American Association of Gynecologic Laparoscopists, 11239 S. Lakewood Boulevard, Downey, California, 90241 USA

2. Bronstein ES: *Laparoscopy for Sterilization*. Year Book Medical Publishers, Inc., Chicago, 1975

3. Cohen MR: *Laparoscopy, Culdoscopy and Gynecography*. WB Saunders Co., Philadelphia, 1970

4. Engel T, Harris FW: The electrical dynamics of laparoscopic sterilization. J Reprod Med 15:33, 1975

5. Frangenheim H: *Laparoscopy and Culdoscopy in Gynecology*. Butterworth and Co, London, 1972

6. Levinson CJ: Laparoscopy is easy—except for the complications: a review with suggestions. J Reprod Med 13:187, 1974

7. Loffer FD, Pent D: Indications, contraindications and complications of laparoscopy. Obstet Gynecol Surv 30:407, 1975

8. Phillips J, Keith D, Keith L: Gynecological laparoscopy 1973: the state of the art. J Reprod Med 12:215, 1974

9. Phillips JM, Keith L, (Eds): *Gynecological Laparoscopy: Principles and Techniques*. Stratton Intercontinental Medical Book Corporation, New York, 1974

10. Phillips J, Keith D, Keith L, Hulka J, Hulka B: Survey of gynecologic laparoscopy for 1974. J Reprod Med 15:45, 1975

11. Steptoe PC: *Laparoscopy in Gynaecology*. E & S Livingstone, Ltd, London, 1967

12. Steptoe PC: Gynecological laparoscopy. J Reprod Med 10:211, 1973

Editorial Comments

This chapter was written by two of the most respected teachers of laparoscopy in the United States today. It would be no exaggeration to say that physicians have beaten paths to their door from all over the country and, in fact, from all over the world to learn laparoscopy. Their chapter is a model for anyone who wishes to begin to learn this procedure.

There are probably few readers of this book who have not performed laparoscopy. Therefore, I turn the reader's attention to the last sentence of the chapter: please go back and reread it. In essence, Pent and Loffer are saying that even after you have learned laparoscopy, you must continue to reevaluate your technique, accomplishments and complications to maintain proficiency in the operation. This admonition is of paramount importance to everyone interested in the health care of women.

L.K.

Chapter 25

Teaching Laparoscopy

David Pent, M.D.
Franklin D. Loffer, M.D.

"A teacher affects eternity; he can never tell where his influence stops."
Henry Brooks Adams

The explosive reawakening of interest in laparoscopy has resulted in profound changes in the nature of gynecologic practice. Physicians were suddenly faced with the necessity of acquiring and mastering a completely new skill. Many physicians who began performing laparoscopy were ill-trained or not trained at all, and this situation subsequently led to complications. A survey by the American Association of Gynecologic Laparoscopists concerning complications[4] revealed inadequate knowledge of certain fundamentals of laparoscopy by some physicians performing the procedure. A number of physicians answering the questionnaire had no idea of the final intraabdominal pressure which had been achieved or the type of electrosurgical units which they were utilizing despite the fact that the two most common complications concern the pneumoperitoneum and electrosurgery.

Since 1971 we have been involved in a continuous teaching program. As the first physicians to perform laparoscopy in our community, we soon noted that many other gynecologists in the area referred their patients to us for diagnostic and surgical procedures. These physicians rapidly became impressed with the value of laparoscopy and expressed an interest in learning the technique. We therefore arranged for two one-day courses to be held, consisting of didactic but amply illustrated lectures followed by demonstration cases. Practical experience was then obtained on a preceptorship basis, in which we assisted some of the physicians with their early cases and they in turn assisted other physicians in the community as they became involved in laparoscopy. These two courses were well received, and we were encouraged to offer additional ones. By the end of 1975 we had conducted 29 courses, which have been attended by 436 physicians from 41 states, Canada and Australia. At the present time laparoscopy is used very extensively in our community. To date, the experience has been satisfactory, both in terms of patient acceptance and a low rate of complications.

Aim of the Course

The actual mechanics of performing any surgical procedure in a simple and uncomplicated case are, of course, relatively easy to learn. However, the essence of surgery is in determining when the surgery is indicated and when it is contraindicated, in the management of the patient pre- and postoperatively and, most importantly, in preventing complications as well as knowing how to handle complications which do arise. The same principles apply for laparoscopy. The aim of any course of instruction in this technique should be the same as that of all surgical procedures. The student must be given a good, thorough background in the principles underlying the procedure and not just be taught "how to" perform laparoscopy. He or she should be familiar with the basic principles of fiber optics and optics, the physiology of the pneumoperitoneum and the principles of electrosurgical equipment. The student should also have a good working knowledge of his or her laparoscopic equipment, a familiarity with the anesthetic techniques used in patients undergoing laparoscopy and a full awareness of the indications and contraindications, how to avoid complications and how to manage those complications which do occur.

Content of the Course

The formal, didactic portion of the course consists of a series of 18 presentations. The total time required to cover this material is slightly in excess of eight hours, which is spread over the first two mornings of the course. The presentations are:

1. Introduction to the Course
2. Overall View of Laparoscopy
3. Physics of Fiber Optics and Endoscopy
4. Indications and Contraindications for Laparoscopy
5. Physiology of the Pneumoperitoneum
6. Technique and Complications of the Pneumoperitoneum
7. Technique of Laparoscopy
8. Complications of Laparoscopy
9. Interpretation of Laparoscopic Appearances
10. Social and Economic Factors of Laparoscopy
11. Surgical Techniques via Laparoscopy
12. Tubal Coagulation
13. Instrumentation and Care of the Instruments
14. Outpatient Laparoscopy
15. Anesthesia
16. Laparoscopy in the Evaluation of the Infertile Couple
17. Culdoscopy and Hysteroscopy
18. Documentation

A few points should be emphasized. The portion of the program devoted to "Overall View of Laparoscopy" includes a brief movie demonstrating the instrumentation, techniques and findings obtained via laparoscopy. Its main purpose is to acquaint those physicians who have had little or no experience with laparoscopy with the general concept of what is involved in the procedure and what we are talking about when we refer to the pneumoperitoneum, when we discuss the trocar and cannula, telescope and light source, etc. In this way there is a common level of knowledge established for all the registrants at the beginning of the course.

The section on "Indications and Contraindications for Laparoscopy" constitutes a review of the current indications and contraindications as obtained from an extensive review of the literature and personal correspondence.[3] The section on "Physiology of the Pneumoperitoneum" is based not only on a review of the current literature but also on the findings of our own investigative studies.

The presentation on "Tubal Coagulation" discusses not only the various techniques of electrocoagulation of the fallopian tubes but also presents discussions of medicolegal problems, the postcoagulation syndrome, postpartum tubal coagulation, luteal phase pregnancies, the operating telescope, the bipolar instrument and the newer nonelectrical occlusive techniques, such as the clip and band.

The section on "Instrumentation and Care of the Instruments" is used to exhibit, demonstrate and discuss the instruments commonly used in gynecologic laparoscopy. The registrants are afforded an opportunity to actually handle and manipulate the instruments and to ask questions concerning their operation. Much of the information concerning the care of the instruments is given at the time of the surgical portion of the course, with groups of registrants accompanying the scrub nurses into the instrument room to observe the disassemblying, cleaning and reassemblying of the laparoscopic equipment.

Presentation of the Course Material
Audiovisual Techniques

It is vital, when trying to present a large amount of almost totally new material in a relatively short period of time, that maximum use be made of audiovisual techniques. Each registrant receives a printed course outline at the beginning of the course, and this material is reproduced on 35 mm slides which are used during the presentation. This serves to visually reinforce what the registrant already has in front of him or her, and, more importantly, frees him or her from having to copy down the material which is being presented on the slide: many students become so preoccupied with the taking of notes that they miss much of the important material which is being presented. Each text slide contains a relatively small amount of printed material. This makes it easier to grasp and under-

stand what is being presented and results in a rapid turnover of slides, which aids in maintaining interest and attention. The text slides are interspersed with a large number of regular photographic slides illustrating the material being presented. The speakers all talk "from the slides" instead of referring to printed notes in front of them, which makes for a much more stimulating and interesting presentation. Some of the lectures have been put on color video tape. The lectures on "Technique and Complications of the Pneumoperitoneum" and "Technique of Laparoscopy" are ideally suited to this type of presentation.

Use of Repetition

An important aspect of these presentations is the use of repetition. For example, the necessity of always having a clear view of the pelvis and operative field is mentioned in the section on "Technique and Complications of the Pneumoperitoneum" and again in the section on "Interpretation of Laparoscopic Appearances." It is also emphasized in the section on "Surgical Techniques via Laparoscopy" and in the presentation on "Tubal Coagulation." In addition, it is emphasized again during the actual surgical cases.

One cannot reasonably expect any student, in the eight hours devoted to formal didactic presentations, to absorb every statement upon its first presentation. This reemphasis, which quite naturally involves those points which are of major importance, serves to identify the major points to the student as important ones and also makes it easier for him or her to absorb them at the time of the presentation. Several years ago we had our teaching program evaluated by a professional educational consultant as part of an ongoing review of our program. It was his opinion that this aspect of reemphasis was one of the most vital, important and profitable aspects of the lectures.

The Teaching Environment

The number of physicians attending each course is limited. We now accept 15 registrants and five auditors for each course. A lecture room has been selected which can comfortably seat 20 individuals at tables, permitting adequate space on the table for the course outline, cassette tape recorders and the taking of notes.

Questions are encouraged, and more than enough time is programmed into the course to allow for the questions and answers. Questions are encouraged as they arise, and, in addition, time is allowed at the end of each presentation for any further questions or discussion.

The atmosphere at all times is informal, with an "open pot" of coffee always available, as well as a formal coffee break each morning. At the conclusion of the first morning's lectures the students and faculty have lunch together. This has proven to be an excellent opportunity for everyone to become better acquainted with each other.

The Faculty

The curriculum and its presentation obviously are the responsibility of the faculty. It is necessary to have a group of physicians who are knowledgeable in the theory, procedures, instrumentation and implementation of gynecologic laparoscopy. In addition, they must be familiar with the theories and procedures used by their peers in other parts of the country.

The core of the present faculty is a group of three gynecologic laparoscopists who give most of the didactic presentations. The topics are rotated among the various faculty members, and differences in voice modulation and technique of presentation help to sustain a continued interest in the material. The faculty also includes a respiratory therapist, who discusses the "Physiology of the Pneumoperitoneum." The remainder of the faculty is made up of anesthesiologists, who participate both in the formal didactic presentations and are also actively involved with student teaching during the surgical portion of the course. The lecture on "Anesthesia" also discusses outpatient laparoscopy, outpatient surgery and the Surgicenter, which is where the surgical portion of the course is conducted. In addition, there is ample opportunity during the surgical procedures for the registrants to talk with the anesthesiologists concerning the anesthetic management of the patient.

Surgical Instruction

Practical Experience

Some degree of practical experience and exposure to surgical techniques must be an integral part of any good laparoscopic teaching program. (The late Robert Benchley once said that he could build the George Washington Bridge if somebody would only tell him where to turn the first shovelful of dirt!) After the formal lecture presentations the registrants are divided into three groups of five each, with each group having its own instructor. A demonstration case is performed by the instructor, and following this the registrants are afforded an opportunity for practical experience in the performance of a laparoscopic tubal coagulation. The case is performed slowly, under close supervision, with ample opportunity for discussion, questions and demonstration of any interesting pathologic findings as well as various aspects of the surgical technique. Rather than using a teaching attachment, which is somewhat unsatisfactory technically in that the light is reduced, a third incision is made in one of the lower quadrants of the abdomen, and a second laparoscope is introduced.[2] The instructor thus has the opportunity of closely observing any laparoscopic manipulations performed by the registrant.

The relationship between the instructor and the registrant is similar to the relationship between the attending and resident physicians at the hospitals in our community. The ultimate management of the case, and especially the control of the electrosurgical equipment, rests with the attending physician, in this case the instructor. One other registrant scrubs in as an assistant, and the remaining three physicians are then free to observe the overall technique, to peer into the abdomen to see any significant findings and to discuss the various aspects of anesthesia with the anesthesiologist.

The Arizona Family Planning Service

The major problem in any type of "wet clinic" teaching program is, of course, the availability of patients. Very early in our experience with laparoscopy we realized that tubal coagulation as the definitive step in family planning was far more than just another surgical procedure but represented a "right" to which the patient was entitled. At that time insurance coverage for elective sterilization was virtually nonexistent, and so there was a large pool of the truly indigent patients as well as medically indigent patients. Because of this the Arizona Family Planning Service was established. This organization has been able to introduce certain economies into laparoscopic sterilization not normally present in a private physician's office. Prepayment is required, and the fee requested of the patient is determined by a sliding scale based both on income and the number of dependents. The surgeon, the anesthesiologist and the surgical facility, as part of their contract with Arizona Family Planning Service, perform a certain number of cases without any charge. Those patients with virtually no funds are referred to the teaching programs at the local community hospitals. Patients with limited funds are given an opportunity to participate in the course. Under this arrangement the registration fee paid by the physicians for attending the course is entirely given over to underwriting the fees for the surgeon, anesthesiologist and facility. The course faculty does not receive any remuneration for their teaching. The patient knows, of course, that she will have her surgery performed as part of a teaching course, and she signs a statement stating that she is aware that the physicians attending the laparoscopy seminar may be in the operating room and participate in her surgery. She also understands that she will be treated as a regular patient of the doctor (instructor) to whom she was referred initially.

Course Registrants

Course enrollment is limited by the available number of patients and operating room time and because of our desire to maintain the more personalized type of instruction program. When we were the only two gynecologists involved in the teaching program, each course had 10 registrants and the courses were held eight times a year. With the addition of a third faculty gynecologist we now accept 15 registrants for each of five courses given during the year. In addition, those physicians who have had some experience in performing laparoscopy but want to learn more about the various aspects of the procedure can elect to audit the course, attending the lectures and the demonstration surgery case. Auditors are limited to a maximum of five for each course.

Since laparoscopy is a new surgical technique, we felt a primary commitment to the postgraduate education of the practicing obstetrician and gynecologist. Furthermore, it is our opinion that the procedure should only be performed by a physician trained in pelvic surgery so that he or she is better able to interpret what he or she is seeing and is capable of handling any complication which may arise. Because of this, and because the course is continually oversubscribed, we have limited enrollment to those physicians who restrict their practice to obstetrics and gynecology and discouraged family physicians, general surgeons and others from enrolling in the program. We also prefer not to accept resident physicians since we feel that their laparoscopic training is primarily the responsibility of their parent institution.

The presence of physicians unlicensed to practice in the state of Arizona creates a medicolegal problem, not so much with regard to their practicing medicine within the state but rather in the event of malpractice litigation: the presence of the special class of "unlicensed" physicians can virtually be construed as malpractice itself. This problem had not been considered previously, and the American Medical Association could offer us no guidelines. The potential problem was discussed with the Arizona Board of Medical Examiners, and a detailed description of the entire teaching program was prepared for them. As a result, the Board has approved a special form of licensing for all physicians taking the course. They are given a resident physician's license in the State of Arizona valid for the three days of the course. It goes without saying that all course registrants are licensed in their home jurisdiction.

The course is recognized by the AMA's program on continuing education and by the Arizona Medical Association's program on continuing medical education for 18 credit hours and is approved for 25 cognates by the American College of Obstetricians and Gynecologists. Each registrant is given a certificate upon completion of the course. Some hospitals request attendance at a formal course as a requirement for operative privileges in laparoscopy, and indeed the granting of operative privileges is and should remain strictly the province of each individual hospital. Many hospitals appear to be looking for a statement that the registrant has become proficient in laparoscopic surgery. The certificate is no more a guarantee of proficiency than a statement which confirms that an individual has completed three years of residency ensures his or her proficiency in performing a hysterectomy.

Some questions have been raised as to whether a short course, such as our three-day course, can be considered adequate training in laparoscopy. In this regard, some physicians who have attended our course had attended other, prior courses, consisting of two to three days of lectures and only demonstration surgery. They came to us because of the feeling, to which we wholeheartedly subscribe, that practical experience is a *must*. Even having didactic material is no assurance of quality since several registrants had previously attended courses where the didactic portion did no more than show "how to" and gave nothing of the basic principles and background in the fundamentals of laparoscopy. Our own poll of registrants, conducted on a periodic basis, has shown that the vast majority have felt confident in performing their first laparoscopy after having attended our course. In addition, many of them elect to have continued supervision on their home grounds, and therefore feel that the three-day, structured course is adequate.

Other Techniques of Teaching Laparoscopy

A significant and unique concept in teaching laparoscopy is the system utilized by Hulka.[1] This is a regional program. Physicians in the state (North Carolina) are given a package of self-instructional material beforehand and then come to the teaching center for a programmed instruction course at the hospital, including the opportunity of working on plastic models. The second phase of the program is the observation of laparoscopic procedures and then participation in actual cases. This gives the trainee an opportunity to become familiar with the many things which go on simultaneously in the operating room which he or she cannot appreciate adequately if he or she is performing the surgery. The third and final phase of the program is to have one of the instructors go out to the trainee's own hospital and introduce the technique there. This allows the physician to work in his or her own hospital with his or her own equipment. It also allows for the training of a hospital team, which is one of the most difficult aspects of instituting a laparoscopic surgery program. The program is ideal for the state, which indeed is what it was designed for.

Summary

There is a need for courses in gynecological laparoscopy which provide a comprehensive background in all aspects of the technique as well as some degree of practical training. Our experience in teaching gynecologic laparoscopy over the past five years has been outlined. It can be adapted by any interested individuals or institutions to meet their own particular needs. To be sure, there are problems and difficulties to be overcome, but the reward, in terms of professional and personal satisfaction, is great.

References

1. Hulka JF: Regional teaching of laparoscopy. J Reprod Med 10:243, 1973

2. Loffer FD, Pent D: A technique for teaching operative laparoscopy. Am J Obstet Gynecol 117:856, 1973

3. Loffer FD, Pent D: Indications, contraindications and complications of laparoscopy. Obstet Gynecol Surv 30:407, 1975

4. Phillips J, Keith D, Keith L, Hulka J, Hulka B: Survey of gynecologic laparoscopy for 1974. J Reprod Med 15:45, 1975

Editorial Comments

This chapter, unlike the preceding one by the same distinguished pair of authors, addresses itself to a small percentage of the readership of this book, or so it seems on the surface; in reality, however, each physician reading this book is a potential teacher of laparoscopy—a potential teacher to house staff, nursing staff, paramedical staff and his or her own colleagues.

For the uninitiated, teaching may begin in the operating room. It is not unreasonable to tell your colleagues what you are planning to do, why you are planning to do it, how you are planning to use the equipment and why you have selected particular items for use. It is also instructive to tell your colleagues why you are not going to do something and why you have changed or modified your operative technique from the past. All too often, though, the surgeon comes into the operating room and performs surgery with little or no communication with the others working in the operating room. This approach cannot help the patient because everyone surrounding the physician is there with the intention of helping the physician care for the patient.

Many physicians think that teaching requires a formal lecture. They are petrified at the idea of standing with a microphone and a set of slides before a sea of eager faces waiting to be given knowledge. Such activity is not really necessary for adequate teaching. Teaching can take place in the operating room, at the bedside and in the clinic.

L.K.

Chapter 26

Development of an Endoscopy Unit

George Berci, M.D.

The term *endoscopy unit* is difficult to define because the organization and function of a unit is largely dependent upon the person directing the activities. Given a director who is interested in endoscopy in general, the program, new techniques and research can be carried out on a broad scale within the endoscopy unit. The organization of such a unit may vary. In a busy hospital several physicians use the same instruments, and it is imperative to have a specially trained nurse supervising the preparation, maintenance, sterilization and repair of these instruments. If the supporting institution has a residency or postgraduate training program with a heavy schedule, one individual interested in the various aspects of diagnostic or operative endoscopy should take the responsibility of organizing the training sessions within the unit.

The unit described below (Cedars-Sinai Medical Center) has become an interdisciplinary department where many subspecialties using endoscopy are working concurrently. The organizational structure is shown in Table I. Over the years it has become a self-contained department within the hospital.

The following clinical areas are included in our program: bronchoscopy (rigid and flexible), thoracoscopy and mediastinoscopy (Department of Thoracic Surgery); esophagoscopy, gastroscopy, duodenoscopy, with or without cannulation of the papilla, colonoscopy, as well as laparoscopy for liver disease (Department of Gastroenterology); choledochoscopy and laparoscopy (Department of General Surgery); gynecologic laparoscopy (Department of Obstetrics and Gynecology); laryngoscopy and nasopharyngoscopy (Department of Ear, Nose and Throat); laparoscopy in infants (Department of Pediatric Surgery); and cystoscopy or transurethral surgery (Department of Urology).

The activities of the unit can be explained under the following headings:

Patient care

The patients are under the care of the attending staff members who use the departmental facilities, which include specially trained nurses or paramedical personnel. These staff members perform the procedures. Occasionally the residents do the examinations under supervision. If assistance is required, the department provides it. The members (including the director) are on call seven days a week, around the clock, in case of emergencies.

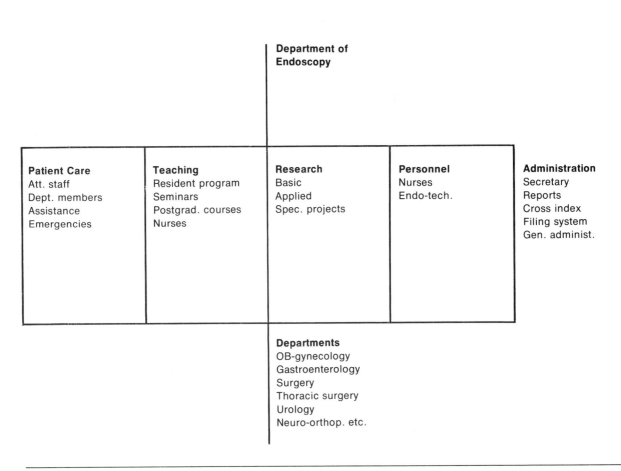

Table 1

Teaching

The attending staff members are periodically informed about new developments, techniques, instrumentation, complications and other changes. If senior members join us from different schools and use new techniques or concepts, we decide on policy in common through the exchange of ideas between the department and the members of the staff.

Teaching programs are available to any new attending member or resident joining the institution so they can receive the necessary training.

Incoming residents are taught procedures and assisted in a number of cases until we feel they have enough knowledge and skill to perform the operation safely. A certain number of cases are required, which vary from individual to individual, until the instructor and student can change places beside the operating room table. During resident instruction the teaching attachment is used to enable the physician in training to follow all manipulations.

We are not only interested in producing technicians but also in teaching clinical aspects of endoscopy as well, including how to recognize indications and contraindications for each procedure and how to deal with complications during or after the operation. We stress that this semiinvasive procedure is not minor surgery that can be squeezed in between the major cases but a type of surgery that must be taken seriously.

Research

In our department great emphasis is given to basic research activities and to specific projects related to clinical work. While a large number of endoscopic examinations are performed in the United States (approximately 10 million per year), it is uncommon to find laboratories devoted to pure research in endoscopy.

In 1952 I became aware of the problems involved in the design and manufacturing of endoscopes. Looking through the old standard lens endoscopes, I found that the image appeared dim. One optical physicist measured the total absorption of the transmitted light, and to my surprise the figures were in the vicinity of 90% to 95%. In other words, only a small percentage of the transmitted light (image) reached the examiner's eye. Practically speaking, our optical design was inherited from Nitze, in 1887, and despite the fact that some improvements had been made during the recent decades, the system remained the same in principle.

Some time later I became acquainted with the activities of Professor H. H. Hopkins. His invention, the rod-lens system,* opened a new chapter in rigid endoscopy. Compared with the standard lenses, rod-lenses transmit more light, with better image quality.[7] They can be decreased in diameter without impunity. If a standard lens system is decreased comparably, the image can hardly be seen.[14]

The rod-lens system triggered many new research and clinical activities in our endoscopy unit, first in urology,[6] then in surgery[10, 17] and gynecologic laparoscopy.[4] There were many pediatric applications, especially in pediatric laparoscopy.[15] The wide-angled view facilitates fast orientation. The crisp, bright image and small size were important factors in promoting laparoscopy. The rod-lens system also helped us document our findings, which had been extremely difficult previously.[1]

Our research endeavors have involved technical areas, resulting in a new teaching attachment,[9, 19, 22] the development of a new high intensity light source,[2, 3, 18] new photographic techniques[16] and still photographic, cinematic and color TV laparoscopy.[5] We extended our radiologic activities into the operating room[11] by introducing the large-sized (10/6 inch) image amplifier with television fluoroscopy and indirect radiology to combine operative hysterography with laparoscopy in cases of suspected tubal pathology[12] and in the differential diagnosis of jaundice.[8]

The introduction of bipolar coagulation, by Rioux and Corson,[13, 21] prompted us to take a closer look at the various instrument designs and the problems in electrosurgery, which are still not solved.[20]

One full-time research assistant is employed in the endoscopic laboratory. Several extramural consultants are involved in these multidisciplinary projects, also.

Instruments

Every new instrument is tested first in the laboratory.[2] The performance of the optic system and accessories is investigated, and a page in the instrument log book is opened. During the life of the instrument information is noted on accidents and changes. With the collection of such information we can follow the performance of the individual instrument and its accessories. Since this policy was instituted and followed through, we have been able to assess our instrument care program and reevaluate the need for improved education of the nurses and/or operators. If there is any failure or consistently inadequate performance, the manufacturer is advised that the design or product needs improvement.

Administration

One secretary takes care of ordering instruments, spare parts and nondisposable items,[1] arranging for necessary repair and exchange, maintaining the inventory and scheduling patients. An endoscopy log book is used in the operating room. Every day the nurse in charge notes the endoscopy procedures with some data (date, log number, patient's name with the hospital I.D. number, type of procedure, assistant, nurse, biopsy and complications). From this log book a cross-index card system has been established. In one card system the patients' names are filed in alphabetical order with reference to the log number and date. In the second card system the patients' names are cross-filed under the type of procedure. In this way it is easy to locate a patient or find out about the procedures.

A copy of every biopsy or specimen report derived from endoscopic examinations is also obtained from the Department of Pathology and filed according to the procedure. If there are some interesting findings or questionable results, the attending physician is contacted and asked to let the department know if he or she followed up the particular patient. Much effort is made to collect data on incomplete sterilizations or the treatment of unusual pathologic findings.

---

* Karl Storz Endoscopy, Los Angeles, California 90048

Table 2
Cedars-Sinai Medical Center
Department of Endoscopy

	Report Date	
No. of procedures	Adults	Private or Clinic
No. of patients	Children	No. of att. staff
Procedures repeated	Biopsies	performing exams
Unsuccessful exams	Emergencies	Complications

Procedure	**Number of cases**	
	private	clinic
Bronchoscopy	_____	_____
Choledochoscopy	_____	_____
Cystoscopy	_____	_____
Culdoscopy	_____	_____
Larynx (direct)	_____	_____
Larynx (indirect)	_____	_____
Mediastinoscopy	_____	_____
Nasopharynx	_____	_____
Neurosurgery	_____	_____
Laparoscopy (gyn)	_____	_____
Laparoscopy (general surgery)	_____	_____
T.U.R.	_____	_____
Colonoscopy + polypectomy	_____	_____
Colonoscopy	_____	_____
Duodenoscopy (ERCP)	_____	_____
Esophagoscopy	_____	_____
Esophagoscopy-gastro	_____	_____
Esophago-gastro-duodenoscopy	_____	_____
Gastroscopy	_____	_____
Hysteroscopy	_____	_____
Sigmoidoscopy	_____	_____
Thoracoscopy	_____	_____
Other (misc)	_____	_____
Total	_____	_____
Comments		

This filing system is available *to every member of the attending staff and the residents.* It is of utmost importance for preparing publications and reports. In addition, many teaching slides and films are on file which can be used by attending staff members for their various classes and seminars.

Having a simple, centralized filing system available is of great help in evaluating our activities. A monthly report is prepared in which the case load is broken down (Table 2) by the various subspecialties, informing both the physicians and hospital administration of the patient population. Since every purchase order is issued through the endoscopy office to the hospital purchasing channels, an account of expenses versus income is also prepared.

Personnel

Personnel is probably the first important subject to consider before an endoscopy unit or department is established. Without specially trained nurses and technicians, a properly conducted endoscopic procedure cannot be completed. Our equipment consists of innumerable accessories that have to be checked, cleaned, sterilized, rechecked and assembled. Spare parts, including endoscopes, must be presterilized and available: nothing is more frustrating than having the patient anesthetized and finding one part missing, thereby extending the examination because the missing piece must be located and sterilized. For this reason, competent personnel are essential.

The active participation of all personnel as a team is of great value. A brief explanation or a quick look through the scope or teaching attachment makes each person feel that he or she is an important participant. Each person should be aware that without his or her contribution the examination could never be done.

Conclusion

A centralized organization or a framework for covering and supervising endoscopic procedures is advantageous in a hospital with a busy interdisciplinary endoscopic schedule. This organization has to be tailored to local circumstances, as our experience at Cedars-Sinai Medical Center has shown.

References

1. Berci G: Peritoneoscopy. Br Med J 1:562, 1962

2. Berci G: Instrumentation. In *Endoscopy.* Appleton-Century-Crofts, New York, 1976

3. Berci G: More light. J Endoscopy 7:201, 1975

4. Berci G, Adler DN, Brooks PG, Pasternak A, Hasler G: The importance of instrumentation and documentation in gynecological laparoscopy. J Reprod Med 10:276, 1973

5. Berci G, Adler DN, Pasternak A: Color television-laparoscopy. Presented at the Second International Congress of Gynecologic Laparoscopy, Las Vegas, Nevada, November 1975

6. Berci G, Getzoff PL, Kont LA: An improved concept in optics applied to cystoscopy. J Urol 104:542, 1970

7. Berci G, Kont LA: A new optical system in endoscopy with special reference to cystoscopy. Br J Urol 49:564, 1969

8. Berci G, Morgenstern L, Shore JM, Shapiro SJ: A direct approach to the differential diagnosis of jaundice. Am J Surg 126:372, 1973

9. Berci G, Panish JF, Olson V: An improved multi-purpose teaching attachment. Gastrointest Endosc 22:30, 1975

10. Berci G, Shore JM: Advances in cholangioscopy. Endoscopy 4:29, 1972

11. Berci G, Steckel R: Modern radiology in the operating room. Arch Surg 107:577, 1973

12. Brooks PG, Berci G, Adler DN: The simultaneous and combined use of laparoscopy and hysterosalpingography using image amplification. J Reprod Med 10:285, 1973

13. Corson SL, Patrick H, Hamilton T, Bolognese J: Electrical considerations of laparoscopic sterilization. J Reprod Med 11:159, 1973

14. Gans SL, Berci G: Advances in endoscopy of infants and children. J Ped Surg 6:199, 1971

15. Gans SL, Berci G: Peritoneoscopy in infants and children. J Ped Surg 8:399, 1973

16. Helmuth J, Hasler G, Berci G: Permanent film records. In *Endoscopy.* Appleton-Century-Crofts, New York 1976

17. Morgenstern L, Shore JM, Berci G: Potentials of a new optical system (endoscope) as a diagnostic aid. Am J Surg 38:312, 1972

18. Olson V: Illumination. In *Endoscopy.* Appleton-Century-Crofts, New York 1976

19. Olson V: Teaching Attachments. In *Endoscopy.* Appleton-Century-Crofts, New York 1976

20. Rioux J-E: Panel on electro-surgery. Second International Congress of Gynecologic Laparoscopy. Las Vegas, Nevada, November 1975

21. Rioux J-E, Cloutier D: Bi-polar forceps for tubal sterilization. J Reprod Med 13:6, 1974

22. Ward PD, Berci G, Calcaterra T: Advances in endoscopic examination of the respiratory system. Ann Otol Rhino Laryngol 83:754, 1974

Editorial Comments

As the reader can see at a glance, not every hospital wants or needs an endoscopy unit. Some of those that want it and even some of those that need it clearly can't afford it. These details aside, there are some points in this chapter which can be easily translated into practice in most hospitals. As I see it, and as the reader will see more clearly in the next chapter, the major advantage of the endoscopy unit is the element of control that the hospital or department has over the activities of the physicians practicing therein. The unit as the mode of organizing endoscopic practice permits control over the care of the equipment, the procedures that are performed and, perhaps more importantly, the calculations of the statistics on what is being done in that unit.

This type of control can do nothing but bring good to everyone concerned. In the first place, it reduces or eliminates the possibility that a new staff member will come into the hospital and practice without the monitoring of his or her performance. Second, it provides an orderly means of educating the house staff and providing continuing education for the paramedical and attending medical staffs. Third, it monitors cost. As everyone knows, the cost of repairing laparoscopic equipment in terms of dollar outlay and down-time is astronomical. Certain malfunctions do occur, and while it is reasonable to expect that some preventive maintenance must be done, it is equally reasonable to request that the staff of a particular hospital take every possible step to avoid the needless destruction of instruments. Last, information on the types of operations and their outcome is available for study by the members of the hospital staff. This becomes an effective means of self-assessment.

L.K.

Chapter 27

Laparoscopy in a Community Hospital

W. Dow Edgerton, M.D.
Richard Kleppinger, M.D.

Introduction

The community hospital, geographically and academically independent of the research-oriented, metropolitan teaching facility, can adequately provide the area it serves with the advantages of modern gynecologic laparoscopy. In most community hospitals new procedures are introduced by one individual who thereafter temporarily carries the responsibility of being the "expert." As such, it is vital that this physician be well versed in every aspect of the project. Although the reasons behind the utilization of laparoscopy are basically the same in any locale, it does not follow that the procedures required for establishing a smoothly functioning hospital program are always similar or that the experience of one group will necessarily be duplicated by another.

The community hospitals represented by the authors are in different parts of the country, have different local problems and serve patients from different ethnic backgrounds. In each instance the authors have been pioneer laparoscopists in the community and have been responsible for organizing and developing their respective programs.

St. Luke's Hospital

St. Luke's Hospital, Davenport, Iowa, is a 275 bed community hospital located in the largest of four cities which comprise a bistate, urban complex straddling the Upper Mississippi River and have a total population of 390,000. Of the five non-profit hospitals in the area St. Luke's has the largest obstetric and gynecologic service and is the only one with a laparoscopy program of any size. Residents in obstetrics and gynecology from the University of Iowa now rotate through the service on a regular basis, and fourth-year medical students from the same institution take electives in advanced obstetrics at St. Luke's. Six staff gynecologists and seven residents contributed to the 62 months (June 1, 1970, through July 31, 1975) of laparoscopic experience.

Table 1
Laparoscopic Procedures
June 1970 to August 1975

	St. Luke's Hospital	Reading Hospital	Combined total
Months	62	41	103
Sterilizations	3,640 (88%)	2,746 (88%)	6,386 (88%)
Diagnostic	517 (12%)	367 (12%)	884 (12%)
Total	4,157 (100%)	3,113 (100%)	7,270 (100%)

Table 2
Pregnancy Rate/Sterilization Failure

	St. Luke's Hospital	Reading Hospital	Combined total
Sterilizations	3,640	2,746	6,386
Operator failure	4	1	5
Method failure		3	3
Gestation type			
Uterine	3	2	5
Ectopic	1	2	3
Failure etiology	2 Round ligament coagulation 2 Incomplete transection	3 Peritoneal tubouterine fistula 1 Incomplete transection	3 Peritoneal tubouterine fistula 3 Incomplete transection 2 Round ligament coagulation
Pregnancy rate as percentage	0.11%	0.15%	0.13%

The Reading Hospital

The Reading Hospital and Medical Center, Reading, Pennsylvania, is the largest of three community hospitals in the area. It has 650 beds and serves a population of 296,000 in the urban-suburban areas of Reading and the large rural areas of Berks County. Referrals from the peripheries of five adjacent counties and the Planned Parenthood Center of Berks County contribute to the patient census. This institution offers an approved residency program in obstetrics and gynecology and a teaching program in obstetrics and gynecology for medical students by affiliation with Temple University Health Sciences Center, Philadelphia, Pennsylvania. Seven senior staff members, eight residents—four of whom were granted junior staff appointments upon completion of their residency—and two courtesy staff members contributed to 41 months (March 1972 to August 1975) of laparoscopic experience at the Reading Hospital.

Procedural Details

At St. Luke's Hospital the majority of laparoscopic patients are admitted and discharged within 24 hours. At the Reading Hospital the majority of patients are admitted the day prior to surgery and discharged within 24 hours postoperatively, but an accommodation (outpatient) program has recently been instituted. In both hospitals all laparoscopies are performed in the operating rooms, and the main recovery room facilities are used afterwards. The majority of procedures have been performed under general anesthesia with relatively light premedication; the technique has been described previously.[2, 3, 4, 5, 6] Almost all procedures for tubal sterilization at the Reading Hospital were performed using a single-puncture technique. Prior to October 1972 all operations at St. Luke's were double-puncture procedures; since that time the majority have been single-puncture procedures. Both institutions use a coagulation plus division technique for tubal sterilization. The results of the programs in both hospitals are summarized in Tables 1, 2, and 3.

Establishing a Program

Feasibility

The question is frequently asked many of us, "Shall we inaugurate a laparoscopy program in our own hospital?" At the 1970 meeting of the Central Association of Obstetricians and Gynecologists one of the authors (WDE) put forth the proposition that the use of the laparoscope in tubal sterilization, by the very numbers of procedures done, would lead to increasing familiarity with the instrument and, consequently, greater use for other purposes. This proposition remains essentially true today.

If one does not plan to use laparoscopy for purposes of sterilization, one probably will not have a successful laparoscopy program. The statistics from the two hospitals described above are remarkably similar in the percentage of diagnostic laparoscopies as compared to tubal sterilizations; these percentages have remained constant over the years. The skills of the operators and the proficiency of the operating room teams are honed to a fine edge by the large number of laparoscopic operations performed for sterilization. In addition, the investment in sophisticated equipment and ancillary instruments is made practicable only by a high utilization rate. Therefore, unless a hospital or a particular staff member has an unusually large infertility practice, the purchase of more than a basic diagnostic laparoscopy set-up is not justified economically.

Before purchasing the initial laparoscopy set careful consideration should be given to the use to which it will be put. If funds are limited but flexibility is desired, an operating laparoscope for single puncture can readily be used in a double-puncture procedure; however, the reverse is not true. In choosing an electrosurgical unit the prospective buyer is faced with an even more bewildering array of possibilities than is the case with fiber optics. Operative laparoscopy, virtually synonymous with electrosurgery, accounts for most of the serious complications reported.[7, 8, 10, 13] In its present state of development the bipolar electrosurgical unit alone will not serve all the needs of a large and sophisticated laparoscopy service; for anyone contemplating a modest number of procedures it should be given preference over the unipolar unit.

Table 3
Major Complications Secondary to 7,270 Laparoscopic
Procedures

Complications	St. Luke's	Reading	Combined
Mortality		1*	1*
Bleeding-Requiring laparotomy			
Mesosalpinx	6	12*†	18*†
Puncture site	1*	1	2*
Uterine artery		1	1
Retroperitoneal hematoma		1	1
Late hematoperitoneum	1*	1	1*
Broad ligament hematoma	3		3
Electrosurgical injury			
Small bowel burn	2		2
Superficial skin burn	1	3	4
Serosal burn of cecum		2*	2*
Serosal burn of sigmoid		1	1
Traumatic injury			
Perforation stomach	2		2
Perforation ileum		2	2
Transverse colon	1		1
Infection			
Pelvic peritonitis (late)	3		3
Bilateral mesosalpingeal abscesses		1*	1*
Pelvic abscess	1		1
Cardiac arrest (CO_2 embolism?)		1†	1†
Total complications (patients)	20	23	43
Total cases	4,157	3,113	7,270
Percent	0.5%	0.7%	0.6%

* Complications in one patient
† Complications in one patient

Equipment Needed

At both hospitals increasing demand necessitated the purchase of a complete second unit within two years. At the Reading Hospital the initial purchases were a unit for performing single-puncture laparoscopy and the ancillary instruments for a second-puncture where indicated. At St. Luke's Hospital the initial purchases provided only for a double-puncture procedure; a single-puncture instrument was added later. Since diagnostic laparoscopy frequently necessitates a second puncture, the authors believe that any laparoscopy program should have second-puncture capability. In an active program, unless an immediate source of supply and repair is available, it is imperative to have "back-up" equipment since breakage and malfunction are to be expected.

Staff Privileges

When a decision has been made to institute a laparoscopy program, the next question which arises is: "What rules shall be adopted to ensure safety, efficacy and efficiency?" Eventually, every physician finishing a residency in obstetrics and gynecology will be trained in the techniques of diagnostic and operative laparoscopy, and this operation will fall under the regulations applicable to all other operations. In the interim, however, there is a problem, which has been recognized by both the American College of Obstetricians and Gynecologists (ACOG) and the American Association of Gynecologic Laparoscopists (AAGL).

The American College of Obstetricians and Gynecologists recommends that in order to be considered qualified to perform gynecologic laparoscopy a physician should be required:
1. to have unrestricted privileges in major gynecologic surgery in an accredited hospital, and
2. to have demonstrated competence in the technique of laparoscopy.

The Board of Trustees of the AAGL has reviewed the question of operating privileges in laparoscopy and feels that the ultimate responsibility to extend such privileges lies with the governing body of each hospital. To aid in establishing criteria for such privileges the Board of Trustees recommends the following:
1. The physician should have privileges in gynecologic surgery and possess the capability of handling unusual abdominal surgical complications.
2. He or she should show evidence that he or she has completed a recognized course in laparoscopy or produce a letter of recommendation from a known preceptor. Attendance at a postgraduate course or at a national meeting does not guarantee competency.
3. A review of each physician's performance in laparoscopy, with attention paid to complications, is recommended before advancing the physician from provisional laparoscopic privileges to permanent ones.

These guidelines and operating privileges of the ACOG have been followed at the Reading Hospital and Medical Center whereas a more detailed set of guidelines has been adopted by St. Luke's Hospital, Davenport, Iowa. In St. Luke's Hospital there is no category of "blanket" or unrestricted staff privileges. Each person must apply to the Credentials Committee for the granting of initial privileges, which are specific in each category, and he or she must request further permission from the Committee in order to go beyond procedures originally approved. Some of the details of the St. Luke's program follow:

Diagnostic Laparoscopy
Privileges in diagnostic laparoscopy will be granted to all interested staff members, regardless of specialty or department, upon presentation of satisfactory evidence of prior experience. An experienced laparoscopist will then be assigned to assist initially, in order to verify skill and ability. Upon written certification by the senior laparoscopist, the staff member concerned will then be allowed to proceed without further supervision, so long as no operative laparoscopy is attempted.

Operative Laparoscopy

Privileges in operative laparoscopy will be granted only to staff members already possessing major surgical privileges, and privileges in gynecologic operative laparoscopy will be granted only to those with major surgical privileges in gynecology. Further, evidence of adequate training must be submitted together with local assistance, supervision and written certification of ability.

Adequate training is defined as one of the following:

1. Approved residency plus local supervision for a minimum of 12 cases. Residency must have included at least 24 cases with primary responsibility.

2. Postgraduate instruction plus the following:

   a. Training with an experienced laparoscopist as preceptor.

   b. Demonstration of competence. This requires a minimum of six cases performed with an experienced laparoscopist as assistant.

   c. Supervision to the point of confidence. This requires scheduling with the knowledge of a single staff member detailed for such purpose and during such times as the senior member is physically present in the hospital and available for immediate consultation. A minimum of 12 cases under such supervision is required, and written certification of competence must be given the Credentials Committee by the supervising staff member before the fledgling laparoscopist is allowed to proceed alone. "Postgraduate instruction" may be either a formal course or instruction pursued locally under a qualified preceptor.

Anesthesiology Privileges in Laparoscopy

A fledgling laparoscopist must use an anesthetist experienced in laparoscopy anesthesia, and anesthesiologists having no prior experience with laparoscopy may give anesthesia for fully trained laparoscopists only.

Operating Room Crew

Personnel in training may be introduced into the team provided an experienced laparoscopist is present. The general rule is: "Green crew—veteran laparoscopist; green laparoscopist—veteran crew."

Courtesy Staff

The Courtesy Staff category is reserved for those physicians "whose use of the hospital is infrequent." "Infrequent" for the surgical specialties has been defined by the Credentials Committee as meaning less than twelve surgical procedures per year. Because the requirement for "supervision to the point of confidence" calls for direct supervision for a minimum of twelve cases, regardless of prior training or credentials, there are essentially no courtesy staff privileges in operative laparoscopy.

Supervision and Education

Formal, recognized and accepted postgraduate courses are available throughout the country. A list of names, courses and locations may be obtained from the American College of Obstetricians and Gynecologists or the American Association of Gynecologic Laparoscopists. The reduction of complications requires a continuous evaluation of how the program is progressing, while the updating of technical advancement, innovations and new procedures necessitates continuous education and review. Because in most hospitals each physician is in private practice, the authority vested in the chain of command is not as all-encompassing as in some institutions. One of us (RKK) requests and receives a copy of every laparoscopic procedure dictated by various operators. This procedure enables hospital data to be current; but, of course, the accuracy depends upon physician integrity and familiarity with what is of statistical importance. At the Reading Hospital staff members and residents of the Obstetrical and Gynecological Department, the medical director, the anesthesia department, operating room personnel and administration are well informed about the "state of the art" of laparoscopy via a "Lap-Letter" (laparoscopy newsletter) distributed at periodic intervals. At St. Luke's Hospital, on the other hand, there is continuing surveillance of the operating schedule and copies of the monthly operation index computer printouts.

A well trained and knowledgeable laparoscopy team is an invaluable asset. Brief, periodic inservice programs efficiently familiarize operating room personnel with electrosurgical and gas insufflation equipment. These programs acquaint personnel with the special care required in instrument handling, cleaning and sterilization, which is absolutely essential to ensure proper function and to keep maintenance costs at a minimum. Visual aids such as slides, movies and television cassettes are a valuable adjunct. If television equipment is available, the head gynecologic nurse should be responsible for the tapes, demonstration equipment and instrument handling. This is of particular value for new members who are introduced periodically into the laparoscopy team.

Administrative Concerns

The Reading Hospital

Facilities for outpatient laparoscopy such as those described by Wheeless[14, 15] were not available at the Reading Hospital in 1972. Most distressing was the lack of beds for the patient who needed laparoscopy. Because of a declining obstetrical census the feasibility of using idle obstetric beds for laparoscopy patients was discussed with the hospital administrator. The following communication from the associate administrator 40 months after implementation is included here to show the efficacy of such policy change and to provide evidence for possible negotiations in other community hospitals:

> When the procedure was first suggested, it was apparent that the potential volume of laparoscopy patients would be limited by the number of available beds. The general medical surgical units have historically maintained a 95% occupancy rate. However, during the preceding years, the obstetrical census following the national trend had steadily decreased from a 77% occupancy rate in 1967 to 63.6% in fiscal year 1973.

> The Department of Public Welfare for the state of Pennsylvania approves the use and occupancy of hospital facilities. Their regulations governing the use of obstetrical facilities preclude their use for nonobstetric care unless a special waiver is obtained from DPW.

> Accordingly, with a decreasing obstetrical census and a potentially increasing volume of laparoscopy patients, approval was sought and obtained for clean gynecological patients to be placed on the obstetrical unit.

During the 40-month study period, this increased the census on the obstetrical unit by an average of 4.5 patients per day with 5,424 days of care being rendered. Because of the relative simplicity of the surgical procedure, the patients normally did not present any complex nursing problems and therefore did not interfere with the nursing personnel's responsibility for obstetrical patient care. Likewise, it was not necessary to add nursing personnel and thus increase the expense of operating this unit. Many of these patients had already received their prescribed admission laboratory and radiology tests through the hospital's pre-admission testing program. This eliminated a considerable amount of clerical work which can prove to be very troublesome, particularly for short term admissions, when a premium is placed on timing in order that the test results are available prior to the surgical procedure.

Based on the average per diem earnings for the Hospital during the study period, this procedure has resulted in approximately $573,900 of additional income for the Hospital from this unit. In view of the continued gradual rise of hospital expenditures and the declining obstetrical census, the procedure enabled this hospital to maintain the present available obstetrical beds which allowed for coping with those unforeseen peaks in obstetrical census. The alternative would have been to increase rates or to change them over to medical-surgical use which would have caused expensive renovation expenditures.

Patient preference and third-party medicine have spurred the inauguration of outpatient (accommodation) laparoscopy at the Reading Hospital. All patients have preadmission testing. Local anesthesia is preferred.

St. Luke's Hospital

When the laparoscopy program first began at St. Luke's, the hospital was already admitting clean gynecology cases to the obstetrical floor. As laparoscopic sterilizations gained momentum, some strains became evident. Because such cases could be scheduled far in advance, the effect of crowding out other elective surgery developed in regard to both availability of beds and operating room time. Since there were no assigned operating days for services or individuals and no operating rooms reserved by service or specialty, general surgical cases seemed to bear the brunt of the crowding. There was no shortage of beds in the community as a whole, but an acute shortage rapidly developed at St. Luke's. Although quite profitable financially to the hospital, laparoscopy appeared to be a mixed blessing.

The first step towards a solution of these problems was to make afternoon surgery popular with surgeons, thereby making full use of operating room facilities. The second step was to gain a full hospital day for each case by late-morning admission and breakfast at home combined with afternoon surgery and early evening discharge. The third step was to simplify admission procedures and to reschedule laboratory personnel time so that blood samples and urine could be obtained quickly upon admission and results made available to the operating room rather than to each floor. Patients could then be assigned to any empty room on any floor except pediatrics.

The benefits of the program were legion: healthy patients were no longer made to feel like sick people, doctors discovered they actually preferred afternoon surgery and morning office hours, and everyone discovered anachronistic practices based only on custom. Patients quickly discovered that they slept better at home than in the hospital the night before surgery, doctors found that many patients really didn't care for (or need) enemata and administrators became aware that much paperwork was not only an unnecessary duplication of effort but sheer nonsense. The way is now paved for true outpatient surgery.

Opportunities

The laparoscopy program at a community hospital provides a fertile environment for research if the physician is so inclined. At the Reading Hospital and Medical Center Dr. Kleppinger, in conjunction with the Richard Wolf Medical Instruments Corporation, had the opportunity to develop and thoroughly test a bipolar forceps which has virtually eliminated the hazards encountered with unipolar instruments. The advantages and safety of bipolar coagulation have been described previously by Corson[1] and Rioux.[9, 10, 11, 12]

Currently under evaluation is the use of direct laparoscopic visualization for the placement of infusion catheters to instill radiocolloids intraperitoneally.

Conclusion

Although gynecologic laparoscopy is a technologically sophisticated procedure, an effective and safe program can be established in any community hospital where adequate physician training, sufficient medical staff interest and administrative cooperation are attainable. Desire alone does not bring a good program into being; responsibility for development of laparoscopic services extends into technical and administrative areas.

Unless tubal sterilizations are to be performed, a laparoscopy program of any size probably will not be economically feasible, nor will the skills of the surgical team be kept at the level of excellence necessary for competent operative endoscopy. The fledgling laparoscopist is urged to begin only after a thorough grounding in basic procedural knowledge and to take the first steps in the company of a capable mentor. He or she is further urged to begin with general anesthesia and an interested, competent and patient anesthesiologist. Outpatient operative laparoscopy should be reserved for the experienced laparoscopist.

Safety cannot be purchased with money alone. The care and maintenance of instruments is essential to success; if many procedures are to be performed, backup instruments are necessary to ensure an efficient program. In capable hands second-rate equipment may prove adequate, but for the inexperienced even the best equipment may not suffice.

Laparoscopy is an inherently unphysiologic procedure. Its potential hazards can be avoided only by the diligent application of knowledge and skill at the cost of relentless personal supervision and meticulous attention to detail.

The satisfaction in providing the invaluable diagnostic and surgical laparoscopic procedures through the community hospital merits the efforts involved.

References

1. Corson SL, Patrick H, Hamilton T, Bolognese RJ: Electrical consideration of laparoscopic sterilization. J Reprod Med 11:159, 1973

2. Edgerton WD: Controversy in laparoscopy. Audio-Digest, Obstet Gynecol 22:5, 1975

3. Edgerton WD: Experience with laparoscopy in a non-teaching hospital. Am J Obstet Gynecol 116:184, 1973

4. Edgerton WD: Laparoscopy in the community hospital: set-up, performance, control. J Reprod Med 12:239, 1974

5. Kleppinger RK: One thousand laparoscopies at a community hospital. J Reprod Med 13:13, 1974

6. Kleppinger RK: The operating laparoscope and the optimal position for tubal coagulation. J Reprod Med 15:60, 1975

7. Loffer FD, Pent D: Indications, contraindications and complications of laparoscopy. Obstet Gynecol Surv 30:407, 1975

8. Phillips JM, Keith D, Keith L, Hulka J, Hulka B: Survey of gynecological laparoscopy for 1974. J Reprod Med 15:45, 1975

9. Rioux JE, Cloutier D: A new bipolar instrument for laparoscopic tubal sterilization. Am J Obstet Gynecol 119:737, 1974

10. Rioux JE, Cloutier D: Bipolar cautery for sterilization by laparoscopy. J Reprod Med 13:6, 1974

11. Rioux JE, Cloutier D: Laparoscopic tubal sterilization; sparking and its control. Vie Med Canada Francais 2:760, 1973

12. Rioux JE, Yuzpe AA: Electrosurgery untangled. Contemp Obstet Gynecol 4:118, 1974

13. Shepard MK: Female contraceptive sterilization. Obstet Gynecol Surv 29:739, 1974

14. Wheeless CR: A rapid, inexpensive and effective method of surgical sterilization by laparoscopy. J Reprod Med 3:65, 1969

15. Wheeless CR: Outpatient sterilization under local anesthesia. Obstet Gynecol 39:767, 1972

Editorial Comments

In my opinion, this chapter is one of the true gems in this book. For me, it is worth the price of the entire volume. My joy in reading it comes from the fact that each author has been able to sit down with his respective hospital administrator and develop a laparoscopic program which fits the needs of the community, gives service to the patients and allows the physicians to practice in a safe and rational manner.

The authors are not ashamed to admit that their respective programs can be operated at a profit. Most hospitals in the United States are set up as nonprofit organizations. In this manner they can receive gifts and donations without paying any taxes on them and can also direct back any unexpended revenue into the hospital operations. In the case illustrated in this chapter, the additional revenues brought in by the laparoscopic patients were able to maintain a department that might otherwise have been closed for insufficient activity.

This chapter should be required reading for hospital administrators throughout the United States.

L.K.

Chapter 28

Laparoscopy in an Academic Training Program

Clifford R. Wheeless, Jr., M.D.

Because the rebirth of laparoscopy has been a contemporary phenomenon, many academic centers did not have the opportunity to plan their laparoscopy unit thoughtfully but rather were thrust into the field. The design of such a unit ideally should begin with an indepth study of the obligations for teaching and patient care for the next decade. Long-range planning and study are efficacious from the point of view of providing the type of unit needed; also, such planning may be required to meet the current and future institutional obligations to regional medical planning committees in various states and Professional Standards Review Organizations (PSRO) representing governmental interests.

The basic requisites for such a study are:

1. The present and projected female population of the geographic area.
2. The current incidence of laparoscopies (diagnostic and surgical) being performed.
3. The teaching responsibility of a given institution (in-service, graduate and post-graduate, community, state, national, and international, paramedical and allied health professionals).
4. An assessment of the facilities for laparoscopy already existing in the geographic area of the institution and the relationship of these facilities to the proposed laparoscopy unit.

The survey should also address itself to the problems of overlapping medical services, overlapping teaching programs and the maintenance of quality facilities which can remain competitive and desirable from the patient's as well as the physician's point of view. When these questions have been answered and approval obtained for further planning and preparation, logistic requirements must be considered, i.e., facilities and personnel for the anticipated volume of patients and teaching responsibilities. In addition to personnel and space, administrative matters, such as patient flow, space utilization, proximity to laboratory and backup inpatient facilities, should be planned.

While these factors are important to the operation of a successful endoscopy unit, the most important area of concern must remain the training of professional personnel. Unfortunately, laparoscopy has been thought of as an easy, simple procedure which can be performed by less experienced pelvic surgeons. Frequently it has been assigned to those department members more inclined toward the medical aspects of gynecology than the surgical aspects. Laparoscopy is an easy, safe and effective procedure in the hands of well trained pelvic surgeons who have taken the time and effort to obtain good training and develop experience in the procedure. Competence in laparoscopy cannot be granted by academic or institutional appointment. It must be earned at the operating table. Failure to recognize this point can result in poor results, major complications and eventual failure of the best-designed laparoscopy unit.

The physical plan of a well designed laparoscopy unit should constantly consider patient comfort and patient flow. Although local circumstances vary, it is frequently undesirable to perform patient counseling or initial history-taking and physical examinations in the laparoscopy unit. These activities should have occurred prior to the patient's arrival at the unit. This is particularly true in sterilization operations since it offers the patient a chance to reconsider her decision and thus avoid the criticism that she has been coerced into having the operation. Similarly, from a logistic point of view it is undesirable to have patients undergoing history and physical examinations mixed with patients undergoing surgery because it drastically reduces the patient flow. Among the criticisms leveled at clinics currently performing large numbers of laparoscopies is that they do not provide appropriate patient dignity. Simply stated, many of these clinics have been set up in the only available facility, and thus patients frequently are required to walk long distances exposed in a hospital gown.

Ideally, the unit should be located as close to parking and (Figure 1) transportation facilities as possible. Administrative activities should be centered at the entrance to the unit. Once the patients have completed these matters, they should be directed to a reception room. This room should be designed with the thought that patients frequently bring one or more family members with them, and adequate waiting space should be provided for all. The waiting space should be comfortable and designed to relieve anxiety and tension (Figure 1A). Adequate toilet facilities should be available in this area for both sexes. The patient flow of the unit should be designed so that the patient has to wait a minimum amount of time in the waiting-reception area (Figure 1A).

The second area of major importance is the patient's dressing room. It should be pleasant and have adequate locker space with secure locks to protect valuables while the patient is dressed in her hospital gown. Toilet facilities in the dressing area are absolutely essential to avoid unnecessary catheterizations in the operating room (Figure 1B). The patient should be required to remain in this dressing area no more than five minutes before being called to the operating room. Otherwise, anxiety and apprehension will frequently cause the bladder to refill, thus requiring catheterization and making the use of local anesthesia more difficult.

The dressing area should flow into the operating rooms and receive traffic from the recovery room in order that the patient not retrace her steps and that two-way traffic patterns be avoided. It is not necessary to take the patient from the dressing area to the operating room on a stretcher, as sedation should not be given in the dressing area. The patient can walk from the dressing area to the operating room escorted by a paramedical assistant (Figure 1C).

The third area of importance in a laparoscopy unit is the operating room itself. These rooms need not be as large as general operating rooms, but if significant teaching responsibilities exist, the size of the room must be appropriate to accommodate students. Ideally, teaching rooms for laparoscopy should be equipped with closed-circuit television, which would allow many students to learn from TV monitors prior to taking their turn at the operating table and learning from experience.

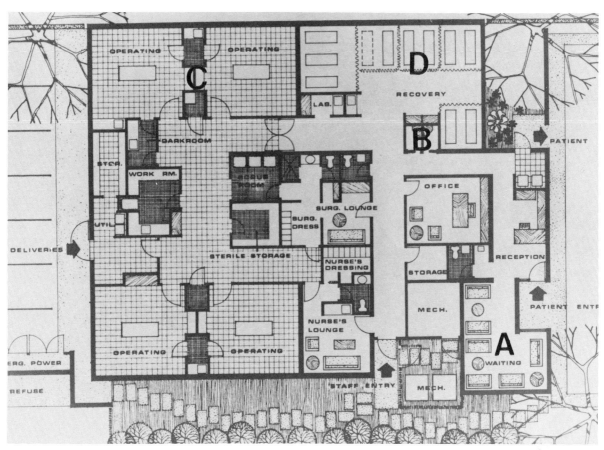

Figure 1
Architect's drawing for outpatient surgical center
ideal for laparoscopy with (A) reception area,
(B) dressing area, (C) operating area, and (D)
recovery area.

We believe that it is not necessary that a laparoscopy operating room be equipped for major intraabdominal surgery. Although some laparoscopists disagree with this opinion, because of the small incidence of perforation of major abdominal blood vessels such as aorta and more frequently the right common iliac artery, the incidence of this complication does not warrant the design of all laparoscopy operating rooms to accommodate major intraabdominal surgery (Figure 2). Such a design would elevate the cost of the laparoscopy unit unnecessarily. However, if possible, the endoscopy unit should be adjacent to the general operating rooms while not an integral part of them. No other complications of laparoscopy other than major vessel perforation are so acute as to require immediate intraabdominal intervention, thus necessitating making all laparoscopy operating rooms into general surgical operating rooms.

The laparoscopy operating rooms should be designed so that an individual surgeon can "ping-pong" cases for maximum efficiency (Figure 1C). That is, while Patient A is undergoing laparoscopy in Operating Room I, Patient B should be placed upon the table of Operating Room II and prepared for the laparoscopy procedure by nurses and nursing assistants. When the surgeon completes the surgery on the first patient, he or she is already to "gown and glove" and make the incision on Patient B by rotating to Operating Room II. Patient A in Operating Room I is then removed from the table by nursing assistants and Patient C is then placed on the table of Operating Room I and prepared for laparoscopy. In this "ping-pong" technique maximum utilization of the unit can be achieved and a minimum of "down" time is experienced, making the unit more efficient. Frequently, patients require removal from the operating room and transport to the recovery room on a stretcher. Therefore, operating room doors and halls should be designed to accommodate stretcher traffic.

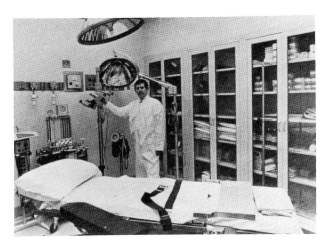

Figure 2
Endoscopic operating area

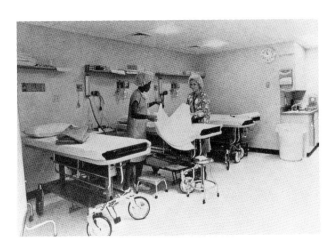

Figure 3
Recovery area

The recovery room should be designed to accommodate patients for a maximum of four hours (Figure 1D). Those patients undergoing laparoscopy under local anesthesia generally require only two hours of recovery. In most cases the unit should not be designed to take care of patients over night. A patient unable to leave the unit adequately and safely by early evening should be admitted to the hospital and discharged the following morning. To maintain a second and third shift in an endoscopy unit is rarely needed and would significantly increase the overhead and cost of such a unit.

The design of the recovery room should be simple and support the following needs of the patients (Figure 3):

1.   An emergency tray or cart for the rare case of cardiovascular respiratory problem.
2.   Drugs for the control of nausea and vomiting (particularly those patients undergoing general anesthesia).
3.   Medication for relief of minor pain associated with the abdominal incision.

The entrance and exit to the recovery room should be designed so that the patient does not have to reenter the operative area to reenter the dressing area. The dressing area should be adjacent to the waiting-reception room in such a way as to avoid traffic congestion and therefore reduce patient flow.

While it is important to have a well designed physical plant for the endoscopy unit, the most important part of any endoscopy unit is personnel. The endoscopy unit should have a director of gynecologic endoscopy. He or she should be an accomplished pelvic surgeon, with extensive experience in laparoscopy from the point of view of management of complications and unusual anatomical variations, which would allow him or her to assist those gynecologists working in the unit with less experience. He or she should have a minimum of administrative responsibilities in order to devote the majority of his or her time to proper patient care.

In an academic institution one or two residents are necessarily assigned to the endoscopy unit on a full-time basis. This assignment can be justified if the endoscopy unit performs all forms of gynecologic endoscopy, not just laparoscopy, including female cystourethroscopy, fetoscopy, laparoscopy, culdoscopy and colposcopy, and proctosigmoidoscopy. By having a concentrated exposure to the gynecologic endoscopy unit the resident can be taught the necessary eye-hand coordination which is required for appropriate visualization through an endoscope of any type. In addition, he or she has a greater opportunity to observe complications, anatomical abnormalities and unusual situations which may arise. This training is more difficult to accomplish if he or she is assigned to the endoscopy unit on an occasional basis, such as one hour per day.

Nursing personnel can be held to a minimum in an endoscopy unit. Generally, one or two registered nurses are all that are required to administer injections and supervise the other paramedical personnel. The operating rooms can be staffed adequately with nonnursing operating room technicians, and the recovery room can be supervised adequately by licensed practical nurses. Adequate administrative personnel must be on hand to complete medical record and financial matters in order to avoid delays in the flow of patients through the unit.

Equipment for the endoscopy unit should include the obvious office and clerical equipment needed for the administrative personnel. The waiting room should reduce patient anxiety. The dressing room should have adequate locker space so that each patient can have her own individual locker which can be secured with a key and the key pinned to her patient gown throughout the procedure. Professional equipment should include either gynecologic operating tables or the new gynecologic stretcher/combination operating table which has been introduced in the last few years. Adequate endoscopes should be available to allow for breakage, service and maintenance. If a center is performing ten laparoscopies per day, a minimum of three complete sets of laparoscopy instruments is needed in order to avoid unnecessary delays between patients and to allow for maintenance. Space and facilities for sterilizing the endoscopic equipment are necessary. Heat sterilization rapidly destroys the endoscopic equipment, and all such equipment should be either gas-autoclaved or soaked in one of the standard soaking solutions. Although numerous soaking solutions have been advocated, a 12-minute soak in 10% formalin solution remains the least expensive and most acceptable solution at the present time. The remainder of the surgical instruments will require steam autoclaving, and facilities for it should be available.

Obviously, adequate life-support equipment should also be available, such as oxygen, respirators, cardiovascular resuscitation equipment and so forth. These instruments are rarely needed since patients who are at risk for cardiovascular disease or other serious medical diseases should not be operated upon in an outpatient endoscopy unit but should have their gynecologic endoscopy performed in a regular operating area.

The type of patients and the procedures which should be performed in a gynecologic endoscopy unit may vary according to the local medical standard of practice. In general, an outpatient endoscopy unit should only accommodate patients in reasonable health and of middle age or under, who are excellent candidates for local or general anesthesia.

Editorial Comments

Perhaps the title of this chapter should have been, "Meanwhile, Back in Academia...." Having worked at both academic teaching hospitals and community hospitals, I sometimes feel some degree of depression when I think of the inability of each type of institution to learn from the other. Some teaching hospitals do not want to recognize the quality of medicine practiced at the general hospital as anything but inferior to the university variety; at the same time, some community hospitals have become fearful of the term *academic teaching*. This is indeed unfortunate because each could learn from the other.

Dr. Wheeless, as usual, sets the record straight.

L.K.

Chapter 29

Worldwide Program Experiences of the Agency for International Development

R. T. Ravenholt, M.D.
Willard H. Boynton, M.D.
Dorothy N. Glenn, M.D.
J. Joseph Speidel, M.D.
Gerold Van der Vlugt, M.D.
Andrew T. Wiley, M.D.
Gerald F. Winfield, D.Sc.

In moving toward development of "programs relating to population growth," as directed by the Congress in the 1968 Title X Amendment to the Foreign Assistance Act of 1961, the Office of Population of the United States Agency for International Development (AID) has given priority to the development of new and improved means of fertility control and to the rapid dissemination and utilization of these methods throughout the developing world.

In addition to providing substantial support for research and development in general (Table 1) and female sterilization in particular (Table 2), AID has purchased large quantities of contraceptives and surgical supplies for distribution to family planning programs in developing countries (Table 3) and has supported the training of thousands of family planning personnel, including the training of 315 selected gynecologic surgeons from 58 countries in advanced techniques of fertility management. Among the main sites of AID-sponsored training of family planning personnel in the United States since 1965 has been the Johns Hopkins University in Baltimore.

Development of Outpatient Laparoscopy at Johns Hopkins

For many years Johns Hopkins University has been a pioneer in the fields of obstetrics, gynecology and public health. A natural extension of this tradition led Dr. Clifford Wheeless of Johns Hopkins to demonstrate in 1968 that the laparoscopic technique of sterilization by tubal electrocoagulation popularized in 1967 by Steptoe[5] of England could be used successfully on an early discharge or outpatient basis.[7] Responding to the admonition of his then chief, Dr. Alan Barnes, that any potentially useful surgical procedure overseas would have to be done as an outpatient procedure under local anesthesia, Dr. Wheeless in 1969[8] demonstrated that laparoscopic sterilization could be done under local anesthesia and that diazepam (Valium) (a sedative) and meperidine (Demerol) (an analgesic) were the only other medications needed. To facilitate the use of local anesthesia Dr. Wheeless developed a simplified, one-incision technique[6] and began to apply this simplified approach to female interval sterilization in Baltimore.

Table 1
AID-Sponsored Research for More
Effective Means of Fertility Control
Fiscal Years 1967–1975

	1967	1968	1969	1970	1971	1972	1973	1974	1975	Total
Research to Develop New Means										
Corpus Luteum Studies:										
Worcester Foundation	–	109,000	–	–	99,000	–	–	–	–	208,000
NICHD-CPR	–		1,510,000	53,000	–	–	–	–	–	1,563,000
Antiprogestins:										
Population Council	–	–	3,000,000	–	–	–	–	–	–	3,000,000
Prostaglandins:										
Worcester Foundation	–	–	–	2,980,000	–	–	–	–	–	2,980,000
University of Wisconsin	–	–	–	–	227,000	–	–	–	–	227,000
Washington University	–	–	–	–	293,000	–	–	128,000	186,000	607,000
Makerere University	–	–	–	–	821,000	–	–	–	–	821,000
University of Singapore	–	–	–	–	–	–	475,000	–	–	475,000
Other	–	–	–	–	217,000	150,000	–	–	–	367,000
Gonadotropin-Releasing-Factor Inhibitors:										
Salk Institute	–	–	–	2,255,000	–	–	2,150,000	–	–	4,405,000
Subtotal										14,653,000

Table 1—*continued*

	1967	1968	1969	1970	1971	1972	1973	1974	1975	Total
Research to Improve Current Means										
Intrauterine Devices:										
Battelle Memorial Institute	–	–	–	150,000	495,000	–	874,000	–	–	1,519,000
Other	–	–	–	–	12,000	–	–	–	–	12,000
IFRP, Inc.	–	–	–	–	–	–	–	–	210,000	210,000
Contraceptive Safety:										
Southwest Foundation	–	–	–	913,000	–	–	1,226,000	–	–	2,139,000
Contraceptive & Disease Prophylaxis Agent:										
University of Pittsburgh	–	–	–	581,000	–	–	138,000	–	–	719,000
Sterilization and Surgical Equipment and Training:										
Battelle Memorial Institute	–	–	–	–	830,000	199,000	–	392,000	–	1,421,000
University of North Carolina	–	–	79,000	–	135,000	–	–	–	–	214,000
Johns Hopkins University	–	–	–	–	–	1,954,000	158,000	–	–	2,112,000
University of Colorado	–	–	–	–	–	–	76,000	–	–	76,000
Small Grants Program Applied Research on Fertility Regulation:										
University of Minnesota	–	–	–	–	–	3,350,000	–	–	–	3,350,000
Other	97,000	107,700	103,000	99,000	182,000	66,000	48,000	100,000	–	803,700
Subtotal										12,575,700
Field Trials										
International IUD Program:										
Pathfinder Fund	194,000	–	1,289,000	–	–	–	–	–	–	1,483,000
International Fertility Research Program:										
IFRP	–	–	–	–	3,106,000	1,800,000	–	1,500,000	2,695,000	9,101,000
Conventional Contraceptive Studies	–	346,000	440,000	340,000	–	–	–	–	–	1,126,000
Subtotal										11,710,000
Total	291,000	562,700	6,421,000	7,371,000	6,417,000	7,519,000	5,146,000	2,120,000	3,091,000	38,938,700

Table 2
AID-Sponsored Research for More
Effective Female Sterilization

	1969	1970	1971	1972	1973	1974	1975	Total in $
U of N Carolina Tubal Clips and other Techniques	79,000		135,000					214,000
Batelle Memorial Institute Transcervical Tissue Glues				199,000				199,000
Johns Hopkins University Tantalum Clips and Silastic (Falope) Ring Tubal Occlusive Method			50,000	123,000	25,000			198,000
University of Colorado Transcervical Cryosurgery					76,000			76,000
International Fertility Research Program (IFRP) Clinical Trials in Developing Countries				6,000	69,000	181,000	215,000	417,000
Northwestern University Hysteroscopy and Transcervical Methods					112,000	80,000	53,000	248,059
Totals	79,000		185,000	328,000	282,000	261,000	268,000	1,406,959

Table 3
Contraceptives Purchased by AID
Fiscal Years 1968–1975

Oral Contraceptives	$62,010,510
Condoms	24,987,145
Intrauterine Devices	2,830,326
Sterilization Supplies	2,818,323
Other Surgical Supplies	2,407,569
Vaginal Foam	3,479,941
Other	811,073
Total	$99,335,887

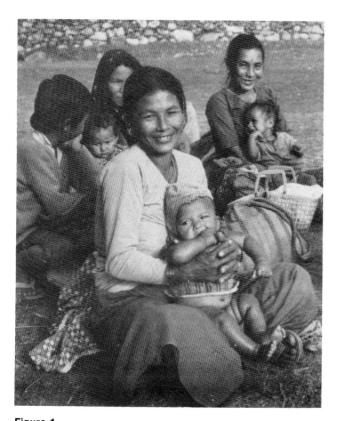

Figure 1
Women awaiting their turns for sterilization at a laparoscopy camp in Nepal.

AID Action on Laparoscopy

In late summer of 1971 Dr. Wheeless presented his experience with laparoscopic sterilization under local anesthesia to Dr. Ravenholt and staff of the Office of Population, AID. It was agreed that this method probably had potential for application in developing countries.

To obtain a consensus on this matter the Office of Population called together an ad hoc committee of experts on September 28, 1971. This group included Drs. Ben Branch, John Marlowe, John Levinson, J. F. Hulka, Alan Siegler, Anne Southam and C. R. Wheeless. They affirmed the judgment that action should go forward to fully explore the potential of laparoscopic sterilization as an outpatient service in developing countries.

At about that time Dr. Kanti Giri, a leading obstetrician-gynecologist in the rugged mountain country of Nepal, observed the procedure at Johns Hopkins during a 1970 United States tour. She subsequently invited Dr. Wheeless to Kathmandu to demonstrate the technique. In November 1971 Dr. Wheeless carried a laparoscope to Nepal, where he demonstrated and taught the procedure to Dr. Kanti Giri. She quickly adopted the procedure and has since pioneered in the provision of laparoscopic sterilization services in camp settings in the remote high valleys of Nepal. In such primitive settings as Pokhara Valley (Figure 1) she has performed as many as 43 sterilizations in one day.[2] She has done over 1,500 laparoscopic sterilizations and is now training other doctors in this technique.

International Sterilization Training Project

The Nepal experience was reported by Dr. Wheeless at an AID/Battelle Conference on female sterilization in December 1971, held at Airlie, Virginia.[1] On the basis of this and related favorable developments AID provided a $50,000 grant to Dr. Wheeless to set up an International Sterilization Project (ISTP) to train developing-country personnel in such advanced techniques of female sterilization. Carrying laparoscopic equipment, Dr. Wheeless traveled to El Salvador, Thailand, Panama, Malaysia, Equador and India, where he trained colleagues in this new technique and provided them with AID-supplied laparoscopes. Later he was joined by other pioneering laparoscopists such as Drs. Bruce Thompson, Philip Pelland and John Levinson. Soon many requests for laparoscopic instruments and training were directed to AID, Johns Hopkins and other training institutions.

Many of these requests for special training and equipment followed a conference on "Advances in Human Fertility" held at Johns Hopkins in June 1973. The deans of 80 Latin American medical schools were asked to nominate physician representatives to attend. One hundred and forty-four professors from 17 countries attended, representing 72 universities. This AID-funded conference undoubtedly marked a turning point in the acceptance of sterilization by many Latin American teachers of obstetrics and gynecology.

Development of an Improved Laparoscope Package

The problem facing the Office of Population at this crucial stage in the overseas acceptance and use of the laparoscope was development of a simpler, better-packaged instrument capable of withstanding the rigors of transportation and use in developing countries.

Dr. Gerold Van der Vlugt, Chief of Technical Services and Commodities, Office of Population, began working with US industry to achieve necessary improvements in design and the substantial production needed to make worldwide dissemination of supplies feasible. The equipment needs of the Office of Population were specified to potential manufacturers in the fall of 1972, and 10 prototype laparoscopic kits were ordered from American Cystoscope Makers Incorporated (ACMI) and Medical Technology International, Inc. (MTI) for field testing in the United States and overseas. Because of strong initial demand, 10 second-generation sets were ordered subsequently from MTI so that altogether 30 scopes and kits were obtained for the initial field testing phase.

Discussions of field test results and required changes in equipment were held with various investigators at the Association for Voluntary Sterilization (AVS) and Agency for International Development-sponsored Second International Sterilization Conference, Geneva, Switzerland, in February 1973. Field testing resulted in suggestions for numerous modifications and changes, one of which was from straight to offset scopes. An expert committee was formed to provide advice on specifications for the laparoscope kit. The committee included Drs. Ira Lubell, Bruce Thompson, G. Van der Vlugt and C. R. Wheeless. After much discussion the specifications were finally agreed upon

and requests for bids issued in December 1973. An order for 150 laparoscopes and kits was placed early in 1974 on the basis of the lowest bid. This order included the option to buy an additional 70 laparoscopes and kits, if desired. The process moved rapidly: by mid-1974 the kits were being produced in quantity. The option to purchase the additional kits was exercised, and by the end of the initial contract period a total of 250 laparoscopic kits had been purchased by AID. The cost of the laparoscope and kit is approximately $3,000.

Program of International Education in Gynecology and Obstetrics

Beginning in 1972 the Office of Population and especially Dr. Gerald Winfild, Chief Manpower and Training Division, worked with Johns Hopkins University and other universities to form the Program of International Education in Gynecology and Obstetrics (PIEGO). Its primary purpose was to provide short-term training for overseas physicians in laparoscopic sterilization techniques and other methods of fertility control and to arrange for distribution of laparoscopic and other equipment to qualified trainees. This program was an outgrowth of the early Johns-Hopkins-based training program in laparoscopy and other fertility control techniques; it now included the University of Pittsburgh and Washington University in St. Louis. Later it expanded to include the American University in Beirut, Lebanon, and the initials *JH* were put in front of the acronym *PIEGO* to indicate that the consortium headquarters would be based at Johns Hopkins. The organization itself is now known as *JHPIEGO*, but the training is called *PIEGO* training.

The funds provided by AID to the individual PIEGO centers are listed by year in Table 4.

PIEGO training at these four centers consists of four to six weeks of didactic and clinical work in all aspects of fertility control, of which laparoscopy training is an important part. The physicians are selected carefully to ensure that they will be able to put their training to good use. Those who complete the course are given certain basic operating equipment.

Table 4

PIEGO Expenditures for Equipment and for Training in Laparoscopic Sterilization and Other Forms of Fertility Control (by center)

	FY 1973	FY 1974	FY 1975	Total
John Hopkins University	328,000	492,000	533,000	1,350,000
University of Pittsburgh		186,000	356,000	542,000
Washington University		350,000	491,000	841,000
American University at Beirut		65,000	192,000	257,000
JHPIEGO Corporation			636,000	636,000
Totals	328,000	1,093,000	1,708,000	5,129,000

Distribution of Laparoscopic Equipment

A few weeks or months after the trainee returns home, he or she is visited by one or two trainers from one of the PIEGO training centers. The trainer brings the laparoscopic equipment or sends it beforehand to be assembled upon arrival. A significant number of supervised laparoscopic sterilizations are performed by the trainee over a period of several days. When the trainer is satisfied with the trainee's skill, a laparoscope is given to the trainee's institution. Three hundred and fifteen physicians from 51 countries have been trained in this manner to date, and 175 laparoscopes have been provided to institutions of those who best qualify (Table 5).

International Project of the Association for Voluntary Sterilization

In May 1972 the Office of Population, AID, made a grant of $876,000 to the Association for Voluntary Sterilization in New York to create an international project for promoting voluntary sterilization in developing countries by means of international conferences, training, supplies and support for development of National Associations for Voluntary Sterilization.

This organization, under the leadership of Dr. Ira Lubell, moved quickly to promote and extend sterilization services in developing countries. An important, early activity of this organization was the joint creation by AVS and AID of the Second International Conference on Voluntary Sterilization, held in Geneva, Switzerland, in February 1973, and chaired by Dr. Nafis Sadik of the United Nations Fund for Population Activities. This conference congregated 370 surgeons, family planning directors and leaders, representatives of relevant organizations and equipment manufacturers. The Association for Voluntary Sterilization also moved with great speed to strengthen sterilization activities on a global basis by means of regional conferences, by sponsoring training, by distribution of AID-purchased laparoscopes and other surgical supplies and by formation of National Voluntary Sterilization Associations (currently in 14 countries). The Third International Conference on Voluntary Sterilization was held in February 1976 in Tunisia.

Table 5
Physicians Trained and Laparoscopes Placed
by PIEGO
(by region and country)

	Physicians Trained	Laparoscopes Placed		Physicians Trained	Laparoscopes Placed
Latin America			Guyana	1	1
North America			Peru	3	4
Mexico	22	3	Surinam	1	
Costa Rica	2	4	Venezuela	1	1
El Salvador	2	2	**Africa**		
Central America			Gambia	2	2
Guatemala	3	3	Ghana	1	1
Haiti	2	2	Kenya	4	
Hondurus	2	2	Nigeria	9	5
Nicaragua	1	1	Sierra Leone	1	
Panama	2	2	Sudan	1	
Antigua	1	1	Zaire	1	1
Barbados	2	2	**Near East and West Asia**		
Grenada	2	2	Afghanistan	1	1
West Indies			Bangladesh	4	1
Jamaica	3	1	Egypt	3	7
Netherland An-tilles	1	1	India	65	19
Santa Lucia	1	1	Iran	7	3
St. Kitts	1	1	Jordan	3	2
Trinidad	2	2	Lebanon	4	2
South America			Nepal	2	1
Argentina	8		Pakistan	14	13
Bolivia	22	2	Saudi Arabia	2	1
Brazil	2	1	Sri Lanka	2	
Chile	6	3	Turkey	4	9
Columbia	5	3			
Ecuador	1	1			

Table 5—Continued

	Physicians Trained	Laparoscopes Placed
Far East and South Asia		
Figi	1	
Hong Kong		
Indonesia	5	6
Korea	11	11
Kymer Republic	1	1
Malaysia	8	7
New Guinea	1	1
Phillipines	31	21
Singapore	1	1
Taiwan	7	5
Thailand	17	9
Tonga	1	
Vietnam	6	1
Totals		
Latin America	98	45
Africa	19	9
Near East and West Asia	107	59
Far East and South Asia	91	62
Total	315	172

Other Distributors of Laparoscopes

AVS, like PIEGO, has distributed substantial quantities of laparoscopes to qualified surgeons. Through October 1975 AVS had placed 101 laparoscopes with trained gynecologic surgeons in 17 countries. Family Planning International Assistance (FPIA-CWS/PPFA) has distributed one, the Pathfinder Fund has distributed six and the International Fertility Research Program of Chapel Hill, North Carolina, has distributed four laparoscopes to trained surgeons.

Total Distributions of AID-Purchased Laparoscopes

Altogether, as shown in Table 6, 375 AID-purchased laparoscopes have been distributed to trained gynecologic surgeons in 52 countries during the four years 1972 to 1975. The total cost of this laparoscopic equipment came to approximately $1,000,000. The widespread distribution of these scopes is shown by the dotted areas on the world map (Figure 2).

Tubal Clips and Bands

At the AID/Battelle sponsored conference on female sterilization held at Airlie, Virginia, in December 1971 it became clear that there was a crucial need to improve the safety of laparoscopic sterilizations by use of a tubal clip or band which could replace electrocautery as the means of blocking tubal functions.[1] Activity in this area has moved rapidly since then, with development of the Hulka Clip[10] and the Yoon band (Falope-Ring),[11] both of which can be applied either through the laparoscope or independently of that instrument, e.g., through a minilaparotomy incision.[9]

Drs. InBae Yoon and Theodore King of Johns Hopkins University were assisted by Drs. Gerold Van der Vlugt and Joseph Speidel of AID's Office of Population in the development and testing of the Falope-Rings and the ring applicator. This development proceeded swiftly at Johns Hopkins University under the direction of Dr. King.

At this writing, the Yoon band shows the greatest promise as a nonthermal means for tubal occlusion through the laparoscope. This method is being tested in 13 countries with AID-International Fertility Research Program (IFRP) support, and findings from 20 centers through October 1975 show[3] only two pregnancies in 2,000 patients, neither of which was due to Yoon band failure.

Table 6
AID-Funded Laparoscope Placements by Year

Country	1972	1973	1974	1975	Total
1. Afghanistan				1	1
2. Antigua				1	1
3. Bangladesh		1	3		4
4. Barbados			2		2
5. Brazil		2		3	5
6. Bolivia			3		3
7. Chile		2	3	1	6
8. Columbia		5	23	2	30
9. Costa Rica	2	3	13		18
10. Ecuador	1	2			3
11. Egypt			6	1	7
12. Gambia			1	1	2
13. Ghana			1		1
14. Guatemala		4	3	4	11
15. Grenada			1		1
16. Guyana			1		1
17. Honduras		1		1	2
18. Haiti			2		2
19. India	3	6	14	3	26
20. Iran		2		2	4
21. Indonesia		1	3	2	6
22. Jordan			1	1	2
23. Jamaica		4	7	4	15
24. Kenya			2		2
25. Kymer Republic			1		1
26. Korea		4	3	5	12
27. Lebanon		1		1	2
28. Liberia			1		1
29. Malaysia	1	1	4	2	8
30. Mexico		1	2	1	4
31. Nepal	1	1	3	12	17
32. Netherland Antilles			1		1
33. New Guinea			1		1
34. Nicaragua			1		1
35. Nigeria				5	5
36. Pakistan		1	6	7	14
37. Peru		1	5	2	8
38. Panama	1	1			2
39. Philippines		7	36	12	55
40. Saudi Arabia			1		1
41. Santa Lucia			1		1
42. Senegal			1		1
43. Singapore		2	3		5
44. St. Kitts			1		1
45. El Salvador	3	4	1	9	17
46. Taiwan		2	6		8
47. Thailand	1	3	19	14	37
48. Trinidad			3	1	4
49. Turkey		2	7		9
50. Venezuela			1		1
51. Vietnam			1		1
52. Zaire			1	1	2
Total	13	64	187	111	375

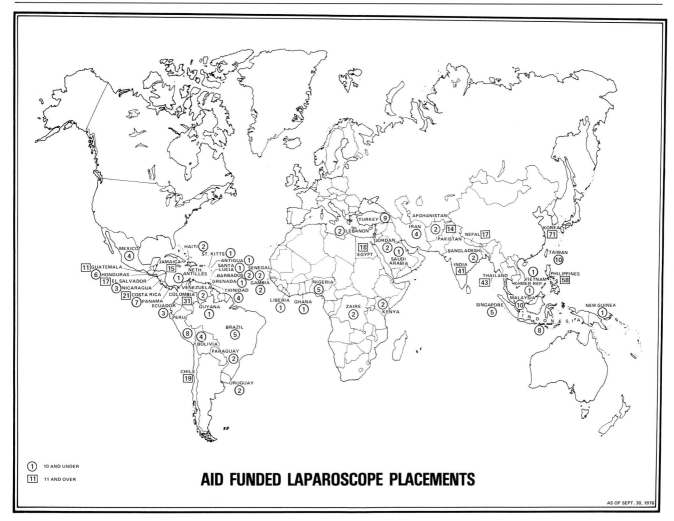

AID FUNDED LAPAROSCOPE PLACEMENTS

1 10 AND UNDER
11 11 AND OVER

AS OF SEPT. 30, 1976

Figure 2
Worldwide distribution of 509 AID-funded laparoscopes.

Significance of Laparoscopy for Developing-Country Sterilization Programs

It is clear that development of outpatient laparoscopic sterilization has brought about a remarkable acceleration of the evolution and application of female sterilization services.

The necessarily complex, high-precision and expensive laparoscopic equipment, requiring a high degree of skill for use, has served to rivet the attention of outstanding gynecologic surgeons upon female sterilization. Much has already been accomplished, and much more will certainly be accomplished by further provision of laparoscope training, supplies and services. The several hundred laparoscopes distributed to date have already been used to perform more than 1,000 sterilizations.

In many countries where AID-purchased laparoscopes introduced the technique three years ago, it has been taught extensively and new scopes have been supplied. At the same time national associations have assumed the responsibility for fur-

ther training and certification. These countries include Thailand, the Philippines, Costa Rica and Korea, where second- and third-generation trainees are now capable of doing the procedure in many smaller hospitals. Dr. Dorothy Glenn, who has been serving as an AID specialist/advisor in many countries, played a particularly strategic role in the demonstration and utilization of laparoscopy in Korea. In that country, in 1975, over 100 physicians received formal training in laparoscopy by the new Korean PIEGO training organization.

An illustrative example of the seeding effect which laparoscopic training for overseas physicians can have is that of Dr. Virgio Oblepias, who was given a laparoscope and trained to use it. In 1973 he opened the first sterilization clinic in the Philippines at the Mary Johnson Hospital, located in a poor section of Manila. He and his group have now done over 6,000 laparoscopic sterilizations as well as many sterilizations using other methods. He has formed mobile teams who have taken the technique to remote areas, and he has trained many other physicians. He is, at present, a member of the Philippine Board of Laparoscopy Certification.

Sterilization is now rapidly gaining acceptance in the Philippines and will undoubtedly play a major role in that country's family planning program. Dr. Oblepias' dramatic performance with the laparoscope has helped trigger this favorable development.

Minilaparotomy

An even greater dividend of the intense interest aroused in female sterilization may derive from the related development of minilaparotomy procedures,[4] which can also be performed under local anesthesia but with much less expensive equipment and by less highly trained surgeons. This technique is now widely used in Thailand and the Philippines and is rapidly gaining acceptance in many other countries.

Minilaparotomy utilizes a simple uterine elevator, inserted per vagina, to push the uterine fundus against the anterior abdominal wall, thus permitting tubal ligation through a very small suprapubic incision under local anesthesia. This technique is particularly well suited to slender Asian women and is currently being used in 15 different countries. AID has made two types of minilaparotomy sets available. The first, a kit, containing all the surgical instruments necessary for the operation, costs $118.00. The second, a packet, containing the uterine elevator and a tubal hook, costs $16.00. The tubal hook is helpful in bringing the fallopian tube into the operative field.

AID has distributed over 1,000 of these surgical kits and more than 6,000 of the packets in the past six months and plans greatly expanded distribution of these kits and packets during the next year.

Worldwide Availability of Sterilization by 1980

Experience to date in countries such as India, Pakistan, Bangladesh, Indonesia, Thailand, Philippines, Korea, Nepal, Tunisia, Egypt, El Salvador, Costa Rica, Panama, Colombia and other countries has demonstrated an extraordinary demand for sterilization services, especially female. We estimate that at this time there are more than 50 million couples in developing countries who would control their fertility by sterilization if these services were appropriately and readily available.

With available technology, building upon training programs already substantially advanced, and with adequate planning and monetary and commodity support, it should be feasible to extend sterilization services throughout the developing world by 1980.

References

1. Duncan GW, Falls RD, Speidel JJ: *Female Sterilization. Prognosis for Simplified Outpatient Procedures.* Academic Press, Washington, 1972

2. Giri K: Experience of outpatient laparoscopic sterilization in Nepal. *Proceedings of the Second International Conference on Voluntary Sterilization.* Excerpta Medica, Amsterdam, 1974, p 36

3. Kessel E: Personal communication

4. Osathawondh V: Suprapubic mini-laparotomy, uterine elevation technique: simple, inexpensive outpatient procedure for interval female sterilization. Contraception 10:251, 1974

5. Steptoe PC: *Laparoscopy in Gynecology.* E & S Livingston, Ltd, London, 1967

6. Wheeless CR, Jr: Elimination of second incision in laparoscope sterilization. Obstet Gynecol 39:134, 1972

7. Wheeless CR, Jr: Outpatient laparoscope sterilization. Obstet Gynecol 36:208, 1970

8. Wheeless CR, Jr: Outpatient laparoscope sterilization under local anesthesia. Obstet Gynecol 39:767, 1972

9. Wortman JS: Female sterilization by mini-laparotomy. Population Report, series C, 5:53, 1974

10. Wortman JS: Laparoscopic sterilization with clips. Population Report, series C, 4:45, 1974

11. Yoon IB, Wheeless CR, King TM: A preliminary report on a new laparoscopic sterilization approach—silicone rubber band technique. Am J Obstet Gynecol 120:132, 1974

Section 10

Special Aspects

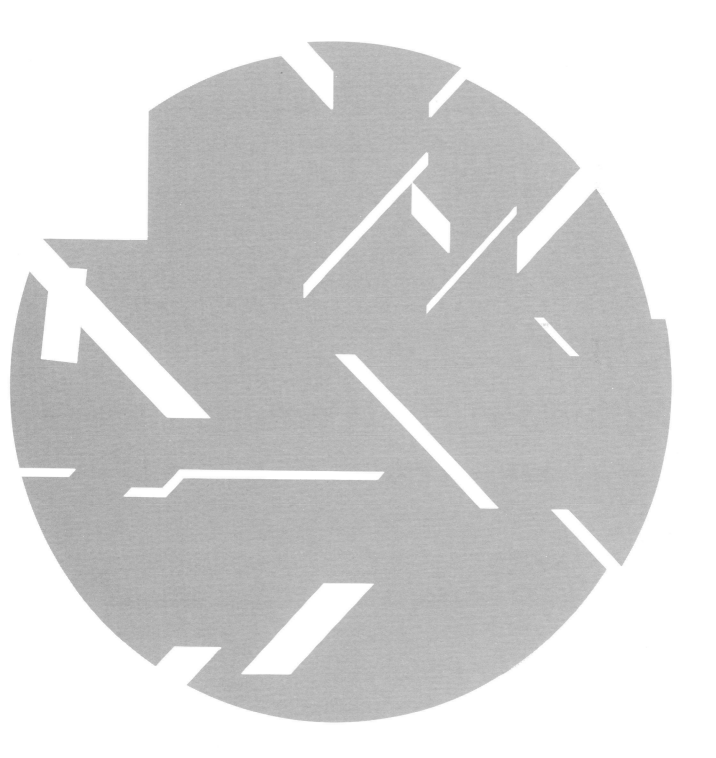

Chapter 30

Pediatric Laparoscopy

Michel A. Cognat, M.D.

The improvement in the technique of peritoneoscopy and the large experience acquired in a wide range of illnesses in adult abdominal and gynecologic pathology has led to its use for pediatric patients. Laparoscopy allows direct observation of the pelvis (Figure 1). Although this procedure appears to be a very useful means for investigating the internal genitalia and ovaries (even in the young infant), pediatric reports on this subject are still rare. Some gonadal troubles can only be assessed by observation during the prepubertal and adolescent periods. In these cases, laparoscopy can be a valuable method in investigation, diagnosis and sometimes treatment, thus avoiding exploratory intervention.

This chapter deals with:
1. Technical details of the method.
2. Indications and characteristic findings.

This experience is based on 100 pediatric laparoscopies performed over a period of five years. The decision for laparoscopy in these young patients was made by their attending pediatricians or endocrinologists at the University Medical Center. We felt capable of performing them on the basis of a large experience in adults. Our youngest patient was six months old.

Technical Details
The requirements are the same as those for any laparoscopic procedure:
1. Operating theater with the same aseptic conditions as for laparotomy.
2. General anesthesia, intubation and electrocardioscopic control.
3. Pneumoperitoneum with carbon dioxide (as used for adults). Insufflation must be done much more carefully to a maximum pressure of 10 to 12 millibars—a short Veress needle and a small caliber endoscope (Wolf 6 mm or Storz 4 mm) must be used (Needlescope is not recommended).
4. Abdominal transumbilical approach is employed.
5. A blunt probe (2 mm diameter) allows the retraction of small bowel and mobilization of the internal genitalia.
6. Catheterization of the bladder before the start of the procedure is specially advisable. A Foley catheter is left in place during laparoscopy.

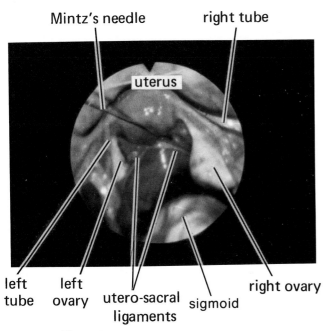

Mintz's needle   right tube

uterus

left tube   left ovary   utero-sacral ligaments   sigmoid   right ovary

Figure 1
Normal pubertal internal genitalia

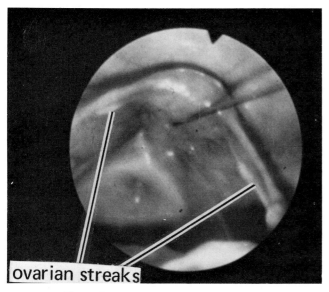

ovarian streaks

Figure 2
Typical Turner Syndrome

All pediatric patients were hospitalized in the surgical gynecologic department one day before the laparoscopy was scheduled and were kept one or two days afterward. There were no complications.

Indications

Gonadal dysgenesis

Laparoscopy allows the assessment of the degree of gonadal development in infancy and allows a more accurate prognosis of future pubertal sexual development and fertility.

It has been demonstrated that in a certain percentage (8%) of "typical" Turner's syndrome cases some ovarian function exists, which is manifested by menstruation or (very exceptionally) by a pregnancy. Furthermore, in "atypical" Turner's syndrome with chromosomal mosaicism, a certain degree of ovarian development, viewed as small ovaries, is often encountered.

It is evident that laparoscopy is not required in the diagnosis of Turner's syndrome, but it is essential to know the status of the ovaries before puberty to know whether or not estrogenic therapy is to be administered. There were 15 cases in this group: nine were "typical" Turner's syndromes with classical clinical features and a 45 X chromosomal constitution and bilateral gonadal streaks (Figure 2); six were "atypical" Turner's syndromes with classical features but chromosomal mosaicism: three of these showed typical streaks, and three had small ovaries of normal gross appearance, supporting the value of laparoscopy in this syndrome.

Primary amenorrhea

Laparoscopy is of great help for the etiologic diagnosis of primary amenorrhea: this already has been established by several authors. Nine patients were seen for primary amenorrhea, all with normal development of all secondary sex characteristics and normal chromosomal constitution (46 XX). A uterine cause for the amenorrhea was found in seven cases: in four the uterus appeared obviously underdeveloped, with no other abnormality. This hypoplasia may either be a congenital abnormality or the result of failure to respond to ovarian hormones (and, as in one patient, a failure to respond to intermittent estrogenic therapy). In three cases there was congenital absence of the uterus as described in the Rokitansky-Kuster-Hau-

ovary

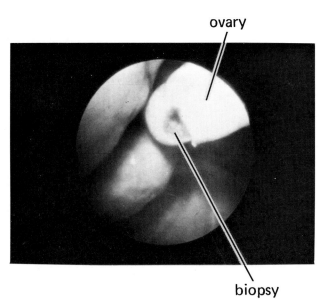

biopsy

Figure 3
Ovarian biopsy of pubertal ovary

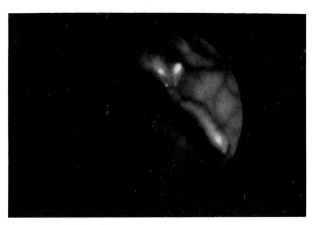

Figure 4
Appendix

ser syndrome. Laparoscopy is a very important tool for confirming the clinical diagnosis, ascertaining that no functional uterus exists above the vaginal aplasia and designing the best treatment for this congenital abnormality.

Secondary amenorrhea

Laparoscopy is done after the biochemical and endocrinological studies are completed. The usefulness of laparoscopy in the study of secondary amenorrhea has already been widely demonstrated. Ovarian biopsy may be performed to obtain a histologic study, but generally the gross findings alone allow a very good approach to diagnosis, especially in the Stein-Leventhal syndrome; thus, in our patients the diagnosis was evident on laparoscopic examination: on three occasions typically enlarged and pearly polycystic ovaries were found; the other seven patients had ovaries which were quite normal, suggesting a psychogenic cause of the amenorrhea. In all the cases biopsy was confirmative. Perlaparoscopic ovarian biopsy, which is a simple and easy procedure for a well trained laparoscopist, confirms the diagnosis and sometimes has a therapeutic effect on ovum release.

Precocious puberty

The routine investigation rules out cerebral (neurological and hypothalamic) or adrenal etiology for this condition. An ovarian etiology is best determined by laparoscopy: there might be an ovarian tumor requiring surgery or a cyst. Several cases of precocious puberty provoked by a luteinizing ovarian cyst have been reported in which unilateral cystectomy or ovariectomy was followed by regression of the sexual precocity. In such cases laparoscopy may have a therapeutic value in permitting puncture and complete aspiration of the cyst; cytological and biochemical studies may be done on the fluid obtained. We did not encounter this condition. All cases were of idiopathic origin with gonadotropic stimulation of the ovaries and no ovarian lesion.

Ovarian biopsy confirmed gonadotropic stimulation. Nevertheless, in young infants it must be done with great care and is often unnecessary (Figure 3). There were 13 patients investigated for precocious puberty. The youngest was 14 months and the oldest four years of age.

Delayed puberty

After the routine workup, a laparoscopy is sometimes indicated.

In our statistics one was performed at the age of 14 on a girl who had a congenital virilizing adrenal hyperplasia due to C 21 hydroxylase deficiency. The diagnosis had been made at the age of one month, and treatment was started at that time. Surgical correction of ambiguous genitalia (Prader's Type IV) had been achieved before the age of four. She had no evidence of puberty at the time of the investigation. Laparoscopy showed quite normal, immature ovaries and an infantile uterus. A gonadal biopsy was done which demonstrated, at histologic examination, typical aspects of the prepubertal ovary. This patient menstruated a few months after the laparoscopy.

Hirsutism

Our study concerned three cases referred by endocrinologists for searching of an ovarian tumor: one was found.

Intersexuality

In some intersexuality cases one must visualize the internal genitalia as early as possible in order to be able to rear the child according to the proper gender. Laparotomy is often indicated and might be replaced advantageously by laparoscopy.

There were four patients with abnormal sexual differentiation, among whom were three cases of male pseudohermaphroditism. The first (three years) was a male pseudohermaphrodite with 46 XY chromosomal constitution and ambiguous external genitalia (Prader's Type III). Laparoscopy showed a total absence of female internal genitalia but revealed the presence, behind the bladder, of a large flaccid membranous cyst implanted on the urethra. This cyst was removed surgically and appeared to be bladder-like on histologic examination. The second patient was an 11-month-old boy with Klinefelter's syndrome (47 XXY chromosomal constitution) associated with ambiguous external genitalia (Prader's Type IV). Laparoscopy demonstrated normal male internal genitalia. The third patient (eight months old) had been operated on one month before for bilateral cryptorchidism. The surgeon had found a uterus with bilateral tubes and two gonads which resembled ovaries. Unfortunately, no biopsy was done at that time. The patient's karyotype was 46 XY. Laparoscopy was used to biopsy the gonads, which looked like cryptorchid testes; the histologic findings confirmed this impression. There was one case of testicular feminization. Laparoscopy was done to ascertain the testicular nature of a sole gonad and the absence of Mullerian derivatives. The diagnosis showed a testicular feminization syndrome in a 16-year-old adolescent whose karyotype was 46 XY. A subsequent laparotomy confirmed this.

Congenital uterine abnormality

A preoperative accurate assessment of the entire internal genitalia is necessary in some cases of double uterus or unicornis uterus.

Miscellaneous

In addition to the indications of the preceding group (almost specifically endocrinological and genetical), there is one other group of pelvic diseases which sometimes requires laparoscopy for the following reasons:

1. Acute or subacute pelvic (or pelviabdominal) pain or dysmenorrhea.
2. Pelvic mass.

By this means one can discover:

1. A diseased uterus: menstrual retention (at times unilateral) with hematometria and associated hematosalpinx.
2. A diseased ovary: an ovarian cyst which can be punctured and which is responsible for pelvic pain or menstrual troubles: laparoscopy can replace laparotomy, minimize it or else delay it.
3. Benign or malignant ovarian tumor, already operated upon, which needs to be checked regularly.
4. Ovarian or tubal or adnexal torsion: laparoscopy permits an early diagnosis and an early treatment, avoiding mutilation or spontaneous necrosis.
5. Diseased tubes: exploration of subacute or chronic salpingitis, laparoscopy making possible: a. early and positive identification of a true salpingitis. b. accurate identification of the concerned organism (per laparoscopic aspiration of fluid from pelvis for culture and sensitivity). c. proper treatment of the salpingitis of the teenager (sometimes of tuberulosic origin) (long and sometimes unnecessary antibiotic treatments are avoided in case of unproven salpingitis or adnexitis).
6. Acute pelvic inflammatory disease: one personal case of bilateral, suppurative salpingitis responsible for persisting menorrhagia in a 15-year-old adolescent.

7.   A diseased appendix: a laparoscopic "coup d'oeil" permits: a. avoidance of unnecessary appendectomies, chiefly at the pubertal or prepubertal period. b. an early diagnosis of true appendicitis and early surgical treatment, which would prevent problems of future infertility associated with late diagnosis of the same condition. c. inspection of the peritoneal cavity and the internal genitalia certainly more thoroughly than through a MacBurney's incision (Figure 4). d. endometriosis, which can be encountered in teenage patients. e. a negative exploration: a sample is given by the case of a girl operated on for appendectomy who still complained of right iliac pain: a negative workup led to an exploratory laparoscopy. The diagnosis of pain from psychogenic origin was most likely after the negative endoscopy.

Conclusions

1.   In infants and adolescents, laparoscopy allows: direct and accurate visualization of internal genitalia, with documentation by photography; ovarian biopsy (in selected cases) for histologic examination; cytologic and bacteriologic examination of the peritoneal fluid; therapeutic procedures, such as the puncture and complete aspiration of a functional ovarian cyst.

2.   Laparoscopy can be performed even on the very young child by using extreme gentleness and care, providing one has a vast experience with laparoscopy in adults.

3.   The indications for laparoscopy in the infant should be decided upon by a pediatrician or an endocrinologist and not necessarily by the gynecologic laparoscopist himself or herself.

4.   Laparoscopy avoids many unnecessary laparotomies.

Additional Reading

1. Bahner F, Schwarz G, Harden DG et al: A fertile female with XO sex chromosome constitution. Lancet 2:100, 1960

2. Bove KE: Gonadal dysgenesis in a newborn with XO karyotype. Am J Dis Child 120:363, 1970

3. Bullock JL et al: Symptomatic endometriosis in teenagers. Obstet Gynecol 43:896, 1974

4. Burgio GR, Argara G: La coelioscopia nello studio della pathologia del sesso in eta infantile a prebuberale. *Proceedings of the First International Symposium on Celioscopy.* I.R.E.S., Palermo, 1964, p 285

5. Chartier M, Dubost M, Cornu C: *La coelioscopie en gynecologie pediatrique: l'appareil genital feminin avant la puberte.* Masson et Cie, Paris, 1971, p 87

6. Chartier M, Dubost M, Cornu C et al: La coelioscopie en gynecologie pediatrique. Ann Pediatrie 74:315, 1967

7. Cohen MR: *Laparoscopy, Culdoscopy and Gynecography: Technique and Atlas.* W B Saunders Co, Philadelphia, 1970

8. Conen PE, Glass IH: 45 XD Turner's syndrome in the newborn: report of two cases. J Clin Endocrinol 23:1, 1963.

9. Cognat M: *Coelioscopie Gynecologique.* Simep Editions, Villeurbanne, 1973

10. Cognat M: Gynecological laparoscopy in infants and adolescents. In *Gynecological Laparoscopy: Principles and Techniques.* (JM Phillips, L Keith, Eds.) Stratton Intercontinental Medical Book Corp, New York, 1974, p 269

11. Cognat M: *Laparoscopy in Infants and Adolescents.* Year Book Medical Publishers, Chicago, 1975

12. Cognat M, Papathanassiou Z, Gomel V: Laparoscopy in infants and adolescents. J Reprod Med 13:11, 1974

13. Cognat M, Rosenberg D: La coelioscopie dans l'enfance et l'adolescence. A propos d'une statistique personnelle de 30 cas. Comptes Rendus Soc Fr Gynecol 8:1, 1970

14. Cognat M, Rosenberg D, David L, Papathanassiou Z: Laparoscopy in infants and adolescents. Obstet Gynecol 42:515, 1973

15. Eberlein WR, Bongioani AM, Jones IT, Yakovac WC: Ovarian tumors and cysts associated with sexual precocity: report of three cases and review of the literature. J Pediatr 57:484, 1960

16. Espiner EA, Veale AMO, Sands VE et al: Familial syndrome of streak gonads and normal male karyotype in five phenotypic females. N Engl J Med 283:6, 1970

17. Ferguson-Smith MA: Karyotype-phenotype correlations in gonadal dysgenesis and their bearing on the pathogenesis of malformation. J Med Genet 2:142, 1965

18. Gans SL, Berci G: Advances in endoscopy of infants and adolescents. J Pediatr Surg 6:199, 1971

19. Gordon RI, O'Neil EM: Turner's infantile phenotype. Br Med J 1:483, 1969

20. Jones HW, Jones GES: The gynecological aspects of adrenal hyperplasia and allied disorders. Am J Obstet Gynecol 68:1330, 1954

21. Lippe BM, Scalley JR, Wong SR et al: Pelvic pneumography in the diagnosis of endocrine and gynecologic disorders in children. J Pediatr 78:779, 1971

22. Prader A: Wachstum und entniwichlung In *Klinic der Inneren Sekreton.* (A Labhart, Ed.) Springer-Verlag, Stuttgart, 1957, p 645

23. Siegler AM: Trends in laparoscopy. Am J Obstet Gynecol 109:794, 1971

24. Steptoe PC: *Laparoscopy in Gynaecology.* E & S Livingston, Ltd, Edinburgh and London, 1967

25. Sternberg WH, Barclay DL, Kooepfer HW: Familial XY gonadal dysgenesis: a family showing characteristics with XY karyotype in three female members. N Engl J Med 278:695, 1968

Editorial Comments

The experience presented by Dr. Cognat will prove to be invaluable to those physicians performing laparoscopy on children. I agree wholeheartedly that a "needlescope" will provide inadequate illumination and would suggest the use of a 6 mm (preferable to a 4 mm) laparoscope since it provides much better illumination and a better opportunity to take photographs. It should be stressed that ovarian biopsy in cases of precocious puberty is unnecessary and that the risk appears to outweigh the benefit. On the other hand, with problems of intersexuality, a karyotype done from ovarian tissue may prove to be valuable.

On several occasions the author mentions puncturing ovarian cysts with the laparoscope; I am afraid that the postoperative effects (particularly adhesions) of such a procedure may be more detrimental than letting the usually functioning cysts resolve themselves.

C.J.L.

Chapter 31

Photography

Melvin R. Cohen, M.D.

Equipment for photography is available for all laparoscopes, culdoscopes and hysteroscopes manufactured or distributed by ACMI, Eder Instrument Company, Karl Storz Endoscopy-America, Inc., and the Richard Wolf Instrument Company. It is the purpose of this chapter to describe the equipment available—viz, fiber optic power supplies, flash equipment, cameras and type of film—in order to obtain the best possible color photographs for documentation of diagnostic endoscopy.

General Principles of Photography

The gynecologic laparoscopist uses rigid rather than flexible endoscopes and also utilizes glass optics. Therefore, images obtained through the telescope are "in living color," with excellent resolution. Fiber optics are utilized for light transmission only. As a general rule, the optics in both the 8 mm and 10 mm laparoscopes are identical. The advantage of the 10 mm laparoscope over the 8 mm is in the employment of additional fiber optic bundles so that there is more intense light transmission. Thus, the 10 mm laparoscope is preferred for cinematography and for still photography. Miniaturization of telescopes is possible. For example, Storz has produced an endoscope of 2.8 mm and a more practical one of 4 mm which is utilized especially for hysteroscopy.

For still photography, as well as cinematography, through-the-lens reflex cameras are essential. Such cameras must be modified by removing the ground glass focusing screen and replacing it with a clear glass screen, the purpose of which is to increase visibility. Focusing is unnecessary inasmuch as the optics of the endoscopes are utilized rather than the optics of the camera lens. The camera lens is set at infinity and opened wide since the size of the aperture is limited by the diameter of the lens system of the endoscope. The camera lens is usually of the telephoto type and varies from 65 to 110 mm. The smaller lenses will reduce the size of the transparency obtained, and hence less light will be needed. The larger lenses permit larger transparencies but, of course, more light is needed.

Electronic Flash (Strobe)

Electronic flash generators are available and are the preferred light source. Although it is possible to obtain satisfactory still photographs using a blue-type light source obtained with either the 300 watt General Electric (GE) lamp incorporated in several fiber optic power supplies or the xenon light source incorporated in the Storz power supply, these light sources are more ideal for cinematography, TV, etc.

Table 1 gives the various types of film ASA rating and lighting balance. Ektachrome film is preferred because it is easily processed, better when reproductions are needed in color and can be force-processed usually by a factor of two and one-half. However, when this processing is used, it results in a very grainy-looking transparency.

Camera equipment is expensive, and a great deal of thought should be given to purchasing the equipment best suited to the individual needs of the gynecologist-endoscopist. Because it would be impossible to test all cameras available in the United States, I will limit my recommendations to those cameras with which I have had experience and rely upon material supplied me by distributors and manufacturers of gynecologic endoscopes. My camera preference is the Leica with an MDa back, a Visoflex III attachment with the ground glass removed and a 90 mm lens combined with a universal focusing mount. This lens needs an adaptor, obtainable from all the manufacturers or distributors, to fit the endoscope used.

Another camera which I have used successfully is the Olympus OM-1. With this new through-the-lens 35 mm camera a Zuiko 85 mm telephoto lens with the proper adaptor is used. Also, it is necessary to modify this camera by removing the ground glass focusing screen and substituting a clear screen. One of the advantages of the Olympus OM-1 is that the focusing screen is removed easily. The flash capabilities of this camera are enhanced further by a hot shoe.

For cinematography a through-the-lens movie camera is essential. I have used the Beaulieu 16 mm camera (Figure 1) but the new Beaulieu Super 8 mm camera (Figure 2) is also easily adaptable to any of the endoscopes. A 38 mm lens is recommended for both the 16 mm and the Super 8 mm camera.

Table 1
Photographic Film Available

Still Photography

| 35 mm Ektachrome X | ASA 64 | Daylight |
| 35 mm Ektachrome High Speed | ASA 160 | Daylight |

Cinematography

| High Speed Ektachrome 7241 | ASA 160 | Daylight |

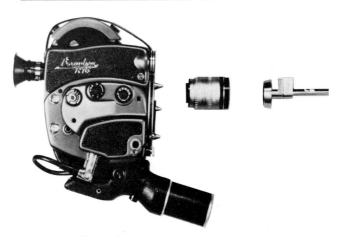

Figure 1
Beaulieu camera for 16 mm cinematography.

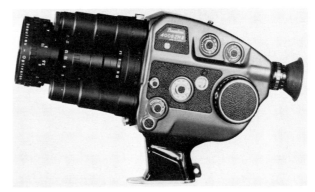

Figure 2
Beaulieu Super 8 camera for cinematography.

Table 2
Cameras and Accessories

Mfg.	Camera	Lens	Image Size
ACMI	Olympus FT (Half frame)	Zuiko 70 mm	10 mm
	Asahi	75 mm	
	Pentax	90 mm	
Eder or R. Wolf	Leica MDa back with	65 mm	15 mm
	Visoflex III	90 mm	20 mm
	Universal focusing mount	110 mm	25 mm
	Olympus OM-1	85 mm	20 mm
Storz	Icarex	Storz zoom	
	Rollei	70–130 mm	
	Robot with Storz Mirroreflex		

Other cameras are available (Table 2) from Karl Storz Endoscopy-America, Inc.; Robot camera with special Karl Storz Verio-lens, from 70 mm to 130 mm; Rollei camera with special Karl Storz Verio-lenses from 70 mm to 130 mm; Polaroid camera with special Karl Storz Verio-lens from 70 mm to 130 mm. American Cystocope Makers, Inc. recommends the Pentax ES-2 as well as all Minolta camera bodies. This manufacturer suggests the Minolta XK, in which the standard focusing screen type P can be replaced with the screen type S, of perfectly clear Fresnel glass. The Eder Instrument Company and Richard Wolf Instrument Company carry both the Olympus OM-1 and the Leica camera with the Visoflex focusing mount and lenses. Each of these companies, however, has special adaptors to fit its own endoscopes.

Fiber Optic Light Sources
Fiber optic light sources are available from all the gynecologic endoscope suppliers in the United States. Some of these sources are diagnostic only and usually employ a 150 watt lamp of the type used in many slide projectors. All of these suppliers have a combination diagnostic and photographic fiber optic power source (Figure 3). The photographic capabilities require either a xenon light source or the 300 watt GE lamp. Some of the manufacturers have bifid cords to attempt to increase illumination; it is even possible to obtain an integrated light bundle which is attached permanently to the endoscope. Although some of the manufacturers call their sources *cold light,* it is obvious that this term is a misnomer since the light projector itself creates a great deal of heat and requires a fan, and, of course, some of this heat is transmitted through the light-transmitting cable. When using the photographic capabilities of fiber optic light sources, high speed Ektachrome daylight ASA 160 film is necessary. The shutter speed is usually set at approximately 1/15 of a second.

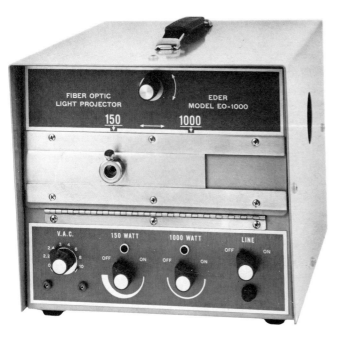

Figure 3
Fiber optic light projector for diagnostic and photographic use.

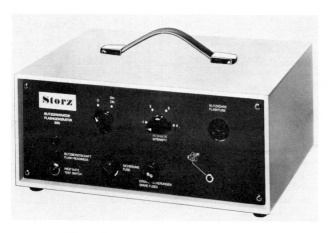

Figure 4
Storz flash generator.

Flash Generator

Flash generators (Figures 4, 5, 6, 7, 8, 9, and 10) are available from all the major instrument companies. My original color transparencies were obtained with the Wolf internal electronic flash (strobe). However, there is great risk in inserting an optical instrument with an electronic flash bulb into the body cavity. Because of possible complications from electric shock and problems of breakage in the plastic housing over the strobe bulb, this type of laparoscope cannot be used in the United States.

Most flash generators employ flash tubes within a plastic mount which is connected to a light pipe attachment to the endoscope. At least two of the manufacturers (Storz and Wolf) (Figure 8) have incorporated electronic flash capabilities into the flash unit itself. With this method a flash is projected through the cable to the endoscope. Obviously this latter technique, although theoretically safer, is certainly less efficient as well as much more expensive to manufacture.

I have had very satisfactory experience with the Storz strobe unit (Figures 4 and 5), which has power increments from one to four. I have found that No. 2 is sufficient for close-up photography, while the No. 4 setting is excellent for panoramic shots. An insulated, completely enclosed plastic housing attaches to the laparoscope, and with this system I have had no electronic problems. With my present Storz flash generator it is necessary to use a separate fiber optic power supply for visualization. Although the Storz flash unit was made specifically for Storz endoscopes, I have been able, with adaptors, to employ it with a 10 mm Eder and Wolf laparoscope, using Ektachrome X film, ASA 64, and we have obtained excellent transparencies, measuring 20 mm in diameter. This same technique, utilizing the electronic flash generator with a plastic enclosed flash tube, may be used to obtain excellent 10 mm diameter transparencies via hysteroscopy.

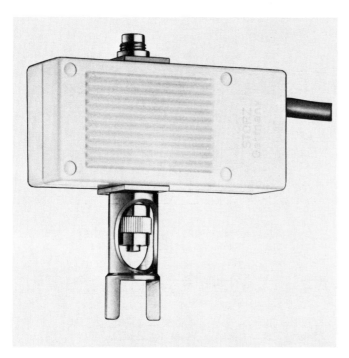

Figure 5
Plastic housing and adaptors containing a flash tube for attachment to Storz electronic flash generator.

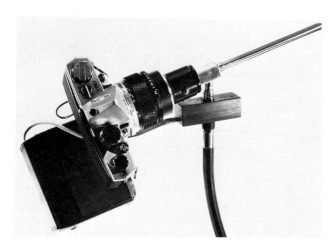

Figure 6
Eder mini-flash attached to OM-1 camera with adaptor to Eder 180° laparoscope.

The Mini-Flash

The Eder Instrument Company has developed a mini-flash (Figures 6 and 7) which can be used with the Vivitar with a charger converter. When fully charged, this very portable unit will deliver from 60 to 80 flashes before recharging is necessary. It is attached to the camera via a synchronization cord. Should the Olympus OM-1 containing the hot shoe be available, the "sync" cord is unnecessary. There also is a setting of *HI* and *LO*. The *HI* is used for panoramic views and the *LO* for close-ups. The quality of transparencies obtained with this portable mini-unit is equal to the proximal flash units supplied by the Eder or Storz companies and is far superior to that obtained with the completely external units.

Fogging of Optics

Obviously, if the optic is fogged with blood or moisture, it is impossible to obtain satisfactory photographs. Before performing laparoscopy and certainly before obtaining photographs it is absolutely mandatory that the optic be inspected, cleansed carefully with a cotton applicator and then warmed with hot towels prior to the insertion of the instrument. Remember, a soiled or foggy endoscope will result in hazy transparencies. Fortunately, no focusing is necessary, and the pelvic organs are always defined clearly.

Conclusions

The problems inherent in endoscopic photography have been solved with the use of improved optical systems with better resolution and better definition. Modern endoscopes employed by gynecologic laparoscopists have more light-transmitting glass fibers of a proper optical density for better light dispersion. Excellent cold light power supplies are available for both routine viewing and cinematography. Reflex cameras can be adapted to all laparoscopes, culdoscopes and hysteroscopes. With the use of electronic flash (strobe), quality transparencies can be made routinely during any endoscopic procedure.

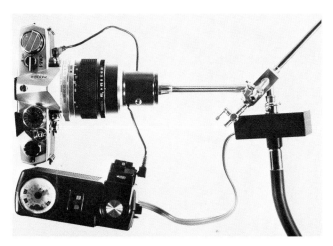

Figure 7
Mini-flash (Eder) attached to OM-1 camera and Eder hysteroscope.

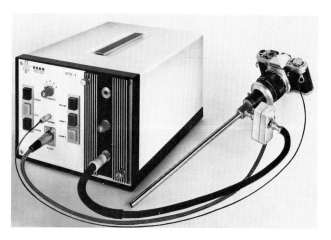

Figure 9
Eder proximal flash generator with fiber optic light source with flash cubicle attached to laparoscope. The camera used is an Olympus OM-1.

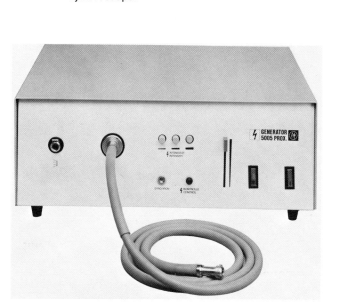

Figure 8
Richard Wolf generator for flash as well as fiber optic light source.

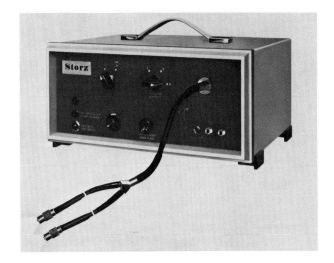

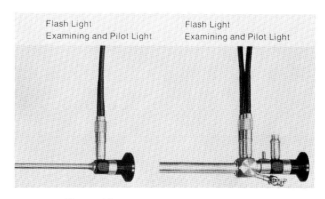

Figure 10
Storz flash generator with fiber optic power supply and twin fiber optic light cables.

Chapter 32

Television in Laparoscopy

A. Albert Yuzpe, M.D.

Laparoscopic visualization of the abdomen and pelvis offers the operator a panoramic view, but this view remains the monopoly of the viewer. This problem can be overcome in part by the use of teaching attachments or sidearms (Chapter 5, Figure 26). However, some or all of the following drawbacks exist with these instruments: (1) a decrease in illumination and image clarity, (2) prolongation of the procedure, depending upon the number of viewers, (3) an inability to obtain photographic records when the "sidearm" is attached, and (4) fragility of the device.

The development of compact and efficient video cameras, first in black and white and subsequently in color, has introduced a new dimension in laparoscopic viewing, instructing and case recording. When the video camera is connected directly to the laparoscope, the number of people capable of simultaneous viewing is limited only by the closed circuit broadcasting facilities and the space necessary to accommodate the viewers. Furthermore, with proper illumination, adequate image definition can be maintained and a permanent record of the findings and surgical techniques can be made. Cost and technical expertise, however, still remain the two major drawbacks to the widespread use of television in laparoscopy.

Criteria for TV Equipment in Laparoscopy
1.   Telescope
2.   Light source
3.   TV camera
4.   Lens system
5.   TV monitor and video recording unit

There are few people who have had any appreciable experience with the routine use of television in laparoscopy. Certain biases are inevitable since when one particular system is found to be suitable, the evaluation of other systems often ceases. The following discussion in part reflects the bias of the author.

Telescope

The largest-diameter telescope, 10 mm, has been the most suitable since the image size and light transmission are greatest.

It is known that each linkage point, or site of discontinuity between the light source and the end of the telescope, results in an appreciable loss of effective light intensity. Thus, the 10 mm laparoscope with an integrated bundle (i.e., permanently attached and sealed to the laparoscope) has been our choice (Figure 1).

The telescope is gas-autoclaved from day to day; when utilized for more than one case per day, it is soaked in cold sterilizing solution in the fashion described in Chapter 6.

Light source

Adequate illumination is essential for obtaining image definition, clarity and true color. In general, two types of light sources are available. The "standard" light source (Chapter 5, Figure 11) is derived from a 150 w bulb, the intensity of which, in most units, may be varied by means of a rheostat which operates independently from the cooling fan. High intensity 1,000 w and xenon light sources, temperature-corrected for "true" color, are also available (Chapter 5, Figure 12). These light sources provide much greater illumination but in our experience have proven more powerful than necessary. In the presence of the moist, intraabdominal serosal surfaces, these high intensity light sources produce glare and reflection which interfere with the vidicon system in the camera, causing "picture wash-out" and possibly damaging the camera.

We have found no necessity for utilizing more than the standard 150 w light source set at full intensity. The high intensity light source is five to 20 times more expensive than the 150 w one. There are some people, however, who feel that for their particular video system the high intensity light source is necessary.

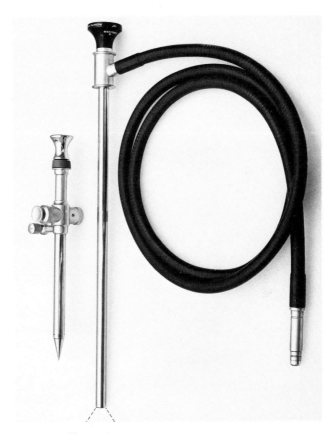

Figure 1
Integrated bundle laparoscope—10 mm.

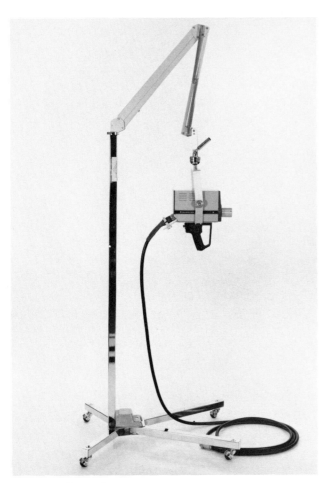

Figure 2
Shibaden HV 1500 TV camera with supporting stand
and counterbalanced arm.

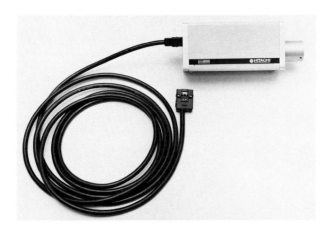

Figure 3
Hitachi HV 9015 TV camera

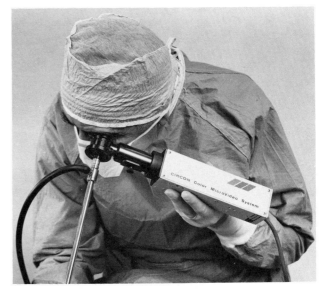

Figure 4
Circon MV 9270 TV camera

TV Camera

Numerous technological advances in circuitry have markedly increased the applicability of television to medicine. One of the major steps is the trend toward solid state design. Consequently, the necessity for large, bulky cameras and receivers has been eliminated. In addition, the high currents and voltages, inherently dangerous, are no longer necessary.

The major criteria that must be met for a video camera to be adaptable to laparoscopic use include:
1.   Small size
2.   Light weight
3.   Ease in handling
4.   Image brightness
5.   Color fidelity
6.   Image clarity and resolution
7.   Low cost

When I first became interested in this aspect of laparoscopy, few compact cameras were available. Constant improvements have resulted in decreased camera size and weight. Although there are numerous color cameras now available, this discussion will be confined to three systems: (1) Shibaden HV 1500, (2) Hitachi HV 9015, and (3) Circon MV 9270 (Figures 2, 3 and 4). The specifications of these units are listed in Table 1. We have had clinical experience only with the first two cameras; the third became available only recently.

The Shibaden HV 1500 was the first camera we evaluated extensively. Because of its weight and size it was not practical to hand hold while operating. Therefore, a counterbalanced sidearm was designed to support the camera and yet allow for a full range of mobility. We also added a pistol grip with an integrated pause control switch for selective recording of video and audio (Figure 2).

With the smaller cameras, such as the Hitachi and Circon, the camera cables connecting the camera to the camera control unit are smaller and lighter. These cameras can be hand held although they may become cumbersome during a long operation.

Lens System

The choice of lens focal length determines the size of the image produced on the monitor and the amount of the monitor screen occupied by the image, i.e., the degree of magnification.

Our choice of a 40 mm lens* is based primarily upon the fact that at the usual working distance from the laparoscope to the anatomical site there is enough of a panoramic view to permit proper orientation and also adequate image magnification, illumination and clarity. This is extremely important during surgery in order to avoid injury to adjacent structures that lie outside the visual field or are visualized inadequately.

The 40 mm lens is employed with both the Shibaden and Hitachi cameras. It is a doublet, binocular lens designed to match the vidicon target area to the exit field angles of the laparoscope eyepiece. This provides optimum coverage of 80% of the monitor screen and maintains the circular format already familiar to the laparoscopist. Unfortunately, there is no built-in iris diaphragm in this lens, and thus no automatic compensation for variation in light intensity is possible. No focusing of the lens is necessary once it is prefocused at infinity, when it is mounted on the camera. The Circon lens does have focusing capabilities.

In our system the lens is attached directly to the eyepiece of the laparoscope, and therefore there is no way for the operator to see through the camera-laparoscope unit (Figure 5). Instead, the operator must view the image on the monitor screen along with the others in the operating theater. Thus, an entirely new dimension in laparoscopic technique is introduced and must be mastered.

An alternative to this technique is available through the application of a beam-splitter unit, which permits direct viewing by the operator while simultaneously televising the procedure. This feature is available with the Circon unit. Such a device could have been adapted to the other units, but the cost would have been prohibitive. Once the operator develops the capacity for operating by observing the monitor, an entirely new concept in visual-spatial appreciation, the necessity for the beam-splitter unit is obviated.

---

* Sterisystems, Ltd., 47 Baywood Road, Rexdale, Ontario M9V, 3Y9, Canada

Table 1
Equipment Specifications

Camera	Camera dimensions (inches)	Weight* (lb)	Camera control unit dimensions (in)	Lens mount	Video system
Shibaden	3.5×4.1×9.3	5.5	13¹/₇×11¹/₄×6¹/₈	C-mount	Single tube vidicon
Hitachi	3¹/₈×3⁵/₁₆×8¹¹/₁₆	3.96	18⁷/₈×5⁵/₈×10⁵/₈	C-mount	Single tube vidicon
Circon	2×2×8	1.25	3.3×19.3×10.5	Type S with C-mount adapter	Single tube vidicon

*excluding lens system

Attachment of the lens to the eyepiece can be accomplished either by a bayonette mount or by means of a collar and screw arrangement. The latter system prevents the lens from becoming dislodged from the eyepiece with sudden lateral motion of the camera: this problem can occur with the bayonette connection in both television and still cameras. The collar is fitted to the laparoscope by unscrewing the plastic eyepiece, placing the collar over the telescope and then replacing the eyepiece. The collar hangs loosely around the instrument but cannot pass beyond the point of the attachment of the fiber optic cable (Figure 6). It need never be removed and is sterilized along with the telescope.

The collar is fitted with a screw thread, as is the inner diameter of the front of the lens (Figure 7). When the lens is placed over the eyepiece of the telescope, the collar is approximated to the lens and screwed tightly into place, thus securing the laparoscope (Figure 5).

TV Monitor and Recording Unit

A compact monitor providing a sufficiently large yet clear image is necessary. We have chosen the Sony CVM 1710 for this purpose. The recorder player unit is a Sony VO 1800. They are mounted on a mobile cart together with the camera control unit (Figure 8) and need never be removed from this unit even during use.

Three-quarter-inch videotape is used because of its size, cassette form, easy storage and handling and good image reproducibility.

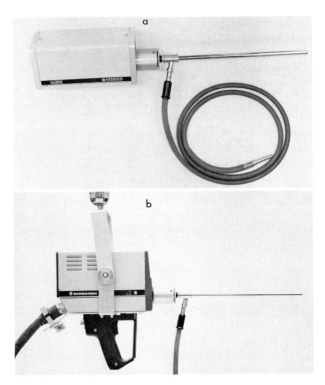

Figure 5
The TV camera lens is attached directly to the laparoscope: (a) Hitachi, (b) Shibaden

Cost

The price of the various components varies considerably. However, it costs about $10,000 to obtain acceptable video recordings with the units discussed. A complete Circon "endo-video unit" package, MV 9890, is available at a similar cost. Additional monitors and video players obviously result in escalated costs.

Conclusion

There is no doubt that constant advances in television technology will provide us with increasingly practical cameras for adaptation to laparoscopy. We consider this medium to be essential in the training of laparoscopists and other medical personnel. Furthermore, it provides a permanent record of any procedure.

Television has added a new dimension to laparoscopy. The laparoscopist can now share his or her findings and operative skills with others by means of this dynamic process, either during surgery or afterwards, as still photographs have never permitted. Television has overcome the visual monopoly of the laparoscopist.

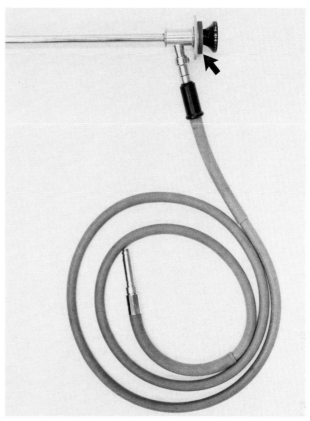

Figure 6
The lightweight collar (arrow) is placed over the laparoscope by first removing the plastic eyepiece. The collar hangs loosely around the laparoscope.

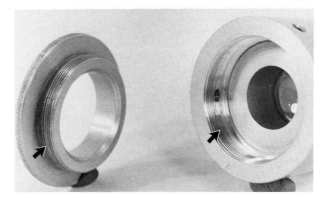

Figure 7
The collar and inner aspect of the lens are threaded (arrows) so that the collar can screw into the lens.

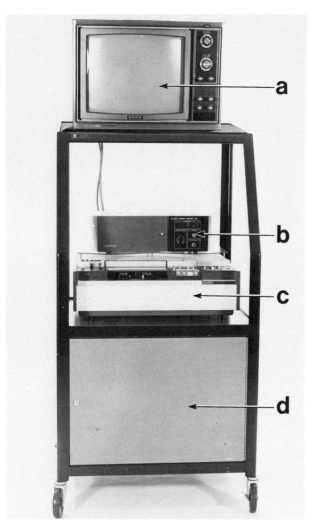

Figure 8
Mobile cart which holds the TV monitor (a), camera control unit (b) and recorder-player (c). A storage compartment is also available (d).

Editorial Comments

The only truly satisfactory television attachment for laparoscopy I have seen was available a number of years ago but unfortunately was priced between $60,000 and $70,000. The newer, lightweight cameras are good but, as yet, far from ideal. The definition on the monitor is not perfect and certainly would not be acceptable on a home television set. Color distinction is adequate but rarely true. The use of a unidirected light makes for highlights and shadows, which tend to distort the picture. Only the Circon camera allows direct visualization through the laparoscope while presenting the image on the monitor. Thus, with all other cameras it is necessary for the operator to learn a new technique: to view and operate while observing the *monitor* rather than looking directly through the camera or laparoscope.

Nevertheless, the television camera is of immense value in teaching laparoscopy. It allows multiple viewers to see the same image, allows permanent recording of procedures and pathology and eliminates the need for a live demonstration during every teaching session. We should look forward to technical improvements that will provide us with pictures as acceptable as those on our home televisions.

C.J.L.

Chapter 33

Legal Liability in Laparoscopy

Jordan M. Phillips, M.D.

There always have been hazards inherent in every medical and surgical procedure. Today, physicians are faced with an ever-increasing probability that their medical judgments and skills will become issues in a malpractice lawsuit, should any complication arise during or following treatment.

This situation applies particularly to relatively new procedures, such as laparoscopy. Whether undertaken for diagnosis or therapy, laparoscopy involves surgical invasion of the human body and therefore is subject to complications and mortality. With many more physicians performing laparoscopy for the first time, there has been a concomitant increase in the number of possible and actual complications, which is resulting in an increasing number of legal actions.

Litigation can be thought of as an octagon (Figure 1): the eight sides are patient, physician, hospital, nurses, anesthesia, medications, instruments and lawyer. The center of this octagon is injury, real or imagined. A legal action may be precipitated from any side. The physician seeking to avoid legal liability will try, of course, to prevent complications. This means anticipating the types of complications that can arise and taking precautions to reduce, if not entirely eliminate, them.

Background: The Malpractice Crisis

A few comments should be made to put the total medical malpractice picture into perspective before we consider specific areas of liability in the practice of laparoscopy.

A review of the literature on malpractice covering the most rapid acceleration in litigation (January 1973–January 1976) reveals virtually nothing current and specific that can help a specialist learn the risks in his or her particular field. Editorials, letters and single-case narratives abound. Most are in state journals, on state experience or legislation. Many are outraged comments; few are detailed studies. The titles are vague and nonspecific or dramatic and attention-getting, such as, "One million dollar award . . . ." There are no easily available or reliable statistical data.

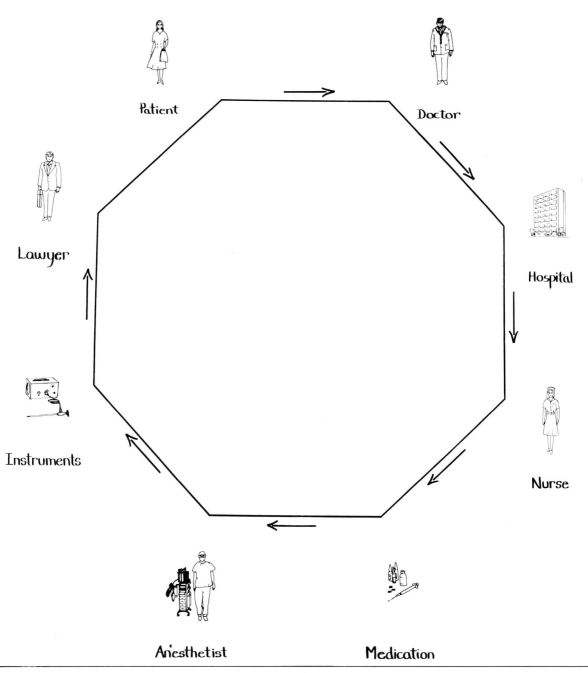

Patient   Doctor

Lawyer

Hospital

Instruments

Nurse

Anesthetist   Medication

Figure 1

In discussions of the medical-legal insurance crisis, many factors have been implicated: great advances in medical technology, with patients expecting cures; an insurance-dependent society that expects compensation for injury; consumerism; the tort system; scared and inadequate insurers; an American public no longer willing to take individual responsibility for illness or recovery; the contingency system for payment of legal costs; greedy lawyers who encourage paranoid patients; punitive and vindictive courts; careless technicians; inadequate manufacturing safeguards. The percentage of blame on each of these factors cannot be calculated, and all may be part of a complex interaction. However, the physician is helpless to change any part of the social and cultural environment surrounding him or her in his or her care of a patient who has a disease: the physician's time is too valuable, and his or her entire attention is needed in the everyday attempts to treat illness and comfort patients.

Physicians almost entirely overlook the common denominator of all malpractice litigation—*injury*. A conspiracy of silence seems to surround this subject. Efforts to define the malpractice crisis point with increasing authority to the subject of injury as the focus for alleviating the crisis.[13] Every study produced to date indicates that there are many times more medical injuries than there are malpractice claims, and the origin of virtually every claim is a physical or mental injury or other adverse result of treatment.[13]

Iatrogenic injury, with death, permanent disability and malpractice judgments as outcomes, must be approached as a disease before it can be controlled. There is reason to suspect that the incidence of medical injury has approached epidemic proportions, which may be another inciting factor in the malpractice crisis.

The initial steps in disease control and treatment are a knowledge of incidence, causes, pathogenesis and predisposing factors. However, no adequate, up-to-date statistics on malpractice are easily available in any field of medicine. Statistics are needed on the incidence of iatrogenic injuries, negligence, compensation, claims filed; percent of claimants judged meritorious, percent receiving payment, percent going to court and percent paid out of court. Data-collecting and data-reporting systems for malpractice information are inadequate. Channels for obtaining this information must be sought, from individual institutions to county, state and national levels. The factors in-

volved must be defined for each specialty and be evaluated repeatedly in each institution. Minimizing the frequency of injuries by obtaining knowledge of their occurrence and risk and thereby reducing their incidence is the surest way to avoid litigation.

In one small, random study of 800 charts from the medical, surgical and gynecologic services of two community hospitals with resident training programs, the overall patient injury rate was 7.5%. Approximately one-third of the injuries were postoperative infections, one-third were other postoperative complications and one-third were adverse drug reactions, treatment errors, falls and other injuries. For each 57 patient injuries, 17 were caused by negligence and one malpractice claim was expected to result. This study provides a model for evaluation of accidents in other institutions.[8]

Figure 2 is a diagram of the outcome in 1,600 malpractice claim files closed by insurers in 1970.[13] (Unfortunately, more recent statistics are not available.) The median payment in that year was approximately $2,000, and only 3% of payments were over $100,000. Thus, the threat is small that a catastrophic claim will be settled against a particular physician. However, we can well do without the expenditure of time, emotional energy and legal fees attendant on every claim.

Infection was the medical emergency of a century ago, and asepsis was the obstetrician Semmelweis's concept that revolutionized surgical and medical practice. Today, medicine's greatest challenges are again in the form of foreign contaminants—not bacteria, viruses or tumors, but machines, currents, power sources and chemicals, elements we as today's physicians understand no better than the physician of old understood bacteria. The past decade and coming ones promise an ever-changing array of mechanical, electronic and pharmaceutical wonders for our use. The potential and theoretical hazards grow faster than the safeguards. Our understanding of each piece of equipment and each chemical we use as well as their synergistic effects is mandatory since we as physicians bear the ultimate responsibility for the patient's safety. The users of this new equipment are also at risk, and employers are liable for injury to employees. Engineers, technicians and surgeons must work together to create *risk-free* environments for our patients and ourselves.

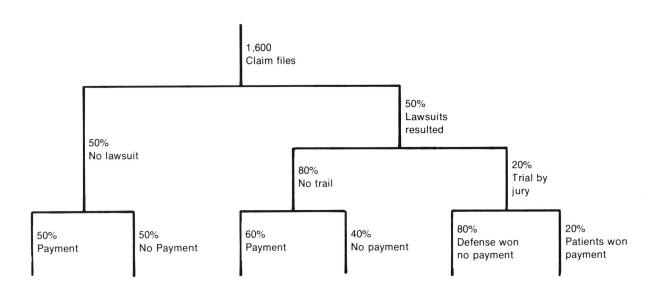

Figure 2
Outcome in 1600 claim files closed in 1970. From US
Department of Health, Education and Welfare.

During his or her hard look at all the causes of the malpractice crisis, the physician's greatest emphasis should be placed where he or she has power and authority to act—in patient safety programs. No matter what course the medical-legal insurance dilemma takes, the malpractice crisis would not exist were it not for injuries, compensable or not, real or imagined. The solution to the problem of patient injury lies within the control of the medical profession.

Litigation Risks Specific to Laparoscopy

A complete list of all complications encountered in laparoscopy would be less useful than mention of the fact that risks attend each phase of a laparoscopic procedure. Periodic review of each institution's experience will point out risks unique to that place and team, while up-to-date knowledge of the literature will familiarize the reader with unforeseen areas of risk. (Several chapters in this book review the most recently collected data and statistics.) A list of the types and incidence of complications should not be considered what any laparoscopist should expect. Rather, it indicates the accidents which special efforts must be made to avoid or preparations made to treat.

Data on malpractice claims involving laparoscopy have not been compiled. However, a general list of potential causes and defenses against legal liability in laparoscopy would include:

Claim or Cause	Best Defense or Deterrent
Electrical—current (shock), heat (burns), static (burns)	Thorough knowledge of principles of current, electricity, electronics. Familiarity with equipment being used. Safety checks of equipment before each use. Alarm systems. Techniques to avoid injury from malfunction. Experience.
Surgical injury of abdominal and pelvic organs, hemorrhage	Immediate recognition and repair or treatment. Consultation by appropriate specialists.
Infection	Asepsis, antibiotic therapy. Recognition of pathology.
Chemical, gas or drug reaction	Knowledge of synergistic action of drugs, current; potentiation of arrhythmias, flammability, embolism, etc. Prevention first, recognition second.
Failure to consult specialist	In event of accident producing nongynecologic complication, consultation with best-qualified consultant available, in addition to complete medical records of event. Remain with patient.
Late complication, especially failed sterilization with pregnancy	Knowledge of potentials, adequate follow-up, informed patient, informed consent on file.
Unnecessary surgery	Informed consent; complete records of indications.
No diagnosis, wrong diagnosis, missed diagnosis, failure to recognize, failure to treat	Complete records of indications, procedures completed and findings, laboratory findings, conclusions. Consultations on file. Careful follow-up.
Psychologic trauma	Careful selection of patient, maintenance of good rapport.
Mechanical injury, including falls, bruises, etc.	Frequent safety checks of premises.

Some injuries are less defensible than others and deserve additional comment. The most common injury encountered during laparoscopy is the burn, of which there are three possible types: external, incisional and internal. The external burn is usually related to inadequate grounding of the return electrode. If the patient is poorly positioned and comes in poor contact with the return electrode, the result can be a skin burn at the limited exit point. A burn around the abdominal incision is probably related to inadequate insulation of instruments. The physician must check the condition of his or her equipment frequently and make use of available safety installations.

The internal burn is still a grey area in terms of lawsuits, but it is safe to assume that there will soon be litigation involving significant burns that led to laparotomy and intestinal resection.[5] Occurring most commonly in the bowel and occasionally in the ureter or a major vessel, this type of burn emphasizes the need for skilled laparoscopists. Williams contends that operative laparoscopy should be attempted only when facility has been achieved in diagnostic laparoscopy.[14] Internal burns also reopen the debate about whether the one-puncture operative procedure is preferable to the two-puncture method. The second incision allows the operative equipment and the telescope to be maneuvered separately, for a wider field of vision and better control of the operative instrument. Physicians using the one-puncture technique (preferred in terms of number of incisions and ease of operation) reported more bowel burns than those using two punctures (Chapter 36).

Each year, several patients receive electric shocks severe enough to warrant emergency resuscitation, and in thousands of hospitals electrical fires are reported. Electrosurgical units are not well understood by many users. In fact, the specific unit in use is often not known by name, and the output power is often unknown, also.[11]

Injury related to pneumoperitoneum is extremely difficult to defend. There is an ever-present risk of embolism, cardiac arrhythmias, cardiac arrest and significant respiratory distress. The physician must be prepared for any or all of these possibilities or he or she will have considerable difficulty defending himself or herself in consequent litigation. Gas tension should be maintained sufficiently to create an adequate space between the abdominal cavity and the abdominal wall throughout the laparoscopic procedure. Devices that permit accurate monitoring of gas pressure and flow will increase patient safety substantially.

Another area of potential liability is aggravation of an injury by delayed diagnosis or treatment of a secondary or tertiary problem. For example, physicians performing laparoscopic procedures are aware that mesosalpingeal hemorrhage can sometimes occur. It may be possible to justify the hemorrhage, but failure to recognize and control it before it causes irreversible damage to the patient is not as defensible. Judge Holder,[2] reporting on a case of cardiac arrest during a laparotomy, showed that the court held the physician negligent for having failed to comprehend the situation.

Closely tied to failure to recognize an injury is failure to treat it rapidly and adequately. This situation can be vulnerable to legal action. A physician may perform a procedure as properly coming within his or her basic training and experience. Even if no liability is associated with the occurrence of an injury, there may be legal liability if appropriate treatment is not instituted in time or if the injury is aggravated. No physician should hesitate to seek consultation or referral for those complications he or she is not adequately trained to handle. Finally, when advice is sought, it should be from the best source available.

Clearly, attempts to avoid legal action should be directed to two areas: (1) avoiding accident, complication or adverse effect; and (2) minimizing the extent of injury once an accident has occurred.

The Litigation Threshold

Any discussion of malpractice should include (but most do not) discussions of reasons for legal action. If many more injuries occur than malpractice suits, secondary factors must influence a claimant's decision to bring suit. The severity of the injury and the financial need of the patient, as well as a breakdown in the rapport between doctor and patient, are known to be determinants.[13] Other areas where the litigation threshold can be raised or lowered can be found in considering the sides of the malpractice octagon.

Patient

Characteristics which might predispose a patient to legal action are: (1) financial need, before or as a result of injury; (2) sex—more claimants are female[13]; (3) misunderstanding of risk or outcome of procedure; (4) frustration with handling of injury or complaint; (5) orientation toward insurance compensation; (6) mental illness; (7) consumerism—patients expecting 100% cures or perfect outcomes.

The careful selection of a patient helps determine the successful outcome of a procedure. We are in the midst of a health care consumerism movement, and there is a growing national trend towards institution of legal action. The physician performing laparoscopy can better protect himself or herself by recognizing that he or she can be sued for doing something wrong *and* for failing to do something. In the report of the Department of Health, Education and Welfare Secretary's Commission on Malpractice, the "human dimension" was given as a common cause of court actions.[13] The reviewers suggested that the quality of the relationship between the patient and the doctor may stimulate the patient either toward or away from filing a malpractice suit. Staying with the patient, even after a consultant has been called in, and adequate follow-up care aid in maintaining good physician-patient rapport.

Physician

Actual malpractice must be acknowledged: it can be due to carelessness, inadequate training, faulty technique, inexperience and other, less definable causes. The physician's first responsibility is to understand what he or she is doing, to anticipate the types of complications that may result from a procedure (despite his or her best efforts) and to be prepared for complications. Specific areas that can influence the initiation or outcome of legal action are: (1) training and experience, (2) medical records, (3) indications and contraindications, (4) informed consent, and (5) negligence.

Training and experience. Complications in laparoscopy usually occur through the operator's inexperience or defective equipment or both. From the moment a physician assumes responsibility for a patient, he or she has a duty to exercise skill and care. Moreover, the physician's practice of medicine implies that he or she is competent according to the accepted standards of the group or specialty to which he or she belongs.[9]

The 1974 survey of laparoscopists detailed in Chapter 36 showed that physicians who had performed fewer than 100 cases had almost four times as many complications as those with greater experience.[6,7] Failed attempts were five times more frequent in those with fewer than 100 case experiences than in those with greater experiences. No matter how many cases he or she has performed or how accomplished his or her technique, the laparoscopist must keep abreast of changes in treatment techniques and should give each procedure the same careful, complete attention. Expertise must not be acquired at the expense of patients or by assuming extraordinary risks of legal action.

Medical records. The physician's medical records on the procedure are vital to his or her ability to offer an adequate defense, should the need arise. A fundamental rule is that good, strong charts equal good, strong legal defenses; incomplete, inadequate or illegible charts equal incomplete, inadequate legal defenses. The State of New York distributed to all licensed physicians a pamphlet entitled "Malpractice Prophylaxis," which stated in part:

> ideal medical records should be kept in every case: a) records that would be acceptable when offered in court; b) records that would clearly show what was done and when it was done; c) records which establish that nothing was neglected and that the given care met with standards demanded by the law . . . .[10]

Ideally, the record of a laparoscopic procedure should document a proper history and physical examination, evaluation of the patient's physical, mental and emotional status, indications and contraindications, meaningful progress notes, accurate and complete surgical reports, the type of anesthetic used and a description of the procedures and instruments used. The patient's chart should indicate the type of gas used, the initial gas insufflation pressure and evidence that gas pressure was monitored continuously during the performance of the procedure. The maximum gas pressure recorded should be included to show that the gas pressure was not excessive. Documentation of every available safety precaution can justify in court that any resultant complication was a "calculated" risk. All complications, major and minor, should be documented properly, with their description, treatment given and consultations requested. Such documentation might prevent malpractice actions from culminating disastrously for the physician: carefully detailed records are viewed as the hallmark of a careful physician.

Finally, the record should show that consent was obtained after adequate disclosure to the patient. The physician is not required to explain every known risk: the law requires that he or she advise the patient of significant hazards that should be evaluated before an informed consent is given.

In malpractice litigation the physician is expected to go into detail about the manner in which he or she treated the patient. His or her competency is going to receive close scrutiny. If the case goes to court, a jury composed of lay people will determine whether a procedure was performed properly and all necessary precautions taken. Therefore, complete notations on the patient's chart, documenting the history of the case from the time of the patient's initial visit, are an absolute necessity.

Indications and contraindications. The indications will be the doctor's best medical justification for performing a laparoscopic procedure. If injuries occur, his or her decision may nevertheless be subjected to malpractice scrutiny. The patient will produce a physician-witness to testify that the procedure was *not* indicated and therefore exposed the patient to unnecessary risk. A controlling factor in the outcome of a malpractice action is whether the procedure was in accord with the medical practice and customs in the physicians' community.

Indications and contraindications have to be considered carefully. For example, laparoscopy may be indicated for an infertility investigation but may be contraindicated because the patient is obese and therefore a prime candidate for complications. If laparoscopy is performed on this patient and a complication develops, a good case can be made for legal liability.

Informed consent. Every state and each country approaches this subject somewhat differently. In New York State the burden is on the plaintiff to prove lack of informed consent.[12] In England, when the patient is made aware of special, known risks before he or she consents to treatment, no liability for any injury results from those risks.[9] German courts consider the patient's consent effective only when he or she was in a position to fully understand the consequences of treatment.[3]

Written consent is required for the performance of surgical operations under general anesthesia. I recommend that consent be obtained in written form for all laparoscopic procedures, including those performed under local anesthesia. The patient's chart should indicate that informed consent was obtained.

The physician should satisfy himself or herself that the patient fully understands the procedure and why it is indicated. In the event of complications, it is difficult to justify a nonindicated diagnostic or surgical procedure. The patient should understand fully that the procedure is not simple. Overplaying the ease of a procedure and the certainty of a cure or outcome is as dangerous as underplaying the risk of the procedure or the possibility of injury. The surgical risks in laparoscopy are somewhat less than for other types of operative procedures (Chapter 14), but the potential for injury or death does exist, and the patient and family should be so informed. The patient should also be fully informed of alternative procedures and their risks and of the consequences of choosing to have nothing done. It full disclosure to the patient is deemed unwise, a responsible family member should be informed and this noted on the chart.[13]

Informed consent should cover the possibility of failure (resulting in pregnancy) when the procedure is undertaken for sterilization purposes. In some states, including California, the parents can institute a "wrongful life" cause of action whereby the physician can be sued to cover the cost of child support and maintenance for 18 years. The physician's protection lies in having informed the patient that the risk of failure, though small, does exist and may even be higher for laparoscopic sterilization than for open tubal ligation. This gives the patient a choice of procedures and the option of deciding which one she wants. If this disclosure does not appear on the consent form, it should be documented on the patient's chart.

Minors cannot give consent. In some states a patient who is 16 years old may give a valid consent; in others he or she must be at least 18 years old. It is expected that every physician in practice will be knowledgeable about the laws of his or her state. In an emergency situation the physician must use his or her judgment about whether performance of laparoscopy on a minor is necessary and then proceed without waiting for consent. To date, the only legal actions decided against the physician involved nonemergency situations.

Negligence. The doctrine of *res ipsa loquitur* can be invoked in the case of burns or other injuries suffered while the patient is under anesthesia.[13] *Res ipsa* applies when (1) an injury is the kind that ordinarily does not occur except for someone's negligence, (2) the conduct or mechanism causing the injury was within the exclusive control of the person from whom damages are sought, and (3) the complaining party is free of any contributory negligence. The law thus permits an inference of negligence, and the physician (to whom the burden is shifted) must prove he or she was not negligent. California courts have extended the use of this rule to apply also in cases of rare medical accidents when there is also some evidence of negligence.

Negligent treatment can take place without resulting in injury; however, if an injury occurs where there is provable negligence, the injury will probably be blamed on the negligence.

Hospital

The physician's choice of hospital and staff is a very important safety measure. The hospital operating room has been implicated as the site of most hospital injuries, and hazard control in the operating room is well defined.[15]

Continuing review of each hospital's safety record and evaluation and control of obvious risks will lessen the frequency of litigation.

Nurses

A carefully trained nursing team is essential to the successful performance of laparoscopy. Nurses aware of potential complications and reasons for litigation can aid in averting legal action. Nurses must be well trained in the use and care of the equipment.

Anesthesia

The risks, necessary precautions and complications of anesthesia are well known. Competent consultants are the laparoscopist's best defense.

Medications

Adverse drug reactions account for a small percentage of medical complications, and their incidence is probably no greater in laparoscopy than in general surgical hospitalizations. Knowledge of every drug used and its synergistic effects is important. Flammable solutions must not be used with electrosurgical units.

Instruments

In this area the injury rate in laparoscopy could be reduced. A recent report has highlighted physicians' ignorance of electrosurgical units.[11] Technical specifications of the 25 electrosurgical generators show many variations in power source, circuitry, output waveforms and frequencies, voltage and watts, and controls and settings. Each laparoscopist is responsible for knowing his or her own unit well.

A Program for Prevention of Laparoscopic Injuries

Laparoscopist

1. Knowledge of potential complications.
2. Thorough knowledge of equipment.
3. Careful selection of patients.
4. Complete patient records, including indications, known risks, unusual occurrences, consultants called in.
5. Discussion with patient and/or family of indications, contraindications, alternative procedures, risks, late complications.
6. Informed consent on file, including discussion with family.
7. Insistence on well-equipped hospital, well-trained team.

Hospital

1. Licensure or certification standards, including continuing education requirements.
2. Training of nurses and technicians in equipment, risks and safety.
3. Thorough check of equipment before each use.
4. Before purchase of each instrument, insistence on safety record, not just sales information.
5. Insistence on equipment industry's taking more responsibility in reducing sources and causes of injuries.
6. Qualified, available consultant staff on call for nongynecologic emergencies.
7. Active medical injury prevention program:
   (a) Analysis of each accident, whether injury occurred or not.
   (b) Development of measures to minimize risk of injuries from accidents.
   (c) Development of alarm systems during use of equipment.
   (d) Safety checklist for preoperative and postoperative evaluation of equipment and premises.

(e) Identification of persons, situation, procedures or equipment likely to give rise to accident and injury.

(f) Involvement of an engineer in safety program.

In law there is no guarantee of the outcome of a malpractice action, just as in medicine there is no guarantee that the patient will survive, complication-free. The physician's safeguard lies in his or her awareness of the variety of events that can bring about legal liability in laparoscopy.

References

1. Curren WJ, Shapiro ED: *Law, Medicine, and Forensic Science.* 2nd ed., Little, Brown & Co, Boston, 1970, p 524

2. Holder AR: Law and medicine: "cardiac arrest." JAMA 216:2217, 1971

3. Knappen FJ: Legal problems of endoscopy. Presented at the 2nd European Congress of Endoscopy, Konstanz, West Germany, April 1975

4. Laufman H: Operating room hazard control. Arch Surg 107:552, 1973

5. Mills DH: Legal implications of laparoscopic complications. Presented at the First International Congress, American Association of Gynecologic Laparoscopists, New Orleans, Louisiana, November 1973

6. Phillips J, Keith D, Keith L, Hulka J, Hulka B: Survey of gynecologic laparoscopy for 1974. J Reprod Med 15:45, 1975

7. Phillips J, Keith D, Hulka J, Hulka B, Keith L: Gynecologic laparoscopy in 1975. J Reprod Med 16:105, 1976

8. Pocincki LS, Dogger SJ, Schwartz BP: The incidence of iatrogenic injuries. In Appendix, US Dept of HEW, Common Med Malpractice

9. Polson CJ, Gee DJ: *The Essentials of Forensic Medicine.* 2nd ed., Pergamon Press, Oxford, 1973

10. Proceedings, 1969 National Medicolegal Symposium, jointly sponsored by the American Medical Assoc and the American Bar Assoc, Las Vegas, Nevada, March 1969

11. Rioux JE, Yuzpe AA: Know thy generator. Contemp Obstet Gynecol 6:52, 1975

12. Trout ME: New York State malpractice legislation. J Legal Med 3:26, 1975

13. United States Department of Health, Education, and Welfare: Report of the Secretary's Commission on Medical Malpractice. Publication No. (OS) 21–25, 73–88.89 Washington, D. C., Government Printing Office, January 16, 1973

14. Williams PP: Avoiding laparoscopic complications. In *Gynecological Laparoscopy: Principles and Techniques.* (JM Phillips, L Keith, Eds.) Stratton Intercontinental Medical Book Corp, New York, 1974, p 117

Editorial Comments

Each and every operative procedure has its legal ramifications, and this is particularly true for laparoscopy. Dr. Phillips has pointed out the potential legal hazards of this procedure.

Several points should be stressed. Care must be given to the selection of the patient, particularly one who is to have a sterilization procedure. There is no substitute for "informed consent," which must be complete; furthermore, the record of such information must be documented for future reference. (A conversation, no matter how complete, is forever lost unless recorded or substantiated by a third party.) Information is best conveyed to the patient by means of some audiovisual technique: a tape, pictures, a printed page. All potential complications must be outlined in such a fashion as to provide information without frightening the patient unnecessarily. Once she has been advised, the patient must convey in written form an understanding and acceptance of the procedure.

The physician must not perform a procedure for which he or she has not been trained properly; there is little defense for inexperience or inadequate training. The equipment must be appropriate and in good working order. Although the hospital may purchase and provide such equipment, it is the responsibility of each physician to understand each element and to be certain of its proper functioning. Reliance on the opinions of others is hazardous since the ultimate responsibility is the physician's.

Once complications occur, they must be recognized, recorded and treated adequately. Consultation must be sought when necessary, and the patient and family must be so informed. An attempt to "cover up" is prima facie evidence of wrongdoing.

In short, to avoid a malpractice lawsuit, try to know your patient; choose the appropriate procedure for the patient; check for contraindications; inform the patient fully, in a fashion that can be documented; be sure to get written consent; be experienced and properly trained in the procedure; know the equipment; pay attention to details; recognize complications; treat complications promptly and adequately; obtain a consultation freely; maintain a good and honest rapport with the patient.

C.J.L.

Chapter 34

Nongynecologic Laparoscopy

Burton H. Smith, M.D.
Arthur I. Goldstein, M.D.

Introduction

In spite of the fact that most gynecologists will explore the upper abdomen manually at the time of laparotomy, all too often the gynecologic laparoscopist will have neglected to direct his or her instrument in a cephalad direction. In an era of over specialization the gastroenterologist can often be accused of the converse. The laparoscope provides the physician with an excellent opportunity to explore a significant portion of the peritoneal cavity, and it is the purpose of this chapter to elaborate on the value of this approach.

Indications for Total Abdominal Peritoneoscopy

It is the opinion of the authors that the entire abdomen should be visualized routinely whenever possible. Indications for pelvic laparoscopy have been discussed elsewhere and therefore will not be reviewed in this chapter. There are several specific indications for directing the laparoscope in the cephalad direction. The use of this technique allows for evaluation of the morphology of the liver, spleen, gall bladder (Figure 1), stomach, bowel, mesentery and parietal peritoneal surface and for the evaluation of ascitic fluid accumulation of undetermined etiology. Observation of these organs may allow biopsy material to be obtained from areas most representative of the potential disease state. This technique also allows for infusion of contrast material in the biliary ductular system for diagnostic studies. It is of interest that laparoscopy may expedite or prevent exploratory surgery when done as an emergency procedure in cases involving intraabdominal trauma in which there is suspected laceration of abdominal viscera, particularly the liver or spleen.

In some hospitals the only individuals who perform laparoscopy are the gynecologists. The gastroenterologist may therefore call upon him or her to define or confirm the existence of some form of infiltrative disease of the liver and/or associated organs and frequently to obtain tissue from these areas for histologic examination. The patient selected for direct visualization and a possible biopsy is one in whom a liver scan may reveal nonhomogeneous uptake of radioactive nuclide with or without hepatomegaly or a homogeneous uptake of the radionuclide with hepatomegaly, or a focal defect observed in an enlarged or normal-sized liver. While the liver scan is a good screening procedure, infiltrative lesions have been found in the presence

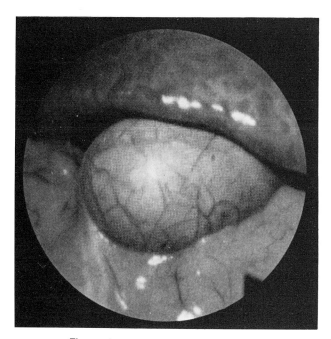

Figure 1
Normal liver and gallbladder

of a normal liver scan in a significant number of cases. Where liver scan may reveal a lesion, it is often difficult to diagnose such specific entities as fatty metamorphosis, tumor (whether it be primary or secondary), granulomatous disease, cystic disease and abscess (whether it be pyogenic or amebic) and/or amyloid infiltration. Obviously, laparoscopy would be ideal for such a situation.

A less frequent indication for the gastroenterologist is the performance of transhepatic cholangiography utilizing the directed vision of the peritoneoscope. This procedure may be extremely helpful in determining the presence or absence of an anatomical obstructive lesion of the intra- or extrahepatic biliary tree. If an apparently normal ductular system is demonstrated in a patient with jaundice, then intrahepatic cholestasis is probably present, and it points toward primary liver disease. The ductular system in and around the hilum of the liver is usually larger than those in the periphery. Under direct visualization the needle catheter may be directed toward the hilum of the liver, and in this manner one may experience a greater degree of success in demonstrating a normal intrahepatic ductular system than by blindly inserting a needle in the liver bed trying to pick up peripheral ducts.

Peritoneoscopy as an adjunct for staging Hodgkin's lymphoma and non-Hodgkin's lymphoma is now being considered. It is argued that percutaneous needle liver biopsy is a valuable adjunct in the diagnosis or staging of such a disease. Directing a needle to an area of abnormality will bring with it a greater degree of accuracy. In the case of Hodgkin's and non-Hodgkin's lymphoma one can also observe the spleen for tumor nodules there. Laparoscopy with guided biopsy of the liver may establish the disease state of Hodgkin's lymphoma with the same degree of accuracy as wedge biopsy of the liver obtained at the time of laparotomy. Bagley[1] and associates have shown that in 46 cases of non-Hodgkin's lymphoma 40% were proven by percutaneous needle liver biopsy. An additional 27% of the remaining cases, after negative percutaneous needle liver biopsy, were diagnosed with positive tissue following peritoneoscopic examination with direct, guided needle liver biopsy.

When one is concerned with metastatic cancer involving the liver (Figure 2), it has been shown that percutaneous blind needle biopsy may permit a positive yield of approximately 31%, which will increase an additional 13% if a second biopsy is obtained at that particular time. Laparoscopically guided needle biopsy should give a positive diagnosis in at least 69% with one single biopsy.[5] Cytologic examination of this tissue will increase the yield by 15%.[4] The yield will be still higher if one obtains representative samples from the right and left lobes of the liver. It should be noted that cancer nodules may not always appear on the surface of the liver. Ozarda and Pickren[7] have estimated that at least 11% of hepatic metastasis is not visible on the liver surface.

Precautions and Contraindications

Much of this subject will be discussed in another part of this book. In the case of patients with suspected upper abdominal disease states there are certain additional, potential problems which must be considered prior to performing the laparoscopic procedure. Many of these patients have some form of liver disease, and a prothrombin time and partial thromboplastin time, therefore, are mandatory. The laparoscopic procedure with accompanying tissue biopsy should not be performed if the prothrombin time and the partial thromboplastin time are greater than 50% of control. A significant number of these patients may exhibit thrombocytopenia, which may be due to hypersplenism, bone marrow disease or subclinical consumption coagulopathy. An absolute contraindication to the procedure with tissue biopsy is, therefore, a platelet count below 50,000. If the information to be obtained may influence the therapeutic course of the patient, fresh frozen plasma may be given during the peritoneoscopic examination to correct the altered partial thromboplastin time. In addition, if indicated, packed platelet transfusion may be given. Obviously, in such cases tissue biopsy is a dangerous procedure. Biopsy would also not be recommended in the presence of multiple cysts of the liver, apparently hemangiomatous lesions and vascular tumors. In the case of the apparently vascular tumor there may be considerable bleeding, which may be difficult to control.

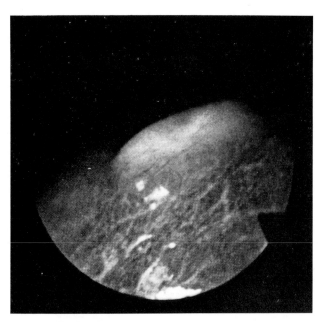

Figure 2
Metastatic cancer involving liver

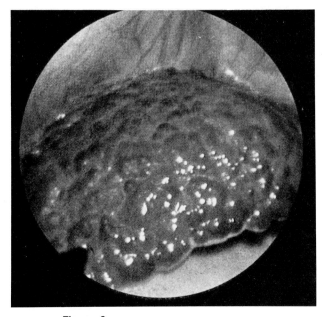

Figure 3
Cirrhosis of the liver

Gynecologic laparoscopists are not infrequently taught that gross ascitic fluid accumulation is a contraindication to the performance of the laparoscopic procedure. The rationale for this statement is that there might be associated adhesions involving the adherence of small bowel to itself and to the anterior abdominal wall which will increase the incidence of bowel perforation when inserting the Veress needle or the trocar. In the experience of the gastroenterologist this has been an infrequent occurrence. For the gastroenterologist, ascites of undetermined etiology is an indication for the performance of laparoscopic examination, provided that caution is employed. It is of particular value in the diagnosis of intraperitoneal tuberculosis and cancer, which may involve the mesothelial surface of the parietal peritoneum. It is not infrequent to find that ascitic fluid accumulation may be due to cirrhosis (Figure 3) of the liver, which may or may not be complicated by superimposed tumor. Klaus[6] and associates reported 19 patients at laparoscopic examination with ascites of undetermined etiology as the primary indication; ten had cancer, seven had cirrhosis, one had tuberculous peritonitis and one had a benign ovarian tumor. It is interesting to note that six patients with a normal-appearing liver upon scan harbored cancer, and in five patients who harbored cirrhosis the uptake on liver scan was reported as normal. Because of the increased danger of perforation of the bowel in the case of cancer or tuberculosis it is recommended that one obtain a small bowel barium x-ray examination. If there is evidence of fixation of intestine by this examination, then one must consider the increased hazard of a laparoscopic examination.

Techniques

Whereas pelvic peritoneoscopy has been performed by the gynecologist in the operating room under general anesthesia with aseptic conditions, the gastroenterologists at our institution employ local anesthesia in a special endoscopic suite. The abdominal wall is prepared and draped, and the laparoscopist scrubs and puts on a gown and sterile gloves. A surgical mask is employed. Analgesia is provided by a drip infusion of a combination of meperidine hydrochloride (Demerol) and diazepam (Valium). Selected skin site is usually in the midline either approximately 2.5 cm above or 2.5 cm below the umbilicus. Location of insertion of the trocar will vary depending upon individual circumstances. For example, if an intraabdominal mass is present in one area, then another area will be employed for the insertion. The selected location is infiltrated with a local anesthetic and a 1.5 to 2.5 cm linear incision is made. A pneumoperitoneum needle is then inserted through this incision. Caution must be exercised when employing the meperidine hydrochloride-diazepam drip. Some of the patients are in the older age group, with coexisting medical problems such as chronic lung disease and/or obesity with hypoventilation syndrome. These people may be very sensitive to the combination of the above-mentioned pharmaceutical preparations which, if not given judiciously, will result in respiratory arrest. The amount of medication given, therefore, will vary greatly depending upon the age and health of the particular patient. The best way to monitor the drip is to allow two to three minutes of time to elapse after a given amount is administered. This allows time to determine the effect of the concentration given prior to continuing with the administration of the analgesia. Room air, compressed air or nitrous oxide is used as the insufflating gas rather than carbon dioxide, for reasons which will be discussed later. After appropriate insufflation is obtained, the pneumoperitoneum needle is removed and a trocar and sheath inserted. The laparoscope is then introduced. Visualization of the abdomen should be performed in a systematic fashion. Blind spots are located primarily on the infradiaphragmatic surface and in the most lateral portions of the right lateral margin of the right lobe of the liver. A probe may be employed to elevate the right and left lobes of the liver in order to see its inferior surface. In this manner one might be able to observe infiltrative disease which may not manifest itself over the anterior aspects of the liver surface. The caudate lobe, as well as the gallbladder, may be observed by this method. The gallbladder should be inspected for evidence of prior pericholecystic disease, tumor infiltration, hydrops and acute inflammation. It should be stressed that in the case of a normal-sized liver the only safe route for needle biopsy of the left lobe is under the guidance of the laparoscope.

When one elevates the left lobe of the liver, it is possible to observe the serosal surface of the distal pylorus of the stomach and follow the distal portion of the body of the stomach. On occasion one may be able to visualize the lesser or greater curvature of the anterior stomach wall up to the diaphragmatic hiatus. The grasping forceps can be employed to pull the omentum in a suitable direction in order to view these areas.

Visualization of the spleen may be difficult. One maneuver which occasionally improves visualization is to tip the patient into the right lateral position and allow the splenic flexure of the colon and omentum to fall away from the spleen. Suspicious lesions in the liver can be biopsied under direct observation. Fluid-filled cavities are best not drained since there may be continued leakage. If echinococcous disease of the liver is suspected, drainage obviously would be contraindicated for fear of spill.

In the case of suspected obstruction of the extrahepatic biliary tree the laparoscope has proven extremely valuable for delineation of primary tumors of the liver and/or metastatic tumor. If liver involvement by tumor is not observed, one can then perform a second percutaneous puncture or even use an operating laparoscope for placement of a needle catheter into the area of the hilum of the liver. One can also insert the needle transhepatically into a dilated gallbladder, decompress it and then infuse contrast material. In the case of obstruction of the extrahepatic biliary tree when the gallbladder is large and metastatic disease is observed on the liver surface and/or parietal peritoneal surface, a needle catheter with a distal inflatable balloon may be placed into the gallbladder bed. Contrast material may then be inserted to try and delineate the level of the obstruction and, by the configuration of the contrast material, the nature of the obstructing lesion. The catheter then may be attached to the skin for drainage.

In the vicinity of the right lower quadrant, although the appendix cannot usually be visualized, one can observe for adhesions which may represent acute or chronic inflammatory reaction. One may also observe for evidence of ischemic bowel disease, Crohn's disease and indirect evidence of pancreatitis. Indirect evidence of pancreatitis has been characterized by waxy spots observed on the greater omentum. Biopsy material obtained from these formations have revealed histopathologic features characteristic of steatonecrosis.[3]

In the past, numerous laparotomies were performed on patients with suspected intraabdominal trauma in oder to determine if bleeding from the liver or spleen was occurring. Laparoscopy of the upper abdomen has been employed at Orange County Medical Center to accurately determine if there is intraperitoneal bleeding, and thus spare the patient a laparotomy, or to hasten a laparotomy if bleeding is observed (Chapter 12). All patients with abdominal trauma have a peritoneal dialysis catheter placed in the abdomen with infusion of 250 to 500 cc of saline. Depending upon the content and color of the return, a decision is made about whether the patient should have immediate laparotomy versus laparoscopy. In the instance of penetrating trauma, laparotomy is usually performed immediately. In all cases the laparoscope is introduced 2 to 3 cm above the umbilicus. The surgeons employ a systematic approach which includes visualization of the right lobe of the liver and gallbladder and then the left lobe of the liver and stomach. The stomach is more easily visualized if nasogastric decompression is performed prior to laparoscopy. The left upper quadrant is best inspected with the patient turned 30° to the right. A second puncture is often made for an instrument which could be used to move the omentum away from the vicinity of the spleen. The bowel is inspected by means of direct overhead visualization. Initially laparotomy was performed on all patients undergoing laparoscopy. As confidence was gained, many patients could be spared the laparotomy. Although the spleen cannot usually be visualized completely, the tip of the spleen is usually identified; if blood is superior to it or under the omentum, splenic injury is usually found. Jejunal perforation is diagnosed by observing small bowel contents along the gutters and small bowel serosal inflammatory changes. In 10 patients with blunt trauma, laparoscopy revealed negative findings, and all 10 were spared a subsequent laparotomy.

Complications of Peritoneoscopy

Complications of pelvic laparoscopy will be discussed elsewhere. This chapter will be confined to complications which are specifically related to exploration of the upper abdomen. Vilardell and associates reviewed complications of pneumoperitoneum for liver biopsy and cholangiography in 1,455 cases.[8] There was a total of 17 major complications, which included: five subcutaneous emphysemas, one pneumothorax, one pneumocolon, one gallbladder perforation, one colon perforation, one puncture of hydatid cyst, four hemorrhages and three hepatic comas.

Prior to the insertion of the pneumoperitoneum needle, complications can be seen in some of the patients receiving analgesia by means of a merperidine hydrochloride-diazepam drip. Respiratory arrests have occurred using moderate amounts of this combination. In such cases, mouth-to-mouth ventilation and intravenous administration of naloxone hydrochloride (Narcan) result in rapid awakening and restoration of normal respirations. Debilitated patients and/or older patients are extremely sensitive to small doses of analgesics. We have also noted patients who developed hypotension and tachycardia supposedly because of hypersensitivity to even small doses of these drugs.

Complications occurring during introduction of the Veress needle, trocar and sheath are similar to those found when performing routine pelvic laparoscopy. The most significant complication incurred by the gastroenterology service occurred when laparoscopy was performed on a patient with a hypogastric vertical midline surgical scar. In spite of the fact that the pneumoperitoneum trocar was inserted in the supraumbilical area, insertion of the laparoscope revealed perforation of the bowel. It was confirmed at surgery, at which time it was noted that there were massive adhesions, with bowel adherent against the anterior abdominal wall. In another case the patient complained of severe abdominal pain at the time of gas insufflation. The procedure was discontinued,

and abdominal x-rays revealed large amounts of air in the intestinal tract. There was no further treatment, and the patient suffered no sequelae. As previously mentioned, room air is used to establish pneumoperitoneum. Many attempts were made to administer carbon dioxide, and almost invariably during the filling period there were complaints of severe abdominal pain and/or shoulder pain by the patient. Some of these patients also developed cardiac arrhythmias. For these reasons room air has been employed successfully. Air is pumped in by hand via bulb, or compressed air is insufflated via automatic insufflator technique. Pain and cardiac arrhythmia have not been a problem when using room air. The only complication to date with room air is that of a patient who suddenly complained of chest pain bilaterally. Auscultation of the thorax revealed diminished breath sounds. The procedure was discontinued, and chest x-ray revealed bilateral pneumothorax. The patient was treated with chest tubes and recovered uneventfully. Subsequent upper gastrointestinal barium x-ray examination revealed a large esophageal gastric hiatal hernia. Of interest is that Chaturachinda[2] used a similar air insufflation technique for laparoscopic sterilization on 1,000 patients in Thailand with negligible morbidity.

Most of the major complications experienced in upper abdominal laparoscopy are related to surgical procedures. Most common is bleeding from the liver following needle biopsy. Usually the bleeding is negligible, but on occasion one may observe pulsatile bleeding from the liver bed for as long as two to three minutes. In all cases to date the bleeding spontaneously stopped, and no patients have required blood transfusions. Biopsies from other areas, such as gallbladder, omental lymph nodes and infiltrative splenomegaly, have not caused significant bleeding. Peritonitis may occur if the gallbladder is entered and there is no decompression of the intracystic contents or if the catheter slips out of one of the major bile ducts. This complication is minimized if the biliary system is decompressed by aspiration and then the catheter is sutured to the external abdominal wall. Bile spillage may be reduced further by using a narrow Foley-type catheter, which can be insufflated, thus making it much more difficult for the catheter to slip out of place. Although spillage of bile is potentially dangerous, we have not infrequently observed anywhere from 100 to 300 cc of bile actually spilled in the intraperitoneal cavity with no unto-

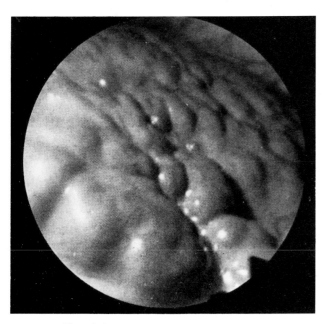

Figure 4
Granulomas over the anterior aspect of the right lobe of the liver.

ward sequelae. Postperitoneoscopy complications are rare. In our experience we have had two patients who have developed elevated temperatures associated with leukocytosis or abdominal pain following the procedure. In both of these cases the liver bed had been entered and contrast material was inserted to study the intra- and extrahepatic biliary tree system. Both cases had findings consistent with stenosing cholangitis, and *E. coli* organisms were cultured from the blood of both patients. Antibiotics were employed with favorable response in both instances.

Discussion

In an era of increasing specialization the gynecologic laparoscopist must not lose sight of the fact that the laparoscope in the abdomen provides a golden opportunity for visualization of the entire peritoneal cavity. Likewise, the gastroenterologist-endoscopist must not neglect the pelvic region. For example, a Mexican female presented with an anesthetic skin lesion over the extremities. Histologic examination of skin biopsy was consistent with Hansen's disease. In the course of the patient's workup an alkaline phosphatase determination was elevated, and subsequent liver scan revealed hepatosplenomegaly. Peritoneoscopic examination revealed tiny, white elevated areas over the anterior aspect of the right lobe of the liver (Figure 4). Biopsy was obtained, and subsequent microscopic examination was consistent with mycobacteria leprae. The gastroenterologist then turned the laparoscope 180°, and a large right ovarian cyst was visualized.

In another instance a white female had abdominal pain and clinical jaundice. Laboratory workup pointed to a diagnosis of extrahepatic obstruction of the biliary tree. Laparoscopy revealed the liver to be greenish and mottled. A transperitoneoscopic cholangiogram was performed which revealed a constricting lesion of the common bile duct. Again the instrument was turned 180° to observe the pelvic region, and an ovarian cyst was noted which, on subsequent resection, turned out to be a benign cystic teratoma.

We recently reviewed our experience with our last 70 female patients, ranging in age from 18 to 79, who underwent laparoscopy for nongynecological indications. Fifteen were discovered to have previously undiagnosed pelvic pathology. The most common pathology noted was ovarian cysts and chronic infection of the adnexa.

Many of the gynecologists on our service have joined in this ecumenical spirit and routinely visualize the liver and gallbladder at the time of pelvic laparoscopy. In some patients with gonococcal salpingitis, perihepatic adhesions have been seen. As previously mentioned, the general surgeons are turning the laparoscope in all directions and have reduced the number of laparotomies heretofore performed routinely after abdominal trauma.

In summary, laparoscopy provides an excellent opportunity for exploration of the entire peritoneal cavity, and this opportunity should not be wasted.

References

1. Bagley CM, Thomas LB, Johnson RE, Chretien PB, DeVita VT: Diagnosis of liver involvement by lymphoma: results in 96 consecutive peritoneoscopies. Cancer 31:840, 1973

2. Chaturachinda K: Laparoscopy: a technique for a tropical setting. Am J Obstet Gynecol 112:941, 1972

3. Cortesi N, Manenti A, Bruni GC: Diagnosis of acute pancreatitis by peritoneoscopy. Endoscopy 2:108, 1971

4. Grossman E, Goldstein MJ, Koss LG, Winawer SJ, Sherlock P: Cytological examination as an adjunct to liver biopsy in the diagnosis of hepatic metastases. Gastroenterology 62:56, 1972

5. Jori GP, Peschle C: Combined peritoneoscopy and liver biopsy in the diagnosis of hepatic neoplasm. Gastroenterology 63:1016, 1972

6. Klaus A, Gluckmann RM: Peritoneoscopy in geriatric patients. J Am Geriatr Soc 22:193, 1974

7. Ozarda A, Pickeren J: The topographic distribution of liver metastases: its relation to surgical and isotope diagnosis. J Nucl Med 3:149, 1962

8. Vilardell F, Seres I, Marti-Vicente A: Complications of peritoneoscopy: a survey of 1,455 examinations. Gastrointest Endosc 14:178, 1968

Editorial Comments

In this chapter Drs. Smith and Goldstein have broadened the outlook of the gynecologist. While some of us routinely explore the upper abdomen, others limit their activity to the pelvis and lower abdomen. Since laparoscopy has not yet become routine with general surgeons, it behooves us to cooperate with them in every way possible.

As the authors pointed out, most visible upper abdominal pathology is related to the liver; the spleen is difficult to locate. Liver biopsy under direct visualization can be of great value to the internist and surgeon. The laparoscope (or peritoneoscope) is indeed a valuable tool to all.

C.J.L.

Section 11

Research and New Developments

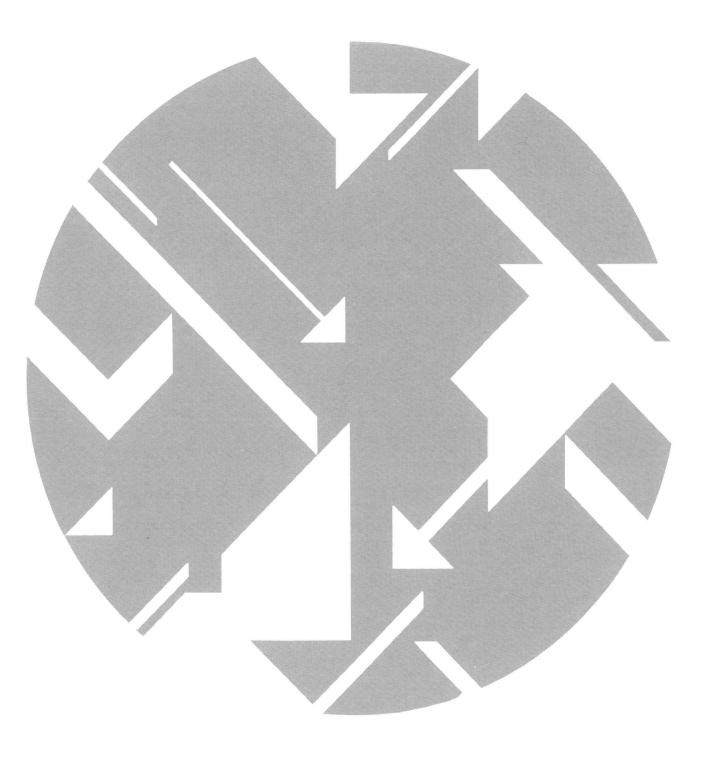

Chapter 35

Laparoscopy in Nonhuman Primates

W. Richard Dukelow, Ph.D.
Satoshi Ariga, M.D.

From the time of the early endoscopic report of Bozzini[3] to the more recent technical advances of Fourestier and associates[8] and Semm,[27,28] people have attempted to peer into the depths of the body to study physiologic function. Human gynecologic laparoscopy has allowed a wide variety of techniques to be applied to this species, including biopsy, tubal sterilization, aspiration, insufflation, lysis of adhesions and coagulation.

In the past six years laparoscopy has become increasingly useful with experimental animals, including the common laboratory species, domestic species and nonhuman primates. Our own studies[6] on laparoscopy in goats and nonhuman primates began in 1969 and, to date, have included laparoscopic examination of the 23 species indicated in Table 1.

This chapter concerns the specific application of laparoscopy to problems associated with reproducing colonies of nonhuman primates maintained for biomedical research applicable to human primates.

Materials and Methods

Animals used: The majority of these studies were carried out on a colony of 104 squirrel monkeys *(Saimiri sciureus)* and a colony of 28 crab-eating macaques *(Macaca fascicularis)* housed at the Endocrine Research Unit at Michigan State University. These nonhuman primates were housed in temperature-controlled quarters at 21 to 26 C. Lighting was controlled on a 12:12, light:dark cycle. The relative humidity fluctuated according to season, varying from 40% to 60%. The macaques were housed individually in 122 cm double-unit modular cages equipped with a squeeze-back apparatus to facilitate animal handling. A visual inspection of the cages was made daily, and the presence and relative amount of menstrual blood was recorded. All data was recorded on a lunar month (28 days, 13 months per year) basis and analyzed on a CDC 6500 computer. A reproductive analysis of this colony after the first four years has already been published.[5]

The squirrel monkey colony was established in 1969 and increased with additional purchases in 1970, 1971, 1974 and 1975. All animals were held, three per cage, in the stainless steel cages described for the macaques until April 1972, when they were transferred to a large community cage 1.2- by 3.0 meters and 2.1 meters high. During

Table 1

Species of Experimental Animals Laparoscoped by Endocrine Research Unit Personnel From 1969 to 1975

Common name	Scientific name
mouse	*Mus musculus*
hamster	*Cricetus cricetus*
rat	*Rattus norvegicus*
tylomys	*Tylomys sp.*
ototylomys	*Ototylomys sp.*
rabbit	*Lepus cuniculus*
mink	*Mustela vison*
chicken	*Gallus domesticus*
dog	*Canis familaris*
cat	*Felis domesticus*
pygmy goat	*Capra hircus*
toggenburg goat	*Capra hircus*
sheep	*Ovis aries*
swine	*Sus scrofa*
cattle	*Bos taurus*
lesser bushbaby	*Galago senegalensis*
greater bushbaby	*G. crassicaudatus*
squirrel monkey	*Saimiri sciureus*
crab-eating macaque	*Macaca fascicularis*
pigtailed macaque	*M. nemestrina*
stumptailed macaque	*M. arctoides*
baboon	*Papio sp.*

the summer and fall of 1975, 24 females and four males were held in two outside compounds, from May 1 to November 10.[15,16] The squirrel monkeys were from two sites of export origin, Colombia and Bolivia.

Limited studies were carried out on a small colony of prosimians, including the greater bushbaby *(Galago crassicaudatus)* and the lesser bushbaby *(G. senegalensis).* In addition to the above, the authors have had the opportunity to utilize laparoscopy in other nonhuman primates at several other laboratories and, where applicable, observations will be included in this paper for comparative purposes. They include observations on the pigtailed macaque *(M. nemestrina),* the stumptailed macaque *(M. arctoides),* and the rhesus *(M. mulatta).*

In addition to the studies described here, the colonies have been used for studies on the adaptation of wild-caught animals to captivity,[13] contraceptive effects of megestrol acetate,[11,12] semen collection[20] and *in vitro* fertilization.[7,22] Complete descriptions of each colony's history, research programs and environmental conditions have been prepared.[10,24]

Laparoscopic technique: Laparoscopic observations were carried out using a procedure first described in 1971[6] and described further in 1975.[5] A 5 mm pediatric laparoscope (Richard Wolf Co., Knittlingen, West Germany) was used for all observations. Initially a Wolf model 4000 light projector was used and later replaced by a Wolf model 5005 proximal light generator. The nonhuman primates were restrained on a tilted laparoscopic table,[18] and abdominal insufflation was obtained with either 5% CO_2 in air or 100% CO_2. Macaques were anesthetized with phencyclidine hydrochloride (Sernylan, Bioceutics, Inc.; 1.5 mg/kg body weight, intramuscular). Squirrel monkeys were anesthetized with 16.2 mg sodium pentabarbital intraperitoneally.

A laparoscopic procedure was developed for the flushing of the squirrel monkey uterine cavity.[1] This procedure, illustrated in Figure 1, consists of inserting the laparoscope midventrally in the normal procedure and laterally inserting a Veress cannula for manipulation of the uterus. A 3.5-inch Kingman alligator forceps (Haver-Lockhart Co.) is then inserted through the Veress cannula puncture site. The forceps grasps the round ligament to steady the uterus while a 25 gauge needle, attached to a 3 ml syringe, is passed midventrally through the abdominal wall. Then 2.5 ml of warmed flushing medium is injected slowly into the lumen. The fluids are recovered through a polyethylene tubing (PE 200, Clay Adams) previously passed through the vagina to the cervical canal. A similar procedure has been described for deposition of eggs into the oviduct.[23]

Ovulation observation and induction: While ovulations have been induced in a limited number of macaques in this colony using clomiphene citrate and various gonadotropin treatments, all data reported here concerns only naturally-occurring ovulations detected by laparoscopy. Conversely, in the squirrel monkey nearly all ovulations have been induced. This species neither menstruates nor shows traditional patterns of cyclical vaginal cytology which permit accurate predic-

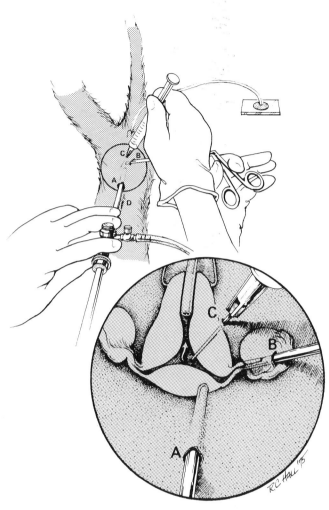

Figure 1
Uterine flushing technique in the squirrel monkey
(inset: A-laparoscope, B-ovary, C-uterus).

tion of ovulation time. Accordingly, a procedure has been developed which allows induction of ovulation in about 60% of the cases.[4] This treatment consists of five days of progesterone (5 mg/day) and four days of follicle-stimulating hormone (FSH) (1 mg/day) with a single injection of 500 international units (IU) of human chorionic gonadotropin (HCG) on the evening of the ninth day. The response to this induction regime is seasonal,[13] and during the months of July, August and September the regime must be altered by increasing the level of FSH.[21] Ova recovered following this regime are normal in appearance, and females receiving the treatment do become pregnant and deliver normal young.[15] Ova recovered following this regime are capable of being fertilized *in vitro* and of developing to at least the eight-cell stage.[7,22]

Results

The mean cycle and menstrual flow patterns for the macaque colony are indicated in Table 2. Also included is an indication of the number of cycles laparoscoped, the total laparoscopic examinations carried out on each animal over a five-year period and an indication of the time of ovulation in those cycles in which it was known accurately. Where the time of ovulation was not known within 12 hours, the data were excluded. Variations in cycle length and menstrual flow length between animals were highly significant (P < .0005). In 1971 the original colony was reduced due to financial pressures. The animals removed were selected on the basis of their variability of cycle and can be identified in the table by their lower numbers of cycles. Of all cycles, 55.6% were subjected to laparoscopy, and an average of 2.3 laparoscopies were done on each cycle.

In over five years of laparoscopy we have seen absolutely no evidence that the procedure interferes with the ovulatory mechanism. Both with macaques and squirrel monkeys, ovulation occurs, fertilization takes place and young are born even during strenuous laparoscopic regimes. As a measure of possible effects we have calculated the mean cycle length (macaques) for the cycle following one in which laparoscopy was or was not used. The results are shown in Table 3. Comparing 586 total cycles, no significant difference in mean cycle length was observed. In an earlier report[25] we emphasized the normal reproductive pattern and return to normal cyclicity of a pregnant animal subjected to a high level of stress with laparoscopy, anesthesia and blood sampling.

Table 2

Reproductive Characteristics of a Colony
of *Macaca fascicularis* Over a Period of Five Years

Female	Mean No.	Cycle Days	Length SE	Mean No.	Flow Days	Length SE	Number of laparoscopies		Days of known ovulation		
							Cycles	Observations	No.	Mean	SE
7	7	28.1	2.5	18	1.6	0.1	9	31	—	—	—
8	3	27.7	0.3	5	1.4	0.2	2	13	1	15.0	0
9	41	34.4	1.0	41	3.1	0.2	18	28	3	16.7	0.9
10	1	27.0	0	1	2.0	0	0	5	—	—	—
11	24	30.2	0.8	34	4.5	0.4	12	15	1	13.0	0
12	32	32.6	0.5	32	4.2	0.4	21	44	3	17.3	0.6
14	21	30.2	0.8	29	2.0	0.2	16	26	1	11.0	0
15	7	33.7	0.6	7	1.6	0.2	5	6	2	18.5	0.5
16	1	29.0	0	3	3.0	1.0	3	5	1	14.0	0
17	17	34.0	2.3	30	2.1	0.2	14	36	—	—	—
18	9	31.4	1.7	12	2.0	0.3	7	38	2	13.5	0.5
25	17	29.4	1.2	28	1.5	0.1	10	38	3	14.7	0.3
26	1	33.0	0	1	1.0	0	11	5	—	—	—
27	7	35.1	1.7	8	2.4	0.3	3	9	1	19.0	0
31	35	29.6	0.5	34	3.4	0.3	13	23	2	16.5	0.5
39	28	36.1	0.8	30	2.9	0.2	12	36	—	—	—
40	33	30.6	0.6	38	3.3	0.2	17	56	3	13.7	0.9
41	36	31.8	0.8	40	2.1	0.1	18	32	5	13.2	1.0
42	39	29.2	0.6	42	3.1	0.2	20	36	4	14.0	0.4
43	46	28.8	0.4	47	3.0	0.2	21	35	4	14.5	0.3
44	48	29.5	0.4	48	3.7	0.2	24	49	6	14.3	0.6
45	1	29.0	0	1	1.0	0	0	0	—	—	—
46	2	30.5	2.5	2	1.5	0.5	1	3	1	13.0	0
51	29	29.4	0.4	39	3.2	0.2	24	69	5	14.0	0.5
52	14	32.2	1.1	27	1.9	0.2	12	42	2	17.0	1.0
53	36	29.7	0.7	39	2.0	0.1	19	38	2	13.5	0.5
54	32	31.4	1.1	33	2.4	0.2	18	29	4	14.8	0.9
55	28	29.9	0.9	34	2.0	0.1	11	19	3	13.3	0.7
	595	30.9	0.2		2.8	0.1	331	766			

Of 138 cycles in which the ovulatory status was known, 124 (89.9%) were ovulatory and 14 (10.1%) anovulatory. The percentage of ovulatory cycles is considerably higher than that reported for rhesus monkeys *(M. mulatta)*, probably due to the tendency for the latter to have anovulatory cycles during the summer months.

Differences in the position of the fimbria relative to the ovary were observed in different species of macaques which have been laparoscoped. In *M. mulatta* the fimbria is in direct apposition to the pole of the ovary and covers it in a cap-like formation. In *M. fascicularis* (and, to a degree, in *M. nemestrina*) the fimbria is more fluid in movement and tends to move towards the ovary as the time of ovulation approaches. No difficulty in the use of laparoscopy was observed in any of these species. *M. arctoides,* on the other hand, is difficult to laparoscope because of its high amount of abdominal fat.

In *M. fascicularis* a definite pattern of follicular development occurs, which we have reported previously.[17] Basically, the start of visual development occurs 24 to 36 hours prior to ovulation at a time concomitant with the luteinizing hormone (LH) surge. At this stage the follicle is characterized by the appearance of a blister-like formation, slightly darkened, with an overall increase in the size of the ovary by about 35%. Later in development a stellate pattern of blood vessels is observed over the surface of the follicle, and at about 10 hours before ovulation the vessels become more pronounced and the follicular cone or stigma is formed. Occasionally the major vessel crosses the center of the follicle, dividing it into two discrete hemispheres, each displaying a localized area of avascular tissue. This type of follicle composed 34.8% of the observed follicles. At eight to ten hours before ovulation the fimbria moves to a position over the follicle, and two to three hours before ovulation a yellowing or luteinization appears at the base of the follicle. Ovulation in this species is not an explosive action but rather a slow release of follicular contents over a 20- to 30-second period. Mass hemorrhage does not occur and, in fact, the blood vessel pattern often persists, without rupture, through the development of the corpus luteum.

Table 3

Effect of Laparoscopy on Subsequent Cycle Length, *M. fascicularis*

	Number	Mean cycle length	SE
No Laparoscopy	334	29.4	0.6
Laparoscopy	252	30.6	0.3

The exact moment of ovulation has been observed and photographed on four occasions in this laboratory.[26] Following expulsion of the cumulus mass the stigmal membrane collapsed. The entire cumulus mass could be seen adhering to the ovarian surface. In one case, after laparotomy to recover the ovum, the viscid properties and adhesiveness of the cumulus mass allowed it to be stretched 1.5 cm before it could be freed from the ovarian surface. Under microscopic examination the ovum was recovered from the cumulus mass.

In the squirrel monkey the vascular changes are not as evident as in *M. fascicularis.* Before stimulation the ovaries are smooth and either uniform in color or slightly mottled. Prior to ovulation the upper portion of the developing blister-like follicle becomes very transparent and, at times, a clear gelatinous peak is seen. Ovulation tends to be more hemorrhagic than with *M. fascicularis,* with the formation of a definite corpus hemorrhagicum. Similarly, in *M. mulatta* ovulation appears to be more hemorrhagic whereas in *G. senegalensis* a pattern more like *M. fascularis* is seen, with vascular development on the follicle.

Using the technique of laparoscopic recovery of uterine fluids from the squirrel monkey, 16 collections have been made, with an average recovery of 73.2% of the fluid injected. To date three ova have been recovered from the uterus at seven days after ovulation. None was fertilized. The procedure can be completed in 10 to 30 minutes and is not difficult despite the small size of the squirrel monkey uterus (8- by 9- by 6 mm; width, length, thickness). One squirrel monkey has been subjected to the procedure eight times without adverse effects.

Discussion

The present studies, initiated in 1969 and carried on continuously to the present time, emphasize the usefulness of laparoscopy as a simple technique to study reproductive processes in a variety of species. Laparoscopy does not exert an adverse effect on ovulation or on subsequent cycle length. An extremely large number of laparoscopic examinations have been carried out in this laboratory on nonhuman primates. Many macaques have been laparoscoped over 40 times, with one animal having been examined laparoscopically 82 times. One squirrel monkey has been laparoscoped 53 times without a bad effect. (For comparative purposes, sheep and swine have been laparoscoped as many as 45 and 25 times, respectively, in this laboratory). Abdominal adhesions rarely occur before 30 to 35 laparoscopies, and even when they do occur they can be corrected by other laparoscopic techniques. As evidence of the soundness of the animals after extensive laparoscopy it should be noted that one animal, laparoscoped 49 times before "retirement," was mated and became pregnant subsequent to the experimental period. Two others, laparoscoped 38 and 47 times, respectively, are pregnant presently.

The usefulness of the laparoscope to study ovulation is evidenced by our studies of normal follicular development, quoted earlier, which have been confirmed by application of the technique to other nonhuman primate species such as the chimpanzee[9] and the rhesus.[2] Koering,[19] using histological techniques, reported that large, well developed follicles appear at about day seven of the normal 28-day *M. mulatta* cycle and have a diameter of slightly over 3 mm. She also stated that at this stage the follicle has a vesicular appearance, with the oocyte located centrally in the follicle. Between days 11 and 13 the follicle diameter has increased to a maximum of 5 mm. At this stage, she states, the follicle has a fully developed antrum and the oocyte is in an eccentric position. At this point the follicle is probably less than three days prior to ovulation and comparable with our report of the final stages of follicular morphology in *M. fascicularis.* In the majority of animals, including macaques, the first maturation division occurs within the tertiary follicle immediately prior to rupture.[14] The heavy precipitate found in preovulatory follicles suggests that the follicular content viscosity is maximal at ovulation. Koering[19] has reported a slow "oozing out" of the secondary oocyte at ovulation, an observation supported by our own observations of four ovulations in *M. fascicularis* and two in *S. sciureus*. The process of expulsion seems to require 20 to 30 seconds.

Summary

Data is provided from more than five years of studies with nonhuman primates using laparoscopic techniques to determine the time and morphology of ovulation. Over 750 laparoscopic examinations were carried out on 55.6% of all macaque cycles (mean of 2.3 laparoscopies per cycle) with no effect on ovulation or subsequent cycle length. Some macaques have been laparoscoped as many as 82 times with no adverse reproductive effect. The usefulness of the procedure has been demonstrated by detailed studies of the morphological development of the follicle in these species as ovulation approaches. A procedure is also given which allows the laparoscopic recovery of uterine flushings (73.2% recovery) and uterine ova.

Acknowledgment

The authors wish to express their appreciation to the Endocrine Research Unit personnel, past and present, who have contributed to the studies reported here. They include Drs. R. M. Harrison, D. A. Jewett, J. M. R. Rawson and D. E. Wildt and Messrs. T. J. Kuehl, D. A. Snyder, C. B. Morcom and J. P. Mahone. This work was supported under NIH grant HD07534, a grant from the National Foundation-March of Dimes and National Institutes of Health Research Career Development Award No. 1-K4-HD35,306. Approved by the Michigan State University Agricultural Experiment Station as Journal series No. 7500.

References

1. Ariga S, Dukelow WR: Nonsurgical (laparoscopic) uterine flushing and egg recovery technique in the squirrel monkey *(Saimiri sciureus).* (Unpublished data)

2. Bosu WTK: Laparoscopic technique for the examination of the ovaries in the rhesus monkey. J Med Primatol 2:124, 1973

3. Bozzini P: Lichleiter, eine Erfindung zur Anschauung innerer Theile und Krankheiten nebst der Abbildung. J der practischen Arzneykunde und Wundarzneykunst 24:107, 1806

4. Dukelow WR: Induction and timing of single and multiple ovulations in the squirrel monkey *(Saimiri sciureus).* J Reprod Fertil 22:303, 1970

5. Dukelow WR: The morphology of follicular development and ovulation in nonhuman primates. J Reprod Fertil (Suppl) 22:23, 1975

6. Dukelow WR, Jarosz SJ, Jewett DA, Harrison RM: Laparoscopic examination of the ovaries in goats and primates. Lab Ani Sci 21:594, 1971

7. Dukelow WR, Kuehl TJ: *In vitro* fertilization of nonhuman primates. La Fécondation. (Collogue de la Société Nationale pour L'Étude de la Stérilité et de la Fécondité, Masson et Cie, Publishers, Paris, 1975, p 67

8. Fourestier N, Glader A, Vulmiere J: Perfectionnements a l'endoscopic medicale: realization bronchoscopique. Presse Med 60:1292, 1952

9. Graham CE, Keeling, M, Chapman C, Cummins LB, Haynie J: Method of endoscopy in the chimpanzee: relations of ovarian anatomy, endometrial histology and sexual swelling. Am J Phys Anthropol 38:211, 1973

10. Harrison RM: Ovulation in *Saimiri sciureus:* induction, detection and inhibition. Ph.D. thesis, Endocrine Research Unit, Michigan State University, East Lansing, Michigan, 1973

11. Harrison RM, Dukelow WR: Megestrol acetate: its effect on the inhibition of ovulation in squirrel monkeys *(Saimiri sciureus).* J Reprod Fertil 25:99, 1971

12. Harrison RM, Rawson JMR, Dukelow WR: Megestrol acetate: II. Effects on ovulation in nonhuman primates as determined by laparoscopy. Fertil Steril 25:51, 1974

13. Harrison RM, Dukelow WR: Seasonal adaptation of laboratory-maintained squirrel monkeys *(Saimiri sciureus).* J Med Primatol 2:277, 1974

14. Hartman CG, Corner GW: The first maturation division of the macaque ovum. Contrib Embryol 29:1, 1941

15. Jarosz SJ, Dukelow WR: Temperate season outdoor housing of *Saimiri sciureus* in the northern United States. J Med Primatol 5:176, 1976

16. Jarosz SJ, Kuehl TJ, Dukelow WR: Vaginal cytology, induced ovulation and gestation in the squirrel monkey *(Saimiri sciureus)* Biol Reprod, 1977 (In press)

17. Jewett DA, Dukelow WR: Serial observations of follicular morphology near ovulation in *Macaca fascicularis.* J Reprod Fertil 31:287, 1972

18. Jewett DA, Dukelow WR: Follicular observation and laparoscopic aspiration techniques in *Macaca fascicularis.* J Med Primatol 2:108, 1973

19. Koering MJ: Cyclic changes in ovarian morphology during the menstrual cycle in *Macaca mulatta.* Am J Anat 126:73, 1969

20. Kuehl TJ, Dukelow WR: A restraint device for electro-ejaculation of squirrel monkeys *(Saimiri sciureus).* Lab Anim Sci 24:364, 1974

21. Kuehl TJ, Dukelow WR: Ovulation induction during the anovulatory season in *Saimiri sciureus.* J Med Primatol 4:23, 1975

22. Kuehl TJ, Dukelow WR: Fertilization *in vitro* of *Saimiri sciureus* follicular oocytes. J Med Primatol 4:209, 1975

23. Kuehl TJ, Dukelow WR: A laparoscopic technique for transfer of embryos in nonhuman primates. (Unpublished data)

24. Rawson JMR: Ovulation in *Macaca fascicularis,* M. S. thesis, Endocrine Research Unit, Michigan State University, East Lansing, Michigan

25. Rawson JMR, Dukelow WR: Effect of laparoscopy and anesthesia on ovulation, conception, gestation and lactation in a *Macaca fascicularis.* Laboratory Primate Newsletter 12:4, 1973

26. Rawson JMR, Dukelow WR: Observation of ovulation in *Macaca fascicularis.* J Reprod Fertil 34:187, 1973

27. Semm K: Gynecological pelviscopy and its instrumentarium. Act Eur Fertil 1:81, 1969

28. Semm K: Das Instrumentarium der gynakologischen Pelviscopie. Endoscopy 2:35, 1970

Section 12

State of the Art

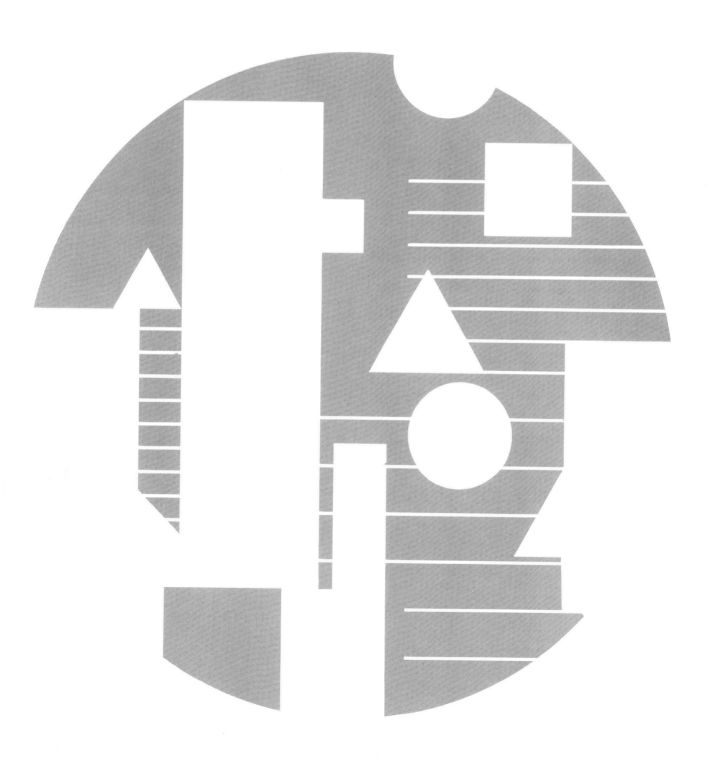

Chapter 36

Survey of Laparoscopy, 1971–1975

Jordan Phillips, M.D.
Donald Keith, M.B.A.
Jaroslav Hulka, M.D.
Barbara Hulka, M.D.
Louis Keith, M.D.

Introduction

The original survey of this Association represented the experience of those individuals who attended the 1972 Congress of the American Association of Gynecologic Laparoscopists (AAGL).[2] Subsequent surveys have taken into account the experience of a growing membership in the United States and abroad.[1, 3, 4] By 1974 the data were the most comprehensive statistical material relating to laparoscopy ever collected and have received international attention. The present report is a continuation of the efforts to monitor the state of the art. The input of all participating members is gratefully acknowledged.

Methodology

Two mailed surveys were utilized along the lines developed previously. The study year of the first was defined as July 1, 1974, to June 30, 1975. Its major sections were: (1) physician experience, (2) preferences in surgical technique, (3) equipment preferences, (4) opinions on equipment, (5) complications and their causes, and (6) other risks.

In order to obtain additional details on pregnancy following laparoscopic sterilization a special questionnaire was utilized in a second mailing. It covered data from 1971–1975.

Sample Size and Response Rates: The first mailing consisted of 1,300 questionnaires. One thousand ten were returned, for a response of 78%. One thousand were received in time for computer processing. As in prior years, all respondents did not complete the entire survey, the result of which was that a varying number of physicians responded correctly to individual questions.

The second mailing consisted of 1,300 questionnaires. Of them, 765 were returned in time for computer processing, for a response rate of 50%. Six hundred and fifty-eight physicians performed sterilizations, and their data are presented in the subsequent analyses.

Results

1. *Physician Experience (First and Second Questionnaire)*

a. *First Questionnaire:* For their entire careers 966 physicians reported 136,094 diagnostic procedures (mean 140.8); 950 physicians reported 241,534 sterilization operations (mean 254.2). Thus, the total experience of these physicians comprises 377,628 operations. For the period under study (July 1, 1974, to June 30, 1975) a total of 113,253 procedures was reported. There were 36,411 diagnostic operations and 76,842 sterilization operations.

b. *Second Questionnaire:* The time of study was 1971 through July 1, 1975. Figure 1 shows that the number of sterilizations in the United States has risen steadily each year. An estimated 76,000 sterilizations will be performed in the calendar year 1975 by reporting members of the AAGL.

2. Preferences in Surgical Technique (First and Second Questionnaire)

a. *Second Questionnaire:* Figure 2 indicates by year the percentage of doctors using different techniques of tubal sterilization. Coagulation, division and obtaining a specimen was the leading technique in 1971 and 1972. Since then it has been superseded by coagulation and division without taking a specimen. Coagulation has shown a steady increase in preference over the years. The percentage of the doctors coagulating, dividing and obtaining a specimen has dropped from a majority of 52% in 1971 and has been replaced by coagulation and division, with a majority (51%) using this technique in 1975. Figure 3 shows increasing utilization of the one-puncture technique. This is in keeping with the increasing use of laparoscopy and the larger numbers of physicians participating in the survey. By 1975 almost one-third of the respondents used a single-puncture technique.

b. *First Questionnaire Data:* Interval sterilizations were greatly preferred to postpartum or postabortion procedures, though 10% of sterilizations were performed in conjunction with pregnancy (Table 1).

Table 2 refers to specific preferences for sterilization operations in 1974–1975. Nonelectric techniques (clip and band) were utilized by 2.1% of the respondents.

Of the physicians who sent presumed tubal tissue for pathologic examination, the majority of respondents (66.3%) stated that tissue confirmation was obtained in more than 80% of submissions. However, almost one-third of the respondents stated that this confirmation was not always bilateral.

Over 95% of all laparoscopies reported as having been performed in 1974 were done utilizing general anesthesia.

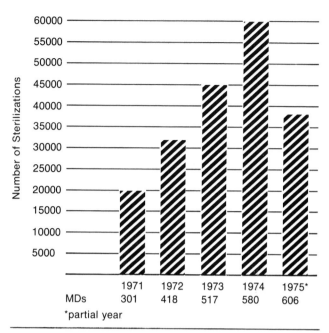

Figure 1
Sterilizations performed annually by AAGL members, 1971–1975

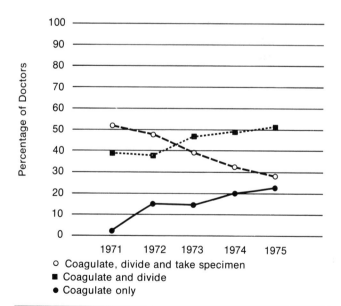

Figure 2
Trends in technique of tubal divisions and/or coagulation by AAGL members, 1971–1975

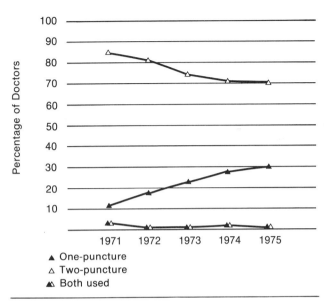

Figure 3
Trends in use of two-puncture versus one-puncture technique, 1971–1975

▲ One-puncture
△ Two-puncture
▲△ Both used

Table 1
Time of Laparoscopic Sterilizations
1974–1975

When Performed	Percent of Procedures
Interval	87.9
Postpartum	5.4
With abortion	5.4
First half menstrual cycle	68.1
Second half menstrual cycle	30.6

Outpatient surgery was accomplished in 24% of the reported diagnostic operations; the remaining 76% were inpatient operations. Such data were not obtained on sterilization procedures.

3. *Equipment Preferences (First Questionnaire)*
Wide variations are still observed in equipment preferences. Table 3 shows that only 17% of the respondents still used spark gap generators; 4% were still unaware of the type of electrical unit utilized in their operative surgery. Bipolar power sources were used by 12% of the respondents.

Cardiac monitors were present in 91% of the operating suites. However, 29% of the respondents did not use them when they were available. Twenty-two percent of the physicians who used monitors have observed cardiac arrhythmias. The occurrence of cardiac arrhythmias was not related to the use of electrosurgical equipment.

4. *Opinions on Equipment (First Questionnaire)*
Table 4 shows that 90% of respondents agree that modern laparoscopic equipment is safe. Eighty-five percent are of the opinion that manufacturers should be liable in case of faulty equipment. Only half (48%) of the respondents were satisfied that the instruction manuals were clear and completely understandable. Even fewer (38.3%) were of the opinion that the persons responsible for the task of laparoscopic equipment maintenance and repair found it easy. Only two-fifths of the respondents (39.4%) were satisfied with the hazard warnings in the instruction manuals. Fewer yet (30.2%) were of the opinion that reading the instruction manuals would readily and easily clarify the potential equipment hazards to patients and doctors.

Laparoscopy   Chapter
36   Survey of Laparoscopy
1971–1975   345

Table 2
Preferences in Technique for Sterilization Operations
1974–1975

Technique	Number	Percent	
Do not perform sterilizations	43	4.3	
Coagulate only, no division	214	21.5	
Coagulate and divide, no specimen	404	40.6	
Coagulate, divide and obtain specimen	306	30.8	
Clip	3	0.3	2.1%
Silastic band	18	1.8	
Other procedure	6	0.6	

(Missing data = 6)

Table 3
Power Source Used
1974–1975

Type Power Source	Number	Percent
Do not perform electrocoagulation	48	4.9
Spark gap	167	17.0
Solid-state	359	36.6
Low voltage	173	17.6
Bipolar	122	12.4
Combination	70	7.1
Don't know	39	4.0
Other	3	0.3

(Missing data = 19)

Table 4
Opinion Regarding Laparoscopic Equipment
1974–1975

Question	No Opinion	Strongly Agree	Agree	Disagree	Strongly Disagree
Modern laparoscopic equipment is safe	27 2.7%	346 35.2%	535 54.4%	65 6.6%	11 1.1%
Equipment manufacturers should be liable in cases of faulty equipment	92 9.3%	336 34.1%	499 50.6%	55 5.6%	4 0.4%
Medical maintenance personnel believe that laparoscopic equipment is easy to maintain and repair	153 15.5%	29 2.9%	349 35.4%	380 38.6%	74 7.5%
Instruction manuals for laparoscopic equipment are clear and completely understandable	173 17.6%	52 5.3%	418 42.5%	294 29.9%	46 4.7%
Hazard warnings are prominently and clearly displayed in instruction manuals for laparoscopic equipment	212 21.5%	33 3.4%	345 35.0%	356 36.1%	39 4.0%
By reading an instruction manual on a piece of laparoscopic equipment you can easily and readily become aware of the potential hazards to both patient and doctor	126 12.8%	27 2.7%	271 27.5%	411 41.8%	149 15.1%

Table 5

Major Complications of Laparoscopy
1974–1975

Complications	Diagnostic Number	Rate/1,000	Sterilization Number	Rate/1,000
Total number performed	36,411		76,842	
Failed attempts	411	11.3	513	6.7
Deaths	4	11	0	0
Laparotomies:				
Bowel trauma	38	1.0	67	.9
Hemorrhage	151	4.1	142*	1.8
Other complications	123	3.4	115	1.5
Total	312	8.5	324	4.2
Bowel burns:				
Recognized	+	+	13	.2
Unrecognized	+	+	25	.3
Total	+	+	38	.5

* Mesosalpingeal tears
\+ No data

Table 6

Techniques Used by Physicians
in Sterilizations Resulting in Bowel Burns
1974–1975

Technique	Number of MDs	Bowel Burns Number	Percent
Coagulate only	175	18	10.29*
Coagulate, divide, no specimen	339	19	4.76
Coagulate, divide, obtain specimen	326	19	5.83
One-puncture	203	17	8.37*
Two-puncture	654	29	4.43

* Significant at a p value of <.05

5. *Complications and their Causes (First Questionnaire)*

Table 5 summarizes major complications experienced in 1974–1975. Diagnostic operations were more hazardous than sterilization operations in most areas of potential complications, including failed attempts, complications requiring laparotomy and death. (Four physicians reported that almost all of their attempts at sterilization ended in failure to complete the procedure; this is so inconsistent with the other physicians' experiences that error in reporting was suspected, and these failures were excluded from this analysis.)

About twice as many bowel burns (25) were unrecognized at surgery compared to those recognized (13). Bowel burns were reported by 71 physicians (7.2%). Ninety-five percent of bowel burns occurred during sterilization procedures. Twenty-one percent of sterilization burns and 33% of diagnostic burns occurred during teaching sessions.

Table 6 shows that sterilization bowel burns were more frequent among physicians using coagulation only compared to coagulation and division and to coagulation with division and the taking of specimens. Physicians using the one-puncture technique had more bowel burns than those using the two-puncture technique; however, this finding was not evident in an analysis of patient data (Table 7). In Table 8 coagulation, division and removal of specimen appears to have the highest rate of mesosalpingeal tears. No other differences between rates of complications and differing techniques were found (Tables 7 and 8).

When complications were related to experience, physicians who had performed fewer than 100 cases had almost four times as many complications (14.7 per 1,000) as those with greater experience (3.8 per 1,000). Similarly, failed attempts were five times more frequent among those with experience of fewer than 100 cases (29.2 per 1,000) than among those with greater experience (5.7 per 1,000). The actual number of physicians with greater (> 100) experience was five times that of those with lesser (< 100) experience—52 versus 87.

Table 7
One-Hole *vs* Two-Hole Technique and Its Hazards
1974–1975

Technique	Number of Patients	Bowel Burns Recognized		Bowel Burns Unrecognized		Other Bowel and Surgical Trauma		Mesosalpingeal Tears		Other Complications	
		Number	Rate/1,000	Number	Rate/1,000	Number	Rate/1,000	Number	Rate/1,000	Number	Rate/1,000
One-hole	13,455	3	.21	2	.14	4	.3	17	1.25	14	1.04
Two-hole	37,605	6	.14	9	.21	10	.27	69	1.83	49	1.30

(Missing data for 342 patients)

Table 8
Technique of Tubal Sterilization and Its Hazards
1974–1975

Technique	Number of Patients	Mesosalpingeal Tears		Bowel Burns Recognized		Bowel Burns Unrecognized	
		Number	Rate/1,000	Number	Rate/1,000	Number	Rate/1,000
Coagulation only	11,298	8	.71	3	.27	4	.35
Coagulation, division, no specimen	30,861	35	1.1	1	.03	4	.13
Coagulation, division, obtain specimen	20,194	34	1.7*	5	.25	4	.20

* x^2 significant at a p value of $<.05$
(Missing data for 263 patients)

Table 9

Systemic Hazards Experienced During
Laparoscopy by Type of Anesthesia
1974–1975

Hazards	Anesthesia			
	General		Local	
	Number	Percent	Number	Percent
Emergence excitement due to hypoxia	70	7.8	9	9.5
Hyperventilation	51	5.7	17	17.9
Hypotension	159	17.7	16	16.8
Hypertension	55	6.1	2	2.1
Cardiac arrhythmias	373	41.5	3	3.2
Cardiac arrest	45	5.0	2	2.1
Biochemical alteration of blood	27	3.0	1	1.1
CO_2 Embolism	15	1.7	0	0

(Missing data = 6)

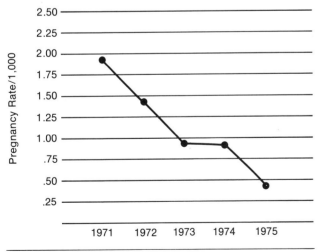

Figure 4
Reported pregnancy rates by AAGL members,
1971–1975.

6. Other Risks (First Questionnaire)

Table 9 shows differences between the chances of experiencing systemic hazards related to the type of anesthesia. This table is based on 879 doctors using general anesthesia and 95 using local. Prominent differences were noted in cardiac arrhythmias (41.5% with general versus 3.2% with local), cardiac arrest (5% with general versus 2.1% with local) and CO_2 embolism (1.7% with general versus 0.0 with local). Hyperventilation, in contrast, was more frequent with local anesthesia.

7. Pregnancies (Second Questionnaire)

Reported pregnancy rates have shown a remarkable downward trend from almost 2 per 1,000 in 1971 to 0.42 per 1,000 in 1975 (Figure 4). However, this trend must be interpreted cautiously. Patients operated on in 1971 have had four years in which to become pregnant; those operated on in 1975 have had barely six months.

There was little difference between the pregnancy rates by technique used, as shown in Figure 5. Somewhat more pregnancies were reported by physicians coagulating, dividing and obtaining a specimen than using other techniques, including coagulation alone. When pregnancy rates were analyzed according to one-hole versus two-hole techniques (Figure 6), no significant differences were observed.

Table 10 reveals that a total of 190 pregnancies were reported to the physicians who performed the procedure, but our membership reported having seen 288 additional pregnant women following the performance of laparoscopic sterilization by other physicians.

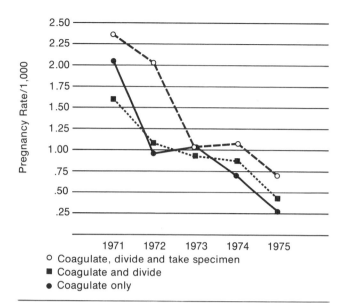

Figure 5
Pregnancy rate by laparoscopic technique,
1971–1975.

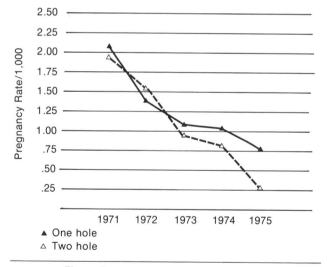

Figure 6
Pregnancy rate by two-puncture versus one-puncture technique,
1971–1975.

Discussion

1. *Steady Improvement in the Art*

This year, for the first time in the history of the Association, there were no deaths reported by our membership in 76,842 sterilizations. Allowing for nonreporting by physicians not members of the AAGL, the estimated total number of sterilizations performed in the US should be about 100,000 a year. As shown in Figure 7, this is in contrast to the death rate reported in 1973 of 13 per 100,000[3] and 7.5 per 100,000 in 1974.[4] This steady downward rate represents a dramatic improvement in our collective technique, in no small part due to the voluntary analysis of our own experience and self-education which the membership of the AAGL continues to provide. Figure 8 illustrates the growing response to this AAGL questionnaire since its beginning in 1972.

Similar trends are not seen, in Figure 7, in the number of laparotomies required subsequent to laparoscopy for sterilization: 5 per 1,000 in 1973, 5.3 per 1,000 in 1974, to 4.2 per 1,000 in 1975. The overall rate for bowel burns has dropped slightly, from 0.9 to 0.5 per 1,000. As in previous years, the more experienced physicians experienced fewer failures, complications and pregnancies.

A major factor in bowel burns and other injuries in 1975 is the difficult process of teaching laparoscopy: 21% to 33% of the burns reported occurred during teaching sessions. Since the teaching of this technique is now done almost entirely in residency training centers, the task of reducing morbidity by developing safe and adequate teaching programs has shifted from the area of private practice, where teaching took place in the early 1970s, to residency training programs.

2. *Changing Techniques of Sterilization*

This year's survey revealed changing trends in physician preference of sterilization technique. The technique originally described as standard in the 1960s and early 1970s was electrocoagulation, division and obtaining a specimen for the pathologic confirmation. This survey indicates that almost one-third of the 1975 respondents still submitting tissue for pathologic confirmation did not obtain bilateral confirmation, rendering this policy of limited legal importance. Of great interest is the fact that there is little difference in pregnancy rates among the three coagulation techniques (Figure 5), with somewhat higher pregnancy rates, if anything,

Table 10
Overall Pregnancy Rate Report
1971–1975

Total sterilizations performed	188,390
Total pregnancies:	478
Same MD	190
Other MD	288
Rate per 1,000 cases in 4 years	2.53

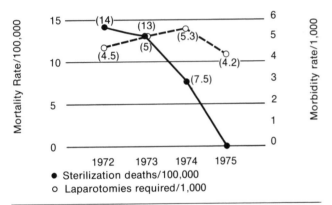

Figure 7
Annual mortality and operative morbidity rates, 1972–1975.

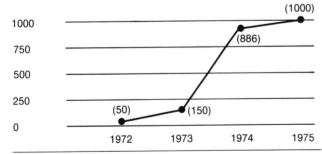

Figure 8
Annual response to AAGL survey by membership, 1972–1975.

among patients whose tubes were submitted for pathologic examination. Moreover, this survey indicates that removal of the specimen carries with it the highest rate of mesosalpingeal tears (Table 8) compared to other coagulation techniques. This raises real questions about relative legal benefits versus medical hazards of such a policy.

The growing acceptance of coagulation only as a technique (20% of all physicians in 1975, Figure 2 and Table 2) appears to have merit in terms of preventing hemorrhage, although somewhat more physicians reported bowel burns with this technique (Table 6) than with others. Similarly, the one-puncture approach is gaining popularity (almost 30% of physicians in 1975, Figure 3), though again a somewhat higher incidence of bowel burns with this method (Table 6) is still reported.

For the first time 12% of physicians indicated the use of bipolar electrocoagulation equipment (Table 3). Also, for the first time the use of nonelectrocoagulation techniques, including the clip or band, has been reported by 2.1% of the membership (Table 2). Continuing surveillance will reveal whether the benefits of minimizing coagulation burns by these techniques will be justified by comparable pregnancy rates.

3. Awareness of Equipment

This year spark gap electrocoagulation sources have been used by a diminishing 17% of our respondents, with 4% still not aware of the nature of the electrical source used. More information about the use and hazards of equipment is wanted by doctors from manufacturers. This seems particularly pertinent since the doctors believe that manufacturers should be liable in case of faulty equipment. Improvement in manufacturer-doctor communication is needed.

Although cardiac monitors were present in over 91% of the hospitals, almost one-third of the respondents did not use them when available. When they were used, prominent differences were noted in cardiac arrhythmias under general anesthesia (41.5%) compared to local anesthesia (3.2%). This suggests strongly that cardiac arrhythmias under general anesthesia will be detected quite frequently if the available equipment is utilized.

4. *The Hazards of Diagnostic Laparoscopy*

One trend first detected last year and which has not changed is the relatively greater hazard of diagnostic procedures compared to electrocoagulation sterilization. In 1974, 11 laparotomies per 1,000 cases were done in connection with diagnostic laparotomies, and in 1975 the figure was 8.5 per 1,000. In each year the rate was double that for sterilization procedures. Unmeasured in this survey, but increasingly apparent to many experienced laparoscopists, is the additional difficulty of knowing, in the subtle problems of pelvic pain and infertility, just exactly what it is one is looking at once the laparoscope is aimed at the pelvic structures. Since one out of three laparoscopies was performed for diagnostic purposes this year, we can anticipate that future training in laparoscopy will pay increasing attention to diagnostic procedures, which are proving to demand more technical and clinical astuteness than had been appreciated previously.

5. *Pregnancy Rates*

A pregnancy rate of about 2 per 1,000 was reported among patients undergoing electrocoagulation in 1971, regardless of technique used (Figures 5 and 6). These rates dropped consistently in subsequent years, but this finding must be interpreted cautiously since patients undergoing the procedure in later years had less time to become pregnant. Moreover, Table 10 reveals a previously undocumented behavior pattern among patients undergoing this procedure: they do not always return to the physician who did the procedure.

Since 1971, 190 women returned pregnant to their AAGL doctors, but 288 additional women came to them pregnant after having had the operation by another physician. If we assume that the same proportion of women sterilized by AAGL members return (or do not return) to their doctors as do women sterilized by non-AAGL members, we see that 1.5 times as many patients do *not* report pregnancies to their doctors as those who do. Since our surveys in the past have been limited to asking physicians about pregnancies reported to them from their own patients of that year, and since pregnancies may take several years to occur after sterilization, the long-term pregnancy rate, suggested in Figures 5 and 6, of about 2 per 1,000 may have to be adjusted to a higher rate over the long term. A need to study the long-term sequelae of sterilization procedures, such as pregnancies, menstrual irregularities and the need for subsequent gynecologic surgery, has been strongly suggested by this year's survey.

6. *Conclusions*

1. Techniques in laparoscopy were in a dynamic evolutionary stage in 1975: coagulation without division, bipolar coagulation and nonelectric clips and bands were beginning to challenge the traditional method of coagulation, division and obtaining a specimen.

2. Judging from the complication rates, diagnostic laparoscopy is emerging as demanding more technical and clinical astuteness than has been devoted to it in our teaching in the past.

3. The burden of teaching and reducing morbidity has shifted from the private practitioner to residency training programs.

4. Dramatic improvements in mortality, continuing low morbidity and a good record of long-term effectiveness are documented in this survey and account for the spontaneous selection of laparoscopic sterilization as a way of maintaining family size by about 100,000 women annually in the United States.

Acknowledgement

Computer analysis was performed by Ms. Barbara Kennedy of the Department of Epidemiology of the School of Public Health, University of North Carolina at Chapel Hill (UNC). Tests for statistical significance, when applicable, were performed by Professor Peter Lachenbruch of the Department of Biostatistics of the UNC School of Public Health. The authors and the AAGL are grateful for their expert contributions.

References

1. Hulka JF, Soderstrom RM, Brooks PG, Corson SL: Complications committee of the AAGL   second annual report, 1973. In *Gynecological Laparoscopy: Principles and Techniques*. (JM Phillips, L Keith, Eds.) Stratton Intercontinental Medical Book Corp, New York, 1974, p 427

2. Hulka JF, Soderstrom RM, Corson SL, Brooks PG: Complications committee of the American Association of Gynecological Laparoscopists, first annual report. J Reprod Med 10:301, 1973

3. Phillips JM, Keith DM, Keith LG: Gynecological laparoscopy 1973: the state of the art. J Reprod Med 12:215, 1974

4. Phillips J, Keith D, Keith L, Hulka J, Hulka B: Survey of gynecologic laparoscopy for 1974. J Reprod Med 15:45, 1975

Chapter 37

Summary
of the
State of the Art

J.F. Hulka, M.D.

Introduction

This chapter must be written swiftly. It will be of practical interest for a brief period of time only and will soon become a historical document in a rapidly changing field. This is a true testimony to the clinical, scientific and engineering ferment so characteristic of the current state of the art. At this point we can only review some of the major trends in gynecologic laparoscopy, describe their present status and attempt to look into the future with the assumption that good things tend to survive and lesser things are soon replaced.

Continuing Self-Surveillance

Gynecologists and obstetricians are among the most compulsive record-keepers in clinical medicine. The significant benefits derived from the study of maternal mortality and cervical cancer statistics are too well known to be recounted here. When laparoscopy appeared as a potentially useful tool, in the mid-1970s, the American Association of Gynecologic Laparoscopists started to collect data about the technique, its complications and its failures. The results of these studies have been reported, and the art has benefitted once again from introspective statistical analyses, as evidenced by a visible decrease in complication, mortality and pregnancy rates in the last five years. The mortality rate of 8 per 100,000, as estimated in 1973–1974, and 0, as recorded in 1974–1975, for this single-event, permanent method of fertility control—sterilization by electrocoagulation—compares well with the continuing risk of mortality in the order of 3 per 100,000 which is associated with birth control pills or IUDs. To a great extent this decrease in morbidity and mortality has been due to excellent instruction in this technique. Once the teachers themselves learned how to perform the operation, they stressed the avoidance of known complications, based on our continuing statistical surveillance.

The Greening of Teaching

In the 1960s a few intrepid American and Canadian physicians crossed the Atlantic to learn modern laparoscopy from the European experts. In the early 1970s this same handful of American students established training programs for other physicians in the US to fill the enormous need for private training in a new and useful surgical technique. By now, the middle of the 1970s, it is pleasing to observe that all major gynecologic-obstetric training centers have laparoscopy as an integral part of their residency program, so the generation of obstetrician-gynecologists emerging into practice in the 1980s will be trained in this technique as thoroughly as they are in all other surgical aspects of our field.

Another trend also emerged in the mid-1970s, that of teaching entire teams of physicians and their assistants to provide the laparoscopic service. These teams include counselors to dispense information and dispel fear, technicians to maintain the equipment safely and efficiently, nurses to help in the special problems of the recovery period and physicians to perform the procedure and act as the captain of the team. Such innovative teaching ultimately will serve to lower the cost of diagnostic and operative laparoscopy and make these operations increasingly available to patients in smaller communities.

The private practice of laparoscopy in the 1980s will no longer have to be a ground-breaking-teaching area for our specialty, as was true in the early 1970s. Improved teaching techniques, such as color television and a more widespread use of photography, inevitably will replace the current, one-to-one teaching method as the appropriate technologies are developed.

The Legal Backlash of Enthusiasm

When laparoscopic sterilization burst upon the early 1970s, the reception was enthusiastic. In their enthusiasm many physicians were so taken by the positive aspects of the operation that they apparently failed to provide patients with full information about hazards as a part of obtaining legal consent. Along with this innocent enthusiasm, physicians were slow to acknowledge complications when they were occurring before their very eyes, and the management of such things as skin burns, bowel burns and the like was sometimes less than adequate when viewed with that marvel-ous instrument, the retrospectoscope. These two factors, failure to inform patients of the risks, and failure to adequately recognize complications as they were occurring, led to a flurry of law suits in the mid-1970s. This in turn led to some abandonment of the procedure: some hospital trustees prohibited the procedure in their units, and even some teaching institutions proscribed the technique for short periods of time. All of these actions were based on the philosophy that "the best way to do no harm is to do nothing." However, the overwhelming popularity of the procedure, the need for sterilization services among American women and the rapid development of safer electric and nonelectric techniques will make this "do nothing" phase short-lived. In view of the genuinely low incidence of complications associated with the skillful performance of the operation, it is reasonable to anticipate that a better alternative to "doing nothing" is to "do it right," when viewed in the light of the alternative methods of fertility control, with their rates of pregnancy, infection, thromboses, discontinuation and death. A more candid informed-consent procedure, a far more compulsive resident training program and a more mature and informed preparation on the part of practicing laparoscopists, acknowledging that complications can and do occur, along with knowledge of proper treatment, will serve to change this situation once again.

More Widespread Use

At this writing it is estimated that about 50,000 diagnostic operations and about 100,000 sterilizations are done annually by laparoscopy. As sterilizations improve, with regard to safety and diminished cost, this level will remain stable or will grow slightly as the percentage of couples who choose female sterilization as a permanent method of family planning increases beyond the 1970 average of 9%.

A far greater increase, however, can be expected in the use of laparoscopy as a diagnostic tool. It already is a standard method for diagnosis in infertility and pelvic pain and may find increasing use in the patient with acute abdominal pain, pediatric problems, and surgical and internal medical conditions such as liver disease, penetrating abdominal injuries and the like. Another possible area for expanding use is the "second look" after such diverse surgical efforts as tuboplasty, ovarian carcinoma and even the more rigorous management of the woman who is a refractory anovulator. Should smaller optics, safe instrumentation and improved local anesthetics continue to develop, as they now appear to be doing, some diagnostic laparoscopy may find its way into skilled gynecologists' offices in the same way as cystoscopy is currently found in urologists' offices.

A further area for the expanded use of laparoscopy will be in the study of basic reproductive physiology. With at least 100,000 patients, presumably normal, now being observed during elective sterilization, we can expect the younger, more curious physicians to question our impressions about what constitutes a normal tube, ovarian morphology and pelvic anatomy, and even to linger a while to observe normal physiologic processes such as uterine contraction, tubal mobility, ovulation, blood flow and the like. With television, tape and photographic techniques for permanent records, the laparoscope conceivably could become as important to gynecologists as the microscope is to pathologists, with original insights into the field of reproductive anatomy and physiology arising from the humbling recognition that the state of the art is always based on this human fact:

We see only what we look for;
We look for only what we know.

A Medical-Industrial Complex is Aborning

This volume is a testimony to the enormous innovative efforts on the part of physicians working independently and together with manufacturers to improve existing equipment. The majority of significant innovations in our field have come from private practice and industry without any governmental support or control. As we go into the last quarter of this century, governmental funding for research is diminishing, but governmental appetite for control is expanding. Enabling legislation is now under consideration to make all development of medical instrumentation as rigidly controlled as is currently the case for drugs.

Rather than passively awaiting the inevitable, the laparoscopists and manufacturers who are contributing spontaneously to the genuine improvement of our art should accept the task of demonstrating ethical, scientific and technical responsibility themselves. They should set up standards for descriptive literature, clinical pretesting of new products and monitoring the complications of techniques and equipment in continuing clinical use. If physicians and manufacturers, now free agents, do not do these thankless, arduous, but ethically necessary tasks now, less qualified, distant bureaucracies will impose standards upon our field, and we will have only our own laziness to blame.

Leaving Mother OR

All new surgical techniques begin in the operating room, where all facilities are available to alleviate the surgeon's anxiety. In these circumstances there is a hospital bed awaiting, an anesthesiologist, all operating room instruments, a recovery room, pathologists, blood bank, etc. Laparoscopy is slowly emerging from this shelter as many sound clinicians and programs have demonstrated that the procedure:

1.   does not warrant a hospital bed but can be done as an outpatient procedure,
2.   can be done, in selected techniques and selected cases, with local anesthesia,
3.   can be done by a few, skilled doctors outside of an operating room.

The state of the art, as described above, is very much like the state of the art of induced abortion in 1970. If we remember, abortion was another new technique thrust upon gynecologists in this decade. It has rightfully emerged from the operating room to the point that it can be done efficiently, safely and at relatively low cost in clinics designed for this procedure. Some skilled physicians are performing abortions in their private offices with hospital backup facilities.

Will laparoscopy ever follow this path? In my opinion it is doubtful that laparoscopy will ever become as widespread an office procedure as abortion currently is. Even the most experienced among us are concerned about the inadvertent vascular injury caused by the insufflating needle or the trocar which would require fairly rapid access to the operating room to avoid death. Even though our record in laparoscopy hemorrhage and death is probably equal to, if not better than, the record of abortion during its days of technical development, it seems fair to analyze the current trends towards outpatient laparoscopy as less strong than those of outpatient abortion and to expect that the majority of laparoscopies will continue to be done in hospital operating facilities or hospital-based clinic facilities in the future with, it is hoped, an increasing number of highly skilled and determined pioneers offering sterilization in non-hospital clinics at lower costs. Similarly, expanded use of diagnostic laparoscopy will be distributed primarily in hospitals, with a few skilled practitioners doing low-risk diagnostic procedures in their offices in a similar way that urologists do selected cystoscopies in theirs.

The Not So New, Not So Brave World of 1984

To summarize these indulgences in predicting the future, based on both the strong and the weak trends of the present, it is safe to say that laparoscopy will be here in 1984, alive, well and more widespread than ever. Hospitals and some offices will be using smaller, safer and simpler equipment for both diagnostic and sterilization operations in a manner probably similar to the current use of cystoscopy by urologists.

The art of photography, which transformed Dr. Roentgen's fluoroscopic technique of exploring the body to one providing permanent, direct medical records, can be expected to have progressed in laparoscopy to the point that diagnostic and operative findings will be recorded permanently as standard care for both patient information and research.

The United States, Canada and Europe will not be the only countries enjoying this expanded interest since our colleagues in the developing countries are equally dedicated physicians, seeking the best diagnostic and therapeutic tools for their patients. Like that of the automobile, the innate attractiveness of laparoscopy will provide the stimulus for developing countries to make up for technological gaps by using this modern convenience. Hopefully, safer techniques of either electrocoagulation or mechanical tubal blockade will emerge from the innovations of the 1970s. By 1984 manufacturing standards and preclinical testing requirements inevitably will have become established by governmental regulating agencies; hopefully, the physicians and manufacturers will

have been given maximal input in order to encourage continuing improvements and innovations rather than stifling them. From the point of view of medical progress, it would indeed be disappointing if the techniques which will be utilized in the 1980s were no better than those presently in use.

Finally, the morbidity and mortality from laparoscopy should level out to an "irreducible minimum" with a full generation of resident-trained gynecologists performing laparoscopy in the 1980s as a routine, compared to the early 1970s, when it was so much of a surgical stunt. The irreducible minimum of complications, including death, is an inevitable part of the fact that surgical techniques must be taught continually and that mistakes are a part of human learning processes as well as part of highly skilled human procedures.

Index

Abdominal
  disease 106
  hernia 53, 57, 148
  mass 53, 58, 327
  pain 53, 104–112, 354
  surgery, previous 147, 170, 220, 225
  trauma, diagnosis of 57, 104, 106, 113–118, 328
  visualization, nongynecologic 113–118, 324–332
  wall
    burns 244
    bleeding 236, 243
    insufflation 93, 225
Abortion
  spontaneous 151
  sterilization combined with 165, 170, 172, 182–186, 190, 343
  therapeutic 10
Abscess (see also Infection)
  from laparoscopy 268
  liver 325
  ovarian 104–112
  pelvic 185, 232, 244, 268
Absolute contraindications 53, 57–59, 155
Academic teaching hospital 275–280
Accident (see also Complications)
  analysis 160, 238, 321
  anesthetic 70–71, 223
  electrical 29, 160, 228–235
  legal liability in 313–323
  occurrence 242–246
  prevention 160, 220–230
  trocar 236–246
Acupuncture 109
Acute abdomen 104–112, 231, 354
Acute adnexal inflammation 105
Adhesions 192–218
  abdominal 55, 79, 106, 176
  after laparoscopy 339
  cauterization of 214
  division of 106, 109, 214
  fimbrial 54, 192, 202
  intratubal 54
  lysis of 52–55, 131, 143, 202, 214
  periovarian 54, 131, 134, 206
  peritubal 52, 131, 134, 176, 193, 202, 206
  postoperative 131, 134, 147
  veil-like 107, 109, 214
  visualization of 106, 212
Adnexal
  inflammation 105
  mass 55, 197, 214
  neoplasm 120
  pathology 120
  torsion 55, 297
Adnexitis 106, 297
Adolescents 55
Adrenal
  hyperplasia 297
  rest tumors 56
Agency for International Development (AID) 281–292
Air
  index of refraction 21
  pneumoperitoneum with 73
    toxicity of 73
  room 38, 100, 327, 329
  under diaphragm 118
Airway 72, 82
Allan-Masters syndrome 55, 108
Allergic reaction 78
Alligator forceps 216, 335
Ambiguous external genitalia 56, 297
Amenorrhea 195–218
  hypothalamic 197
  post-pill 197

primary 53–56, 131, 133, 138, 295
  secondary 53–56, 131, 133, 296
American, historical background of laparoscopy 9–16, 354
American Association of Gynecologic Laparoscopists (AAGL) 3, 4, 10, 11, 31, 166, 252, 269, 271, 342–353
American College of Obstetricians and Gynecologists 159, 269, 271
American Cystoscope Makers, Inc. (ACMI) 20, 35, 37, 286, 300–302
Amnesia 69–86
Amyloid infiltration 325
Analgesia 69–86, 176 (see also Anesthesia)
  local 78
  regional 77
Anatomy
  knowledge of 239
  misidentification of 244
  systematic approach to 99
Androgens 133
Anesthesia 69–86, 89, 93 (see also Specific procedure)
  and bowel burns 232
  agents 69–86
  complications 70–75, 223
    index of 70–71
  consent 320
  epidural 77
  general 9, 65, 69–77, 134, 141, 146, 183, 209, 213
  local 10, 36, 65, 69–81, 162, 165, 168–170, 175
  monitoring 76
  of tube 172
  pain studies 168
  previous complications with 53, 58
  problems 58, 66, 70–86, 224
  recovery 81
  regional 65, 69–78
  spinal 77
  survey of hazards 348
  technique 75–81
Anesthesiologist 69–86, 255
  privileges 270
Anesthetic infiltration of uterosacral ligaments 109
Angle of penetration 92–94, 225, 239
  precautions 92
Angle of view 18, 37–37
Animal studies 167, 334–340
Anomalies 206
  congenital 56, 206, 209, 295–299
  genetic 53–56, 133, 297
  genital 56
  tubal 54
  uterine 55–56
Anovulation 138, 338, 355
Antefixation of uterus 109
Antibiotics 105, 112, 186, 201, 232, 317
Anticoagulant therapy 171
Antihistamines 172, 201
Anxiety 62, 69–86
Aorta 118
  bifurcation of 92, 239
  laceration of 236, 243
  penetration of 92
Apnea 74
Appendicitis 55, 208, 298
  diagnosis of 104–106
Appendix
  previously ruptured 82
  visualization of 55, 99, 298, 328
Arcing 162
Arrhythmias (see Cardiac arrhythmias)
Artery (see also Blood vessel)
  injury 184

puncture 92, 236, 268
Asahi camera 302
Ascites, ascitic fluid 56, 120–125, 324–332
Aspiration
  curettage 182
  of endometrial cysts 53, 54, 59, 109, 131, 212–214
  gastric contents 69–75
  ovarian cyst 54, 55, 109, 296
  peritoneal fluid 53–56, 210
Association for Voluntary Sterilization 287
Atelectasis 73
Atropine 69–86, 94, 164, 168, 172, 188, 224
Audiovisual 254
Autoclave 44–50, 98, 225, 280

Band sterilization (see Ring sterilization)
Barbiturate 78–81
Basal body temperature 138, 195, 201, 207
Basic techniques 88–102, 160, 175
Bayonet type laparoscope 36
Beam-splitter unit 309
Beaulieu camera 301
Berci bipolar instrument 42
Biliary
  carcinoma 125
  disease 125, 324–331
Bioengineering 33
Biopsy 133–139 (see also Specific organs)
  drill 42, 135
  forceps 135, 162
  instruments 120, 134–136
  needle 120, 134
  nongynecologic 324–332
  telescope 36, 98, 134
Biphasic menstrual cycle 214
Bipolar (see also Electrosurgery)
  coagulation 164
  forceps 30, 31, 161, 164, 273
  instruments 31, 42, 164, 228
  sterilization 31, 164
  systems 30, 31, 267, 344, 350
  techniques 10, 164
Birth control (see Contraception)
Bladder
  adhesions 107
  catheterization of 200, 213, 224, 294
  perforation of 96, 97, 99, 226, 244
Bleeder 42, 236
Bleeding (see also Hemorrhage)
  as indication for laparoscopy 55
  control 88, 136, 143, 156, 228
  diagnosis of 57, 328
  during sterilization 66, 162, 164, 165, 181, 236, 243
  following biopsy 120, 135–136, 326
  from aortic penetration 236
    ectopic gestation 56, 130, 155
    epigastric vessels 226
    liver laceration 91
    skin 66, 95, 226
Blended current (see Current)
Blind spot 36, 162, 227, 327
Blood gas
  balance 57
  changes 57, 70–74, 169, 224, 348
Blood pressure 70–80, 243 (see also Hypertension, Hypotension)
Blood vessel
  burn 317
  injury 236–246
  insufflation 70, 225
  laceration 145, 243, 278
Blood volume 70–72, 164, 188
Blunt abdominal trauma (see Trauma)
Bone marrow disease 326

Bowel
    burns 66, 143, 229, 231–235, 244, 268, 346–
        347
    carcinoma 120, 125
    diverticulosis 106
    injuries 147, 181
    insufflation 145, 225, 329
    ischemic disease 328
    obstruction
        contraindication to laparoscopy 53, 112
    perforation 57, 93, 96, 145, 147, 185, 244,
        268, 327, 329
    puncture 91, 241
    resection for thermal injury 232, 244
    strangulation 153
    trauma 113–118, 346
    visualization 324–332
Bradycardia 70, 168, 172
Breast carcinoma 119, 127
Broad ligament 112
    endometrial implants on 131
    hematoma 268
    lacerations 108
Bronchial intubation 70
Burns 21, 25 (see also Specific location)
    bowel 66, 143, 229–235, 244, 268, 317, 346
    course of 231
    electrical 75, 78, 97
    inspection for 143
    litigation 317–323
    precautions 11, 229
    skin 66, 89, 228, 231–235, 268, 317
    theories on production 161, 229, 231
    to operator 228

Cables 39
Calibrated probe 21, 100
Cameras 300–312
    movie 22, 306–312
    still 22, 300–305
Cameron-Miller snare 179
Cancer, carcinoma 119–128 (see also Malig-
    nancy, Metastasis, Specific organs, Tu-
    mors)
    detection 98
    diagnosis 119–128
    extraperitoneal 57, 119
    staging 56, 119–128, 326
    work-up 98
Cannula
    Cohen 43, 79
    Corson 43
    double 38
    for open laparoscopy 145
    Semm 43
    suction 136
Capacitance 24–33, 37
Capacitor 25, 26
Carbon dioxide, CO$_2$ 65, 93, 95, 209 (see also
        Gas, Pneumoperitoneum)
    complications 70–75, 268
    delivery systems 38
    discomfort with 81, 169, 329
    history of use 7–14
    maintenance of delivery systems 49
Carcinomatous peritonitis 104
Cardiac
    arrest 69–72, 94, 243, 268, 348
    arrhythmias 69–74, 95, 224, 243, 317, 329,
        348
    complications 69–74, 171, 279
    compression 243
    instability 243
    irregularity 94
    monitor 88, 350
    murmur 70, 73, 94
    output 72, 73, 116
    puncture for gas embolization 94
Cardiorespiratory disease 53, 57, 76, 120, 223
Cardiovascular
    collapse 73
    complications 69–74, 280
Carts
    for cameras 310

    for instruments 48, 49
    for resuscitation equipment 279
Case filing system 263
Catecholamines 72
Cautery, history 7–16 (see also Electrocoagula-
        tion)
Cellulitis 122
Central venous pressure 72
    catheter 73, 75
Certification 269, 321
Cervix
    carcinoma of 127
    laceration of 185
    mucorrhea 195
    mucus 195–196
Charge 37 (see also Current)
Chemotherapy 56, 19–128 (see also Cancer)
Children, laparoscopy in 294–299
Chloroprocaine 78
Chocolate cyst 197, 206
Cholangiography 325
Cholangitis, stenosing 330
Cholelithiasis 125
Cholestasis 325
Cholinesterase deficiency 74
Chorionic gonadotropin 133
Chromic phosphate P32 121
Chromosomal
    anomalies 210, 297
    mosaicism 295
Chromotubation 192–218 (see also Dye)
    technique of 208
Chronic abdominal disease 106–109
Chronic abdominal pain 106–112
Chronic adnexitis 106
Chronic appendicitis 106
Chronic lung disease 327
Cinematography 39, 261, 300–305
Circon TV camera 308–310
Circuitry 24–33, 309, 321
Cirrhosis 327
Clamps 146, 156
Clip (see also Hulka clip, Sterilization)
    sterilization 10, 165–173, 189, 229, 289, 343,
        350
    studies 168–170, 284
Clomid 197
Clomiphene citrate 131, 133, 192, 197, 335
Coagulation (see also Current, Electrocoagula-
        tion, Generators, Sterilization)
    current 24–33, 156
    errors 227, 266
    for bleeding 120
        endometriotic implants 131, 210
        sterilization 161–165
        tubal pregnancy 130, 156
    forceps 161–165
    historical background 7–16
    necrosis 233
    process 161
    time 161
Coagulopathy 326
Cobalt irradiation 121
Coelioscopy, historical background 8
Cohen cannula 43, 79
Cohen-Eder
    intrauterine cannula 43
    modification of Palmer biopsy forceps 45,
        136
    uterine manipulator 134
Coital history 194 (see also Sexual activity)
Cold light 302
Colicky abdominal pain 107
Colitis 106
Colon
    burns 231
    carcinoma 127
    insufflation 93, 145, 329
    irritable 106
    perforation 145, 241, 244, 268, 329
    puncture 93
Colposcopy 279
Colpotomy 105, 141, 158, 159, 174
Common iliac vessels laceration 236–246

Community hospital program development
        265–274
Complications of laparoscopy (see also Errors,
        Failed laparoscopy, Injuries, Risk,
        Safety, Specific complication, Specific
        organ, Specific procedure) 24, 70–75,
        145, 219–246, 329
    and physician experience 59, 243–246, 319,
        342–352
    catastrophic 3, 229
    committee 3, 10, 252, 342–352
    during training 44, 244, 349
    incidence 148, 242–246
    of diagnostic procedures 120, 122, 243, 346,
        351
    of operative procedures 130–132, 136, 143,
        157
    of sterilization 160, 166, 171, 178, 181, 185,
        346
    rate 160, 185, 353
    requiring laparotomy 97, 120, 132, 171, 178,
        346–350
    statistics 242–246, 268, 342–352
    time of occurrence 242
Conception 194–218
Confidentiality 68
Congenital abnormalities 55, 206, 209, 295–299
Consent 60–68, 160
    document 67, 68
    in mental retardation 63
    in minors 63
    in single adults 61, 68
    informed 60–68, 141, 143, 250, 317–323, 354
    spouse 60–68
    withdrawal 63–67
Consultation 57
    following injury 317–323
    gastroenterologic 106
    orthopedic 106
    psychiatric 106
    staff 270, 321
Continuing medical education 321
Contraception 60–68, 194
    permanent 159–190
    research 334–340
Contraceptive alternatives 61, 66, 159, 281, 285,
        354
Contraindications to laparoscopy 9, 52–59,
        130–132, 176, 220, 223
    absolute 53, 57–59, 155
    inexperience of operator 59, 181, 221
    relative 53, 58–59, 149, 250
    to nonelectric sterilization 229
    to upper abdominal peritoneoscopy 326
Contrast material (see Dye)
Copper 7, T 143 (see also Intrauterine device)
Cornu 161
Cornual
    obstruction 192
    occlusion 206, 217
    spasm 192
Corpus luteum 54, 105, 138, 201, 338
    hemorrhage 55, 105
    ruptured 105
Corson
    acorn cannula 43
    bipolar forceps 31–33, 42, 164
    uterine manipulator 43, 98, 99, 134
Corticosteroids 105, 109
Cost 4, 78, 82, 153, 218, 354
    of equipment 264, 311, 312
    to patient 62, 159
Counseling patients 60–68, 86, 182, 276, 317–
        323
Counselor, role of 60–68, 354
Course of instruction 160, 252–258
    programmed 257
Credentials 269–270
Crepitus 93
Criteria for privileges 269
Crohn's disease 106, 108, 328
Cryptoorchidism 297
Cul-de-sac 136
    metastases 127

nodularity 197
postcoital test 192
Culdocentesis 55, 105, 192
Culdoscopy 20, 61, 159, 174, 279
  contraindications 92
  historical background 8
Culture 201
Cumulus mass 338
Curare 77
Current 24–33, 315 (see also Electricity)
  "bleed off" attachment 37
  blended 28, 135, 163, 181
  coagulating 27, 156
  complications 223, 227–229, 231–235, 244
  cutting 26, 27, 136, 163, 180
  density 89, 161–164
  excessive 131, 223
  high frequency 24, 160–164, 181
  high voltage 24, 42, 160
  historical background 8–16
  low frequency 24
  low voltage 160–164, 181
  misuse 50
  path through patient 90
Cyanosis 70, 74
Cystectomy 296
Cystic
  disease 325
  teratoma 330
Cystoscopy
  from above 96
  historical background 6
  instruments 36
Cysts
  aspiration of 109, 214, 296
  chocolate 197, 206
  dangers of puncture of 299
  endometrial 59, 214
  follicular 108
  liver 326
  Morgagnian 54
  ovarian 104–112, 206, 296, 297
Cytology 9, 53, 56, 100, 120, 296, 326

Dalkon Shield 143 (see also Intrauterine device)
Dangers of laparoscopy 65 (see also Complications, Accidents)
Death (see also Mortality)
  65, 72, 144, 171, 230, 232, 238, 244, 346, 349, 350, 356
Deaver retractors 145
Defibrillator 82
Department of Health, Education, and Welfare
  guidelines 63
Depty of penetration 95
Description of operation 65
Developing countries 4, 38, 89, 281–292, 356
Diabetes 120
Diagnostic laparoscopy 88
  for cancer 119–128
    infertility 191–218
    pelvic pain 104–112
    trauma 113–118
    unruptured tubal pregnancy 155–158
  incidence of complications 243, 346, 351
  survey 194, 342–352
Diaphragm
  free air under 118
  lymphatics 120
  metastatic disease 56, 120
Diaphragmatic
  hernia 57, 243
  hiatus 328
  pain 77
  tumor 121
Diathermy 25–33, 160
Diazepam 76–79, 281, 329
Diffusion hypoxia 74
Dilatation of phimotic tubal ostium 53, 54, 212–218
Distortion 18, 36
Diverticulitis 106, 108
Division of
  adhesions 106, 109

uterosacral ligaments 109
Documentation
  of informed consent 60–68
  of laparoscopic findings 198, 209, 261, 298, 319
  of safety precautions 319
Double cannula needle 38
Double puncture (see Technique)
Draping 90
Drug reactions 315, 321
Dyclone 78
Dye 44, 54, 100, 172, 192–218 (see also Chromotubation)
Dysfunctional uterine bleeding 189
Dysmenorrhea 107, 108, 151, 197, 297
Dyspareunia 108, 151, 194, 197

Echinococcus disease 328
Economics 267
Ectopic IUD (see Intrauterine device, ectopic)
Ectopic pregnancy (see Pregnancy, Ectopic)
Eder Instrument Co., Inc. 9, 20, 35, 37, 145, 300–305
Education 53, 57, 160, 247–292 (see also Training, Instruction)
Ektachrome film 301
Electrical (see also Current)
  accidents 29
  burns 75, 78, 231–235
  capacitance 24–33
  complications 24, 75, 223, 227–229, 231–235
    incidence 234, 244
  energy 31, 160
  fire 75, 318
  hazards 75, 160
  shock 24, 223, 303, 317
  system check 89
Electricity 24–33
Electrocardiogram 70
  grounding electrode 75
  monitor 76, 223
  system 75
Electrocoagulation 24–33 (see also Coagulation, Current, Electrosurgery)
  accidents 69, 75, 160, 227, 231–235
  for ectopic pregnancy 156
    tubal sterilization 160–166, 179–181
  historical background 8–16
Electrocution 75
Electrode 28
  ground 164
  historical background 7–16
  return 30, 31, 90
Electrodessication 29
Electrofulguration 25–33, 160–166 (see also Coagulation)
Electronic flash 301–305
Electrosurgery (see also Generators)
  caution 37
  complications 50, 223, 227, 231–235, 244, 268
  contraindicated 120
  current 24–33, 160, 223
  for bleeding 88
  grounding 30, 31, 160, 223
  principles 24–33, 160, 223
  risk 156, 160, 223
  sterilization 160–166, 179–181
  units 24–33, 40, 160, 223, 321
    ignorance regarding 252, 318, 344
Embolization of gas 69–73, 94, 145, 225, 243, 268, 317, 348 (see also Gas CO_2)
Emergency
  equipment 82, 169, 279
  laparoscopy 104–106, 324
  laparotomy 88, 97, 113–118, 120, 130, 157, 169
  resuscitation 82, 318
Emotional barriers 60, 61
Emphysema 71, 93, 122, 145, 225, 329
Encapsulation of ovary 55
Endobronchial intubation 70–77
Endocrine
  assay 195
  disorders 53–56, 297

evaluation 131, 138
research 334–340
Endometrial 192–218
  biopsy 192–211
  carcinoma 127
  cysts 54, 59, 214
  implants 54, 131
    cautery of 54, 107, 109, 131
    fulguration of 54, 55, 193
  polyps 192
Endometriosis 54, 107–112
  and infertility 192–218
  associated with retroversion 151
  asymptomatic 193, 197
  collaborative studies 54
  diagnosis of 54, 107
  historical background 8
  evaluation 53, 54
  follow-up 53, 54
  hormone therapy 53, 54, 107–112
  teen-age 298
  treatment 53, 54, 107–112, 131
    medical 54, 109
    surgical 53, 54, 109, 131, 212–214
Endoscopes 34–35 (see also Laparoscopies, Telescopes)
  direct view 18–23
  indirect view 18–23
Endoscopy
  closed cavity 7
  historical background 3, 6–16
  open cavity 6
  unit 259–264
Endotracheal
  anesthesia 70–86
  intubation 58, 70–75, 134, 141, 146, 213
  tube 70–75, 82
    misplacement 73
Energy sources (see Current, Generator, Electrosurgery)
England, historical background of laparoscopy 9–16
Enteritis, regional 106
Equipment (see also Endoscopes, Instruments, Laparoscopes, Specific procedure)
  avoiding complications with 70–75, 221–230
  awareness of 350
  defective 46–50, 160, 232, 236, 319, 350
  development 261
  emergency 82, 169, 279
  failure 46–50, 70–75, 165, 174, 221, 261
  hazards of 350
  inspection 42, 46–50, 89
  maintenance 32, 46–50, 160–164, 221–230, 232, 238, 279
  manufacturers 35, 261, 344–350
  preferences 97–100, 342–352
  resuscitation 82
  sterilization of 44–50, 225, 280
Errors 220–246 (see also Complications)
  manufacturing 172
  surgical 172, 178, 181
Esophagus
  carcinoma 119, 126
  intubation 71
Estrogen (see also Hormone)
  biosynthesis 133
  treatment 56
Ethics 167
Europe 89
  historical background of laparoscopy 3, 6–16, 354
Experience 88, 147, 153, 162, 187, 218, 342–352
  (see also Inexperience, Instruction, Training)
  acquiring 249–280
  and complication rate 160, 221, 229, 243–246, 319, 346
  and failed laparoscopy 319
  for hazardous cases 56–59, 155–158
  practical 255
Experimental animals 334–340
Experts 3, 248, 265, 354
Extrauterine IUD (see Intrauterine device)

Eye-hand coordination 279
Eyepiece 37, 47

Failed laparoscopy 145, 147, 185, 190
  and experience 243, 319, 346
  causes 165, 225, 243, 346
  incidence 342–352
Failed sterilization 189, 317, 320, 348–351
  rate 161–166, 173, 190, 266
  with clip 172
  with ring 178
Fallopian tubes (see Tubal, Tubes)
Falope-Ring 165, 174–178
Family planning programs 60–68, 256, 281–292
Fasting state 72
Fatality (see Mortality)
Father of modern gynecologic laparoscopy 8
Febrile reaction 147
Federal guidelines 63
Feminization, testicular 297
Fentanyl 77–79, 168
Fertility 192–218 (see also Infertility, Sterility, Sterilization)
  control 281–292, 353
  surgery 212–218
  survey 195
  work-up 193–211
Fertilization in vitro 3, 57, 335
Fetal loss 56
Fetoscopy 279
Fiberglass sleeves 95, 223, 227
Fiber optics 18–23, 37, 98, 300
  historical background 8
  maintenance 46–50, 99
  power supplies 302–305
  relay systems 19
  teaching extension 78
Fibroids 108, 120, 206
Field of vision 19–21, 34–37
Film (see also Photography)
  documentation 57
  historical background 9
  speed 22
  type 301
Fimbrial
  adhesions 54, 192, 202
  dilatation 53, 198
  hoods 56
  motility 54
  mucus 193
  phimosis 53, 131, 202
  positions 338
Fimbrioplasty 205
Flammable solutions 69, 75, 317, 321
Flash equipment 98, 301–305
Flexible
  laparoscope 37, 120
  teaching instrument 44, 98
Flow ball (see Gas)
Flow rate (see Gas)
Fluid compartment shifts 120
Flying Doctors Teaching Team 10, 31
Fogging of lens 98, 171, 172, 304
Follicle stimulating hormone 131, 197, 207, 336
Follicular
  apparatus 138
  cysts 108
  development 338
Follow-up (see Specific procedure)
Foot pedal 223
Forceps
  alligator 216, 335
  biopsy 120, 135, 152
  bipolar 30, 42, 161–164
  coagulation 161–165
  grasping 99, 134, 141, 151, 156, 161, 179
  maintenance 48
  Palmer 135, 162
  punch 135, 162
  Semm 29, 136
  Siegler 135, 162
Foreign objects 36, 53, 56 (see also Intrauterine device)
Fore-oblique 20, 34

Fourestier, Gladu, Valmier apparatus 8, 9
Frangenheim punch biopsy scissors 162, 164
Frequency (see Current)
Fulguration 25–33, 160–166 (see also Coagulation)
  current 8
  inadvertent 160
  of endometrial implants 53–55, 193, 210
  of fallopian tubes 8
Functional disturbances 106
Future of laparoscopy 353–356

Gallbladder
  carcinoma 125
  hydrops of 108
  perforation 329
  trauma 113–118
  visualization 324–332
Gamete formation 201
Gas 21, 65 (see also Insufflation, CO₂, N₂O, Pneumoperitoneum, Pressure)
  absorption of 97
  amount 94, 97
  complications with 70–75, 82, 222–225, 238, 243
  embolization of 69–75, 94, 225, 243, 268, 348
  flow ball 38
  flow rate 38, 91, 93, 225
  historical background 7–16
  insufflation 38, 91–95
  leakage 97, 163, 222, 225
  preferred 81, 95, 209, 327, 329
  pressure 38
    excessive 70–75, 243, 319
    monitor 38, 318
  reserve tank 97, 222
  selection 81, 95
  system 38, 82
Gastric (see also Stomach)
  contents aspiration 69–75
  dilatation 71–75
  perforation 74, 76
  suction 223, 225
  trauma 113–118
  ulcer 104–106
Gastroenterologic laparoscopy 125, 324–332
Gastrointestinal
  burns 228–235
  complications 71, 74
  pains 106
  perforation 145
  tract carcinoma 125
  use of laparoscopy 324–332
General anesthesia 69–77 (see also Anesthesia)
Generators 24–33, 88, 160–164, 345 (see also Electrosurgical units)
  maintenance 50, 223
  solid-state 26
  spark-gap 25, 160
  vacuum-tube 26
Genetic anomaly 53–56, 133, 297
Genital (see also Congenital)
  anomaly 56
  tuberculosis 108
Genitalia, ambiguous 56, 297–299
Germinal cell count 210
Gestation (see Pregnancy)
Gestational sac 155–158
Glucose 72
Gonad
  biopsy 297
  dysgenesis 131, 197, 295
  hypoplastic 138
  streaks 138, 295
Gonadectomy 131
Gonadotropins 131
  elevated 138
  exogenous 133
  stimulation 296, 335
  therapy 56, 138
Gonococcal salpingitis 331
Graafian follicle 195
Granulomatous disease 325
Granulosa cells 133

Grasping forceps 99, 134, 141, 151, 156, 161, 179
Ground plate 11, 30, 31, 50, 75, 90, 134, 164, 223, 317
  metal objects as 89
Grounded system 31, 160–163 (see also Coagulation)

Halothane 70–86
  avoid 183
Hansen's disease 330
Hasson balloon cannula 44
Hazard 37, 52–59, 65, 220–246, 354 (see also Complication)
  of anesthesia 69–82
  of electrosurgery 75, 160–165
  of operative laparoscopy 130–132
  of pneumoperitoneum 91
  warnings 38, 344–350
Heart (see also Cardiac)
  gas in 70, 73, 243
  mill wheel murmur 70, 73, 94
Hematoma 136, 185
  retroperitoneal 171, 268
  subcutaneous 226
  subfascial 226
Hematometria 297
Hematosalpinx 297
Hemoperitoneum 53, 55, 116, 268
Hemorrhage (see also Bleeding)
  complications 70, 145, 243, 317, 350
  diagnosis of 57, 104, 106
  from anticoagulant therapy 171
    biopsy 136
    blood vessel injury 109, 236
    ruptured tubal pregnancy 130
Hemostasis 27, 59, 95, 100, 120, 131, 135, 156, 163
Hemostatic current 25, 27, 135
Hepatic coma 329
Hepatomegaly 324
Hepatosplenomegaly 330
Hermaphrodism 56
Hernia
  abdominal 53, 57, 148
  contraindication 53, 57
  diaphragmatic 57, 243
  hiatal 53, 329
  incisional 95, 148, 244
  inguinal 55
  umbilical 95
Hiatal hernia 53, 329
High frequency current (see Current)
Hilar rest tumors 56
Hirsutism 133, 138, 297
Histology 56, 120, 131, 133, 296, 324
History of laparoscopy 6–16, 249, 253, 261
Hitachi TV camera 308–310
Hodgkin's disease 123–125
  diagnosis with laparoscopy 123
  staging 123, 325
Holes, One, Two, Three (see Technique)
Hormone therapy
  follow-up assessment of 54
  for endometriosis 107–112
Hospital
  administration 274
  community 265–274
  privileges 257, 269
  program development 248–292
  safety 32, 320
  stay in days 117
  teaching 257, 259–264
  time 62, 168, 171, 182, 187
Hospitalization 60–62 (see also Inpatient, Outpatient)
Hulka
  spring clip sterilization 10, 165, 167–173, 189
    technique of application 168
    follow-up 170
  tenaculum 79
  uterine manipulator 44, 99, 183
Human
  experimentation 3

studies 168
Human chorionic gonadotropin 133, 336
Hydatid cysts 108, 329
Hydrocortisone acetate 214, 217
Hydrosalpinx 55, 107, 108, 198, 202, 206, 209, 217
Hydrotubation 193, 202, 205, 210, 214, 217
Hyfracator 30
Hypercarbia 69–81, 94, 95, 116, 224
Hyperemia of peritoneum 55, 107
Hypersplenism 326
Hypertension 69–75, 348
Hyperventilation 70, 95, 116, 348
Hypoestrogenic state 197
Hypoglycemia 70
Hypoplastic uterus 55, 197, 295
Hypotension 69–75, 116, 122, 168, 172, 185, 188, 329, 348
Hypoventilation 70–74, 243, 327
Hypovolemia 70, 78, 118
Hypoxia 69–81, 348
Hysterography 192, 208, 261
Hysterosalpingography 10, 54, 56, 141, 192–218
Hysteroscopy 20, 56, 61, 140, 141, 203, 208, 284, 300, 303

Iatrogenic injury 315
Icarex camera 302
Ileus, contraindication to laparoscopy 53
Iliac vessel laceration 236
Illumination 21, 221 (see also Light source)
Image
    amplifier 261
    distortion 18, 36
    magnification 20, 36, 98, 100, 120, 309
    minification 20
    transmission 18–23, 57
Immunologic tests 195
Incision (see also Specific procedure)
    burns 317
    closure 148
    hernia 148, 244
    left McBurney point 91
    minilaparotomy 156
    scars 159
    second 99
    suprapubic 99, 156, 158, 181
    trocar 91, 95
    umbilical 91
    vertical midline, in trauma 113
Index of refraction 21
Indications
    for laparoscopy 52–59, 104–112, 191–218, 317–320
        carcinoma 119–128
        two chief 3
    for laparotomy 130–132
Indigo carmine (see Dye)
Inexperience of operator 58, 59, 158, 160 (see also Experience)
    related to complications 221, 238, 243–246, 319, 346
Infants, laparoscopy in 55, 56, 259, 294–299
Infection 78
    complication of laparoscopy 66, 244, 268, 315
    contraindication to laparoscopy 53, 57
    precautions against 47, 174, 201
    wound 147, 185
Infertility 191–218 (see also Fertility, Sterility)
    diagnosis in 8
    documentation of 198–204, 209
    investigation of 9, 52–54, 56, 133, 194–211
    laparotomy indication in 88, 131
    mini-survey 198, 207
    operative laparoscopy for 88, 131
    primary 133
    secondary 133, 194
    survey 194–211
Inflammatory disease
    pelvic 8, 47, 105, 112, 198, 208, 244, 297
    tubal 54
Informed consent 60–68, 141, 143, 250, 317–

323, 354
Infusion catheter placement 273
Inguinal hernia 55
Inhalation agents 81
Injury (see also Complications, Specific organ)
    from laparoscopy 219–246
        avoiding 147, 309
        laparoscopic diagnosis in 113–118
            blunt 104, 106, 113–118, 329
            penetrating 113–118, 354
        thermal 97, 231–235, 244
        to blood vessels 92, 184, 236–246
        to gastrointestinal tract 228–235
Inpatient laparoscopy 60, 183
    anesthesia 69–86
Insemination 208
    donor 192
Instillation of radioactive material 120, 121
Instruction 247–292 (see also Education, Training)
    equipment 34–50
    manuals 32, 34, 344, 350
    self 248–251
    to nurses 46–50
    to patients 81
Instruments 34–45 (see also Equipment, Specific procedures)
    accessory 130, 132
    check list 50
    design 261, 286, 355
    instruction manual 32, 34, 344, 350
    log book 261
    maintenance 44–50, 89, 99, 162, 221–230, 232, 238
    preferences 97–100
    repair 259
    safety record 321
    testing 174, 261
Insufflation 91–95 (See also Gas)
    equipment 38, 93, 97, 222
    erroneous 70–75, 93, 97, 145, 225, 243, 329
    gas 73, 95
    gauges 38, 223
    historical background 7
    in open laparoscopy 147
    inadequate 222
    left subcostal 127
    monitoring during 76
    needle 38, 91
    pediatric 294
    time 147
Insulation
    against arcing 162
    check for defects in 47–50, 227
    defects in 223, 232, 317
    external 164
    internal 164
Intercourse 186 (see also Sexual activity)
Intersexuality 53, 297, 299
Intestinal (see also Bowel)
    cancer 120
    injuries 97, 113–118, 131
    obstruction 104–106, 112
    perforation 57, 96
    ulcers 104, 106
Intraabdominal pressure 38, 70–75 (see also Gas, Pressure)
Intrahepatid cholestasis 325
Intraperitoneal
    bleeding 328
    isotopes for ovarian carcinoma 121
    metastasis 56, 119
    pressure 70–75, 223
Intrapulmonary shunting 70, 73
Intratubal adhesions 54
Intrauterine
    devices (IUD) 62, 66, 140–144, 283
        ectopic 10, 36, 53, 56, 108, 132, 140–144
        removal 53, 56, 140–144, 244
    sound study 140–142
Intravascular insufflation 73
Intubation
    bronchial 70–75
    esophageal 71

tracheal 58, 70–75, 134, 141, 146, 213
Irritable colon 106
Ischemic bowel disease 328
Isolated (see also Unipolar, Bipolar)
    ground circuitry 160–163
    system 31
Isotopes 120, 121
Isthmic block 209

Jaundice 325
Jejunal
    artery 236, 240
    perforation 114, 240, 329
JHPIEGO 286
Judgment, combined with skill 132

Karl Storz Co. (see Storz)
Karyotyping 53, 54, 131, 133, 210, 297, 299
Kidney carcinoma 127
Kleppinger bipolar forceps 43, 164, 273
Klinefelter's syndrome 297

Lacerations (see also Specific organs)
    of abdominal organs 145
    of blood vessels 145, 236, 246
    of bowel 145
    of broad ligaments 55, 108
Laminaria digitata tent 183
Laparoscopes 34–45, 98 (see also Endoscopes, Equipment, Instruments, Manufacturer's name)
    bayonet type 36
    diagnostic 35, 160
    flexible 37, 44, 120
    fore-oblique 34
    maintenance of 46–50, 225
    operating 35, 134, 136, 156, 160–166
    physics of 18–23
    integrated bundle 307
Laparoscopy
    effect on ovulation 334–340
    kit 286
    program in academic hospital 259–264, 275–280
    program in community hospital 265–274
    program worldwide 281–292
    survey 342–352
Laparotomy
    capability of operating room 88, 157
    emergency 88, 97, 113–118, 120, 130, 157, 169
    exploratory 143
    for bowel burns 232, 244
        cancer 119–128
        complications of laparoscopy 97, 120, 132, 171, 178
        control of bleeding 238, 243, 268
        ectopic pregnancy 156, 158
        lysis of adhesions 131, 202
        removal of IUD 141, 143
        uterine suspension 132, 151, 154
    indications for 88, 104, 112–118, 130–132, 141, 212, 226
    previous 147
    rate 349, 350
    set, sterile 88
    unnecessary, in trauma 104, 106, 116
Laryngeal edema 81
Laryngoscope 82
Lavage studies 100, 192
Lawsuits 92, 236, 313–323, 354
Learning 181, 247–292
Legal
    aspects 61–68, 354
    liability 3, 236, 313–323
        manufacturers 344–350
Leica camera 301
Leiomyomata 55, 120, 194
Lens
    camera 300–312
    fogging 98
    relay system 18–23
    systems
        historical background 6–16, 261

Lens—*continued*
  systems—*continued*
    maintenance 46–50, 225
    TV 309
Leukorrhea 194
Licensing 256, 321
Lidocaine 69–86, 168
Life support equipment 280
Ligaments, uterine 151
Light source 18–23 (*see also* Fiber optics)
  adequate 39, 98
  development 261
  for oncologic laparoscopy 120
  for photography 98, 300–312
  Fourestier, Gladu, Valmier apparatus 8, 9
  historical background 6–16
  inadequate 221, 299
  maintenance 46–50, 221
  physics 18–23, 261
  quartz rod 8, 21
Lippes loop 143 (*see also* Intrauterine device)
Lithotomy position (*see* Position)
Litigation 256, 313–323 (*see also* Malpractice, Medical legal)
Liver
  abscess 325
  biopsy 119–123
    direct vision 7, 325
  bleeding 120, 329
  carcinoma 119–128
  cysts 326
  disease 259, 325, 354
  enlargement 91
  hemangioma 120, 326
  laceration 91, 114
  malignancy 56, 119–128
  scan 123, 324
  trauma 104, 106, 113–118
  visualization 324–332
Local anesthesia 69–81 (*see also* Anesthesia)
Low frequency current (*see* Current)
Luteal phase pregnancies 244
Luteinization 338
Lymphatics of diaphragm, tumor 120
Lymphoma 124, 325
Lysis of adhesions 52–55, 131, 143, 198, 202, 214 (*see also* Adhesions)

Machida flexible laparoscope 37
Madlener technique 165
Magnification 20, 98, 100, 120, 309
Maintenance of equipment 46–50, 160–164
Male patient 90
Malignancy 119–128 (*see also* Cancer, Tumor)
  extraperitoneal 56, 119
  metastatic 53, 57, 119
  pelvic 53, 56
Malpractice 4, 256, 313–323 (*see also* Medical legal, Legal liability)
Malpresentation of fetus 56
Manipulators, uterine 43, 79, 99, 134, 158, 183, 213
Manufacturers 162 (*see also* Equipment, Instruments, Specific name)
  error 172
  responsibility 344–350, 355
Margulies spiral 144
Mass
  Abdominal 53, 58, 327
  Adnexal 55, 197, 214
  Pelvic 53, 55, 120, 297
Mechanical occlusion devices for sterilization 165, 167–178, 189, 356 (*see also* Clip, Ring, Nonelectric sterilization)
Meckel's diverticulum 106
Medical legal aspects 3, 162, 236, 254, 256, 313–323
Medical Technology International, Inc. 286
Megestrol acetate 335
Mendelsohn's syndrome 71
Menometrorrhagia 197, 297
Menopause, premature 197
Menotropins 131, 197
Menstrual

cycle 107, 214
disorders 133
history 194
research 334–340
retention 297
period 195
Menstruation, retrograde 105
Meperidine hydrochloride 170, 281, 329
Mesenteric
  insufflation 225
  vessel injury 97, 226, 236, 238
  visualization 324–332
Mesosalpinx
  abscess 268
  bleeding 178, 185, 227, 243, 268, 318
  tear 162, 166, 346
Metastasis 53, 56, 57, 119–128, 326 (*see also* Cancer)
Mesovarium 131
Method (*see* Technique)
Methylene blue (*see* Dye)
Metroplasty 56, 197 (*see also* Uterine)
Microbacteria lepra 330
Mill wheel cardiac murmur 70, 73, 76, 94, 225
Minification 20
Mini-flash 304
Minilaparotomy 132, 165
  historical background 7
  incision 156, 166, 289
  technique 158, 166, 292
Mini-wedge resection 193
Minolta camera 302
Minors 63, 320
Monitoring
  equipment 88, 350
  gas pressure 38, 76, 223, 225, 243, 318
  patient 76–80, 86
  television 310
Monkeys 334–340
Morbidity 153, 155, 182, 234, 349, 350 (*see also* Complications)
Morgagni cysts 54
Morphine 78
Mortality 144, 189, 234, 243, 268, 313 (*see also* Death)
  rate 72, 350, 353
Mosaicism, chromosomal 295
Motivation 60–68
Movie 253
  cameras 22
Mutliple sclerosis 78
Muscle
  fasciculations 76
  relaxants 69–86
Myocardial infarction 171
Myomata 209
Myomectomy 206

Naloxone 81, 329
Narcotic
  antagonist 70–74, 81
  overdose 70–74
  reversal 70–74, 81
  sedation 73–80
Nausea 76, 172
Needle (*see also* Biopsy, Pneumoperitoneum, Veress)
  biopsy 120, 134
  pneumoperitoneum 91–95
    inadequate 225
    injuries 225, 236–246
      rate 243, 244
    placement 91, 225
Needlescope 294, 299
Needlescope 294, 299
Negligence 315–323
Neoplasms 119–128 (*see also* Cancer, Malignancy, Metastases, Tumor)
  Ovarian 56, 133
  Pelvic 8
Neurovegetative disturbances 106
Nidation 201, 203
Nitrous oxide (N$_2$O) 65, 93 (*see also* Gas, Pneumoperitoneum)
  delivery systems, 38

diffusion hypoxia 70, 73
selection for insufflation 81, 95, 169, 209, 327
toxicity 73
Nonelectric sterilization 165–178, 189, 229, 232, 289, 343, 356 (*see also* Clip, Ring, Sterilization)
Nongynecologic laparoscopy 324–332
Nonhuman primates 334–340
Nontherapeutic sterilization 63
Novice 59, 164, 181 (*see also* Inexperience)
  complications of 220
  experience for 160
Nulliparous patients 147
Nurses 222
  training 46–50, 258–292, 321, 354

Obese patient
  angle of penetration in 239
  as contraindication to laparoscopy 53, 223
  incision in 91, 95
  open laparoscopy in 147
  pneumoperitoneum in 38, 91, 92
  position of 90
  problems with 55, 58, 82, 86, 169, 172, 327
Obstetrics and gynecology residency training 10, 248–280, 349, 354
Oligomenorrhea 133
Oligoovulation 56
Olympus camera 301, 302
Omentum
  bleeding 236
  insufflation 225
  puncture 240
  visualization 328
Oncologic laparoscopy 95, 119–128
One hole, one puncture (*see* Technique)
Oocyte recovery 10, 53, 57, 339
Open laparoscopy 10, 145–149
  advantages 132, 148
  complications 132, 147
  technique 146
Operating laparoscopy 21, 134, 136, 156, 160–166, 179, 232
Operating room
  laparotomy capability 88
  personnel 42, 46–50, 86, 160, 242, 247–292
  preparation 88–102, 276
  safety 32, 321
  time 272
  wiring 32
Operative gymnastics 154, 157, 158
Operative laparoscopy 88, 109, 130–158 (*see also* Open laparoscopy)
  complications 130–132
  for ectopic IUD 140–144
  for ectopic pregnancy 155–157
  for infertility 198–218
  for ovarian biopsy 133–139
  for tubal sterilization 160, 162
  for uterine suspension 150–154
Operative privileges 257, 269
Operative time 147, 159, 171, 178, 179
Operator (*see also* Skill, Experience, Instruction)
  experienced 160, 162, 187, 218
  inexperienced 158, 160, 221, 238, 250
  injury 228
  proficiency 88
Optical
  design 261
  distortions 18
  systems 18–23
    for photography 300–305
    historical background 6–16, 261
    maintenance 46–50
Orthopedic pain 106
Oscillating circuit 25
Oscilloscope 27, 28
Outpatient laparoscopy 60, 89, 101, 141, 267, 344
  anesthesia 69–86
  facilities 277, 281–291
  not for ectopic pregnancy 157
  ovarian biopsy 138

sterilization 169, 174, 183, 232
Output waveforms 27, 321 (see also Current)
Ova, ovum
    collection 3, 210, 336, 339
    fertilization studies 334–340
    pick-up 52, 54, 210, 214, 216
    release 54, 296
    transport 160, 198, 201
Ovarian
    abscess 104–112
    artery injury 184
    bleeding 135, 136, 156, 197, 243
    biopsy 54, 120, 131, 133–139, 193–218
        complications 131, 136, 243
        histology 120
        indications 53–56, 133, 296
        instruments 136
        interpretation 138
        technique 134
    cancer 119–128, 354
    cyst 104–112, 206, 296, 297
        aspiration of 53–55, 105, 120, 214
        diagnosis 105
            historical background 8
        luteinizing 296
        puncture, dangers 299
    cystectomy 296
    dysfunction 133, 192–218
    dysgenesis 131, 133
    encapsulation 55
    endometriosis 131, 206, 214
    failure 138, 197
    follicles 138
    function 53
    histology 131, 133
    neoplasm 56, 119–128, 133
    physiology 57
    postmenopausal 55
    resection 3, 131
    rupture 197
    streaks 295
    torsion 297
    tumors 108, 119–128, 133, 296
    wedge resection 53–59, 192–218
        dangers 131
Ovariectomy 296
Ovariolysis 212–218
Ovary 192–218
    adherent 131, 198
    carcinoma 120
    congenital defect of 55
    immature 297
    pathology 120
    polycystic 3, 56, 131, 197, 296
    research 334–340
    steinoid 201, 206
    Stein-Leventhal 56, 136, 206, 214, 296
    streak 197, 295
Overinsufflation 38, 116
Ovulation
    failure 133, 195
    induction of 131, 197, 335
    observation of 54, 335, 338, 355
    pain 55
    research 335
    tests 193–211
    time 54, 194–196, 336
Ovulatory function 55, 192–218
    effect of laparoscopy on 334–340
Oxygen saturation 70–74
    prior to anesthesia 77
Oxytocin 164, 183

Pacemaker 75
Pain (see also Abdominal pain, Pelvic pain,
    Specific organ)
    pelvic 104–112, 297
    studies 53, 55
Palmer drill biopsy forceps 9, 42, 135, 162
    modifications of 136, 162
Pancreatic carcinoma 120, 125, 127
Pancreatitis 328
Paracervical block 78, 79
Paraovarian cysts 54, 104, 105, 107

Partial thromboplastin time 326
Passive regurgitation 71, 74
Pathology
    confirmation of 179, 343
    specimen 162, 181
Patient
    card system 261
    counseling 60–68, 276
    -doctor rapport 60, 61, 318
    ideal 250
    instruction 81
    male 90
    preparation 60–68, 89–90
    selection 88, 170, 317, 318
Pediatric laparoscopy 261, 294–299, 354
Pedunculated cysts 55, 104–105, 112
Pelvic
    abscess 185, 232, 244, 268
    adhesions 55
    congestion 55, 112
    disease 194
    endometriosis 131, 107–112, 212–214
    fracture 114
    infection 53, 57, 201
    inflammatory disease 8, 47, 112, 198, 208,
        244, 297
    malignancy 53, 56, 57, 119–128
    mass 53, 55, 88, 120, 297
    pain 53, 55, 88, 104–112, 297
    pathology 206
    thrombophlebitis 232
    trauma 57, 104, 106, 113–118
    varicocele 107, 108
    varicosities 55
    vascularity 57
Penetrating injuries of abdomen (see Trauma)
Penetration of laparoscope
    angle of 92–94, 225, 239
    complications of 92–97, 236–246
    depth of 95, 240
Pentax camera 302
Perforation during laparoscopy 96–97 (see also
    Specific organ)
Pergonal 197
Perifimbrial adhesions 192–218
Periovarian adhesions 54, 131, 134, 192–218
Perisigmoiditis 107, 108
Peritoneal
    bleeding 243
    fluid 298
        aspiration 9, 53, 54, 56, 210
    hyperemia 55, 107
    insufflation 72, 91–95, 223
    metastasis 56, 119
    trauma 104, 106, 113–118
    tubouterine fistula 266
    visualization 118, 324
Peritoneoscopy
    historical background 6–16
    nongynecologic 324–332
Peritonitis 104–112
    carcinomatous 104
    complication of laparoscopy 268, 329
    contraindication to laparoscopy 53, 57
    from bowel burns 66, 229, 232, 244
    previous 82
    tuberculous 53, 57
Peritubal adhesions 52, 131, 134, 176, 193–218
Personnel training 44, 46–50, 160, 247–292, 321
Pharyngeal injury 71
Phenergan 171
Phimosis 54, 131, 193, 202, 212–218
Photography 22, 261, 300–312, 354
    for record 100, 193, 209, 298, 356
    light source 39, 98, 301
    of ovulation 338
Physics of light and image transmission 18–23
PIEGO 286
Pitocin 164, 188
Planned parenthood 60–68, 267
Plasma
    cholinesterase deficiency 74
    transfusion 326
Platelet transfusion 326

Pleural puncture 120
Pneumocolon 329
Pneumomediastinum 71
Pneumoperitoneum
    complications of 57, 70–86, 93, 94, 222–225,
        238, 318
        incidence 243
    creation of 91–95
    effects on blood gases 169
    historical background 7
    inadequate 220, 222, 239, 246
    in open laparoscopy 132, 147
    intravascular 73
    monitoring 76
    needle 38
        injuries 145, 225, 236–246
    pediatric 294
    research 100, 153
    technique 91–95
    time 132, 147
Pneumothorax 69–86, 93, 122, 225, 243, 329
Polaroid camera 302
Polycystic ovary 56, 131, 197, 296
    ovarian resection for 3
Pomeroy sterilization method 162, 186
Population control 281–292
Position
    basic rules 224
    knee-chest 8
    lithotomy 8, 71, 89, 183
    left lateral decubitus 73, 126
    right lateral decubitus 127
    reversed Trendelenburg 118
    supine 90
    Trendelenburg 7, 70–74, 90, 107, 127, 138,
        169, 188, 312
Postanesthesia 69–86
Postcoital test for spermatozoa 54, 192–195,
    209
Postgraduate education 10, 31, 160, 247–292
Postmenopausal patients 55, 120
Postpartum (see Puerperal sterilization)
    hypotension 72
    patients 72
    sterilization 187–188, 343
Pouch of Douglas 105, 107, 109, 120, 144, 214
Power source (see Generators)
Power supply circuit 25
Preanesthesia 76–80
Precautions 58, 160, 326 (see also Techniques,
    Complications)
Preceptor 248, 252
Prednisolone 71
Pregnancy
    after sterilization 166, 171, 178, 244
    contraindication to laparoscopy 53, 58
    ectopic 53–56, 104, 105, 107, 190, 216
        criteria for laparoscopic removal 56, 130,
            155
        operative treatment 8, 53, 88, 155–158
    rate
        after infertility treatment 193, 214–217
        after sterilization 166, 173, 190, 244, 266,
            317, 320, 348, 353
    termination (see Abortion)
    tubal 56, 130, 155–158
        unruptured 3, 55, 155–158
    uterine 190
Pregnanediol test 197, 207
Premedication 76–80
Preparation
    for training 249
    of operating room 88–102
    of patient 89–90
Presacral neurectomy 109
Pressure (see also Gas)
    airway 72
    excessive 70–75, 243, 319
    intraabdominal 38, 57, 246, 252
    intraperitoneal 223
    maximum 38
    meter 38, 223
    monitoring 38, 76, 223, 225, 243, 318
    regulator 38

Previous surgeries 147, 170, 220, 225
Primary amenorrhea 53–56, 131, 133, 138, 295
Primates 334–340
Prisms 37
Privileges 257, 269
Probe 120
　calibrated 100
Problems with laparoscopy 21, 242 (see also Complications)
Proficiency of operator 88, 250, 257 (see also Experience)
Progestational therapy 131, 133, 214
Progesterone 131, 201, 336
Progestins 133
Program of International Education in Gynecology and Obstetrics 286
Programmed instruction 257
Prolene, self-tying 155, 156
Prostaglandin levels 133
Prothrombin time 326
Pseudohermaphrodism 56, 297
Psychiatric
　consultation 106
　findings 107
　history 107
Psychologic trauma 317
Psychomatic disturbances 106
Puberty
　delayed 297
　development 295
　precocious 133, 296, 299
Puerperal sterilization 10, 164, 187–188 (see also Sterilization)
Pulmonary
　aspiration 69–74
　bleb rupture 71, 74, 76
　disease 120
　embolism 69–73, 232
Punch biopsy forceps 135, 162
Puncture (see also Specific organ)
　of blood vessel 236
　of hydatid cyst 329
　of ovarian cysts 55, 105
　of pleura 120
Puncture technique (see Technique)
Pylorus visualization 328
Pyosalpinx 105, 108

Qualifications 269
Quartz rod light source 8, 21
Questionnaire 342–352

Radiation therapy 119–128
Radioactive isotopes 120
　infusion catheter placement for 121, 273
Radioimmunoassay 201
　of FSH 131
　of luteinizing hormone 131
Radiotherapy 56, 119–128 (see also Cancer)
Recanalization 167
Recoagulation 163, 243
Records 199–204, 319
　photographic 100, 193, 209, 300–312, 353–356
　release 68
　visual 57, 198
Recovery
　from anesthesia 69–86
　from sterilization with abortion 186
　room 81, 168, 267, 278
　time 171, 182, 279
　time, prolonged 76
Rectal polyp snare 156, 163
Rectum carcinoma 126
Referrals 250, 267
Reflective relay systems 18–23
Refractive relay systems 18
Regional (see also Analgesia, Anesthesia)
　analgesia 69
　anesthesia 69–78
Regional enteritis 106
Regurgitation 71, 74
Relative contraindications 53, 58, 149
Relaxation 93, 229

　inadequate 55
　with anesthesia 69, 86
Relay systems 18–23
　fiber optic 19
Reporting form 100, 193, 199
Reproduction research 56, 57, 334–340, 355
Research 53, 57, 334–340
　in endoscopy 260
　in reproductive physiology 56
Resection of uterosacral ligaments 109
Residency training 248–280, 349, 354
Res ipsa loquitur 321
Respirators 74, 280
Respiratory
　arrest 327, 329
　complications 73
　distress 122, 318
　studies 169
　therapist 255
Responsibility for safety 89, 315, 323, 344–350, 355
Rest tumor 56
Resuscitation equipment 77–82, 279, 280, 318
Retractors 145
Retroflexion of uterus 106, 108, 109, 132, 150–154
Retrograde menstruation 105
Retrograde tubal lavage 54
Retroperitoneal
　hematoma 171, 268
　insufflation 225
　perforation 226
Retroversion of uterus 150–154
Return electrode 30, 31, 90, 317 (see also Ground)
Reversible sterilization 165, 173, 189
Richard Wolf Medical Instrument Corp. (see Wolf)
Ring sterilization 11, 165, 174–178, 189, 229, 284, 289, 343, 350 (see also Yoon ring)
Ringers lactate 70, 164, 188
Rioux bipolar instrument 43, 164
Risks 42, 52–59, 65, 220–246, 303, 315 (see also Complications, Specific procedures)
　analysis of 342–352
　of anesthesia 69–86
　of bleeding 56
　of failure 320
　of oncologic laparoscopy 120
　of operative laparoscopy 130–132
　of pneumoperitoneum 91
Rod-lens system 261 (see also Light source)
Rokitansky-Kuster-Hauser syndrome 295
Rollei camera 302
Room air 38, 100, 327, 329
Round ligament
　clip application to 172
　coagulation of 227, 266
　ring application to 172
　shortening 3, 109, 150–154
Rubin's test 54, 192, 207, 208 (see also Tubal patency, Tubal insufflation)
Rupture
　of corpus luteum 55, 105
　of ectopic pregnancy 55, 105, 155–158
　of endometriotic cysts 108
　of hydatid cysts 108
　of ovarian cysts 55, 104, 108
　of pulmonary bleb 71, 74
　of tubal pregnancy 55, 105, 108, 130, 155, 158

Sacrouterine ligament 107 (see also Uterosacral ligament)
Safety (see also Complications)
　anesthesia 69–86
　checks 317–321
　devices 164, 223
　recommendations 32, 38, 219–246
　responsibility 315–323
　review 321
Saf-T-Coil 144
Salpingectomy 3, 130, 162, 202
Salpingitis 9, 54, 55, 104–112, 176, 185, 297
　gonococcal 331

Salpingography 52, 192
Salpingolysis 193, 202, 212–218
Salpingostomy 156, 193, 210–218
Sargis uterine manipulator 183
Scars 53, 58, 62, 65, 92
Second-look procedures in cancer treatment 53, 56, 119–128, 354
Second puncture, trocar (see Technique)
Secondary amenorrhea 53–56, 131, 133, 296
Secondary instruments 36, 42, 160–166
Sedation 75–81 (see also Anesthesia)
Self
　analysis 264
　education 349
　instruction 248–251, 257
　surveillance 353
Self-tying prolene 155, 156
Semen analysis 193–195, 205
　collection 335
Semm
　biopsy forceps 152
　tubal cautery forceps 29
　uterine manipulator 134
　vacuum cannula 43
17-hydroxycorticosteroids 207
17-ketosteroids 197, 207
Sexual (see also Intercourse)
　activity 60–62, 159
　development 295
　precocity 133, 296, 299
Shibaden TV camera 308–310
Shock
　electric 25, 223, 303, 317
　hemorrhagic 130, 155
　hypovolemic 118
Shoulder pain 81, 95, 329
Siegler forceps 135, 162
Silicone ring 165, 174–178, 189 (see also Ring)
Single puncture (see Technique)
Skill 4, 36, 58, 59, 88, 112, 154, 169, 178, 182, 193, 218, 221
　combined with judgment 132
　needed in oncologic laparoscopy 119
Skin
　burns 30, 66, 89, 228, 231–235, 268, 317
　clips 101
　closure 101
　incision 91
　sutures 101
Small bowel
　burn 229–235, 244, 268
　perforation 114, 147, 241, 244
Snare
　complications 181
　sterilization 10
　　technique 163, 179–181
　technique
　　for removal of tubal pregnancy 130, 156
　　for removal of defective clips 172
　　tubal resection 163
Soaking instruments 44–50
Soderstrom snare technique (see Snare)
Sodium thiopental 77
Solid-state
　generators 26
　TV cameras 309
Sonogram 55
Sony TV monitor 310
Spark-gap generators 25, 160, 344
Spermatozoa 54
　aspiration of 53, 56
　reception 194, 203
　transport 201, 209
Spinal anesthesia 77, 78 (see also Anesthesia)
Spinnbarkeit phenomenon 195
Spiral stents 205
Spleen
　enlarged 91
　malignancy 124
　perforation 91
　trauma 104, 106, 113–118
　visualization 324–332
Spring clip (see Hulka clip)
Staging 119–128